Cheryl,
Thanks for the
kind words. I hope
this fits your "view
of epigenesis".
Best wishes,
Gary Novak

Developmental Psychology:

Dynamical Systems and Behavior Analysis

Developmental Psychology:

Dynamical Systems and Behavior Analysis

by

Gary Novak

CONTEXT PRESS
Reno, Nevada

Developmental Psychology: Dynamical Systems and Behavior Analysis
by Gary Novak.

Hardcover. 339 pp.

ISBN 1-878978-25-X

933 Gear Street, Reno, NV 89503-2729

Printed in the United States of America

Preface

What, another developmental psychology textbook? In recent years there has been an explosion of texts in this area, reflecting the enormous popularity of the field. So why another one? I think this one is unique. Here is why:

- A Coherent Approach. I've been a college professor for twenty years. My experience tells me that many students come away from a course in developmental psychology with their heads filled with the facts of development, but without an overall picture of the process of development. Students may know Freud's theory for identification, Piaget's for cognition, and Skinner's for behavior problems. Yet they have no consistent approach to all of development.

Likewise, students may have studied the latest research findings in these areas (many of which appear to contradict each other) but are left without a consistent overview of how the theories and data fit together. In this book I have attempted to provide such a framework, in the form of a coherent approach to development, upon which students can hang the facts of development.

- Dynamical Systems and Behavior Analysis. This approach combines the views of dynamical systems concepts with a behavioral view of development. The dynamical (or dynamic) systems view reflects an emerging consensus in modern developmental theory. It is an approach which incorporates both person and environment influences. It views developmental outcome as a constant process of reciprocal interactions (or transactions) between nature and nurture. The result of these ever-changing transactions is continual reorganization of the person-environment systems.

The behavioral approach has long been under-represented in developmental psychology. Its emphasis on process, on interaction, on environmental influences and on the individual, make it a good fit with a dynamical systems approach. I think the synthesis of these views, which might be called a "Behavioral Systems Approach" provide a powerful and coherent view of the process of human development.

- Emphasis on Process. The two fundamental questions in developmental psychology are: (1) *What* develops?; and (2) *How* does it develop? The "what?" is largely a question of developmental structures and describes development. The "how?" is primarily a question of function or process. It attempts to explain development. I take the latter approach. Developmental psychology has become increasingly concerned with questions of process.

- Developmental Psychology as a Natural Science. My approach views child development as a natural process, one that can be understood from a scientific perspective. Early on, I attempt to place developmental psychology in its relationship to other sciences. I try to analyze the process of development in a way that is consistent with analysis in other sciences. In doing so, I hope to reach our goal of providing a coherent approach to the field.

- Development as a Parallel Process to Evolution. One way I provide a natural science approach is to present the process of child development as paralleling the process of evolution. Developmental psychology focuses on changes in individuals, whereas evolution focuses on changes in species. I try to show how both the person's evolutionary and learning histories interact, but the focus is on natural selection of individual behavior as the process of individual development. This "selectionist" approach carries into the next point.

- Emphasis on Learning as a Natural Process. In recent years developmental texts have ignored or de-emphasized the role of learning in human development. It has often been relegated to the status of a special process reserved for use by parents and teachers to deal with behavior problems. I choose to emphasize the role of learning as the key process, which in interaction with genes and other person variables, determines developmental outcome. I think learning is a key thread that unifies this approach to understanding child development.

- A Non-linear Approach. I view human development as an open system simultaneously involving many influences. Furthermore, the product of the interaction of these influences changes the process in complex ways. I believe approaches that view development as a set of simple interactions among factors are doomed to failure. Development must be viewed as involving ever-changing dynamic systems whose effects result in a reorganization of the systems involved. For this reason I am interested in some of the developments in a new field called Chaos Science.

- A Contextual Approach. In a dynamical systems approach, when systems are reorganized, the context of development is constantly changing . Development is affected by the current context as well as past.

- Development Should be Analyzed at Different Levels of Systems. I have found that students have difficulty grasping how the different content areas covered in developmental textbooks relate to each other. For example how does learning relate to cognition? How do both relate to schools? I think the key to understanding these relationships is to understand that we are analyzing interlocking systems at different levels. Thus I have organized this book based on four system levels, from basic processes to society and culture. I use the metaphor of a painting by Seurat to illustrate how it is our perspective which determines on which of the simultaneously present systems I choose to focus.

- Systematic, not Encyclopedic. If you look at the majority of other developmental textbooks you are impressed by their sheer size. Each appears to try to outdo the other in the number and recency of the studies they cite. My goal is more modest. I would like students to come away from reading a book with a good understanding of how children develop. My experience is that only a limited number of concepts may be reasonably mastered by students studying each chapter. Much of the rest gets lost in the enormous task of trying to retain it all for a test. Often the forest is not seen for the huge growth of underbrush. My goal is to provide a framework for understanding the process of development. I think such a framework will be more useful to students in the long term. As research discovers new facts and revises others I think this approach will continue to provide a structure for understanding the process of human development.

Finally, I think this book offers faculty and students an alternative approach to the study of development. By focusing on issues, rather than on details, I provide flexibility in how child development is taught. I have found encyclopedic texts constraining. The shear amount they cover (and cost) makes assigning readings or other material nearly impossible. I think these more limited goals open up exciting (and more flexible) possibilities for the study of child (or human) development at both the undergraduate and graduate level.

Acknowledgments

Throughout this text I use the word "we." Very early on, the plural was necessary because I had the assistance of a co-author, Ted Schoneberger, a former student and a current colleague of mine. We spent many hours discussing the material and revising early chapters of mine. Parts of Chapter 6 on habituation and Chapter 11 on empathy remain largely Ted's. Unfortunately, developments necessitated Ted to devote himself to more financially fulfilling pursuit's and the writing of this book again became the endeavors of a single individual.

However, the "we" remains appropriate, for without the input and assistance of many, the project would have never reached its current state. Many of the ideas were formed and clarified in discussions with students and colleagues. Students also had a significant impact through their encouragement and feedback.

Two students were particularly critical, and receive my deep gratitude for their assistance. Emily Branscum and Gena Martella are responsible for the glossary entries and much more. Many ideas contained in these pages were clarified in discussions occurring over the past year. Emily has taken on major responsibility for recruiting a team of student assistants to review and edit sections of the book. In addition, both Emily and Gena have worked tirelessly in getting versions of this book ready for use in my class and to the publisher. They have my deeply felt thanks.

Other students, too, deserve special recognition. Among these are Margaret Winklemann Walker whose early encouragement and work on the initial glossary were critical in the beginning stages of this book. Candy Branson and Brian Williams assisted in the taking of photographs to illustrate issues in these pages. Brian Williams also took the photograph of Shawn Cook on the cover. Vicky Eden contributed her artistic expertise on several drawings and tables, and to the cover design. Lynn Ostrander, Lynde Carrington, Elyse Hamilton, Lawrence Ruiz, Rita Rush, Mike Higuera, and Rick Sheppard. All helped in reviewing parts of the manuscript. Finally, there are many others, including students in my courses who discussed the material and provided me feedback. I must give them credit for making this manuscript better. I accept the blame for its failings.

Like the process of development itself, the approach described in the following pages is the result of many factors coming together. As many know, this project has taken a long time to reach this stage, but it needed the state of developmental psychology at this time, with the emergence of dynamical systems, for it to come together. Like development itself, this work too is a work in progress.

Developmental Psychology:

Dynamical Systems and Behavior Analysis

Table of Contents

Chapter 1

Introduction

Who am I? This is one of the central questions that psychologists answer. *How did I get to be me?* This is the question that developmental psychologists answer. The task of this book is to provide an answer to the second question. It examines the

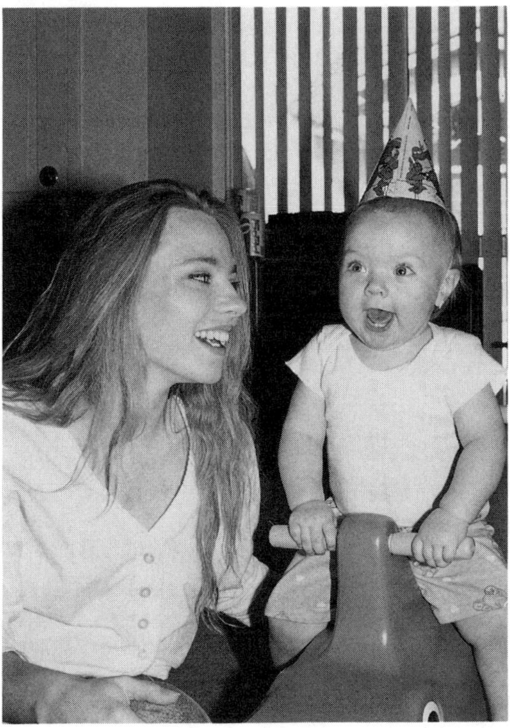

processes that underlie the complex changes individuals undergo during their lifetimes. It tells the story of the amazing transformation of each individual from a simple, single-celled organism to a mature adult comprised of billions of cells. But this book is about much more than physical development. It is primarily about the development of increasingly complex and diverse relationships between what a person does and the environment in which she does it. As a single celled organism, the individual's interactions with the world are limited to primitive, life-maintaining activities. However, as an adult, a person possesses a rich repertoire of actions. For example, we can watch the TV news, read a book, go for a jog, or think about what we'll do this weekend. Which action is performed at any given time depends, in large measure, on the person's past history of interactions with the environment. Your present acts of reading and (hopefully) understanding these words are examples of such action. They require not only that you have undergone a certain level of physical development. These acts also require a certain level of psychological development defined in terms of a history of interactions with your world.

A Dynamical Systems Approach

In our view, development involves ever-changing, or dynamical, systems. These systems involve the ever-changing person in constant and reciprocal interaction with a continually changing environment. This environment both is affected by, and effects changes, in the person. In turn, the person both is affected by and effects changes in the environment. In dynamical systems, the person and the environment are in reciprocal interaction, or transactions. This book will treat psychological development as the outcome of progressive interactions, or "transactions," between the person and the environment. Neither nature nor nurture alone is responsible for development; both are. The structures of biology interact with the effects of the environment over the life span of the individual. From the moment of conception, *who you are* is determined by these ever-changing, dynamic interactions. A dynamical systems approach attempts to view development from this perspective.

A Behavioral Systems Approach

The approach taken in this book is to combine dynamical systems principles with principles of behavior analysis. By focusing on behavior-environment relations as the main phenomena of psychology, behavior analysis has discovered many powerful principles relevant to human development. In recent years behavior analysis has expanded its provence to include the analysis of larger units of behavior, and in doing so, has recognized the importance of dynamical systems principles (See Galbicka, 1992; Marr, 1992). This book seeks to combine those principles from both dynamical systems and behavioral perspectives which are relevant to human develoopment. The result is a natural science approach to development that emphasizes constant, reciprocal interactions between behavior and environment called a ***behavioral systems approach***.

What is Development?

According to the dictionary, ***development*** means change over time. Therefore, if we were interested in studying physical development alone, we would be interested in the changes occurring in an individual's body over time. Since we are interested in ***psychological development***, we need an adequate definition. Bijou and Baer (1961,

1978) viewed psychological development as ***progressive changes in the interactions between the behaviors of a person & and the events in his/her environment.*** Thus, there are three important aspects in defining psychological development. First, there are changes in interactions. Second, these changes are progressive. Third, these changes occur over the lifetime of the individual.

Changes in Interactions

Psychologists study behavior. In studying psychological development we are not only concerned with changes in behavior, but with changes in the person/environment relationships. Not only does behavior change, but behaviors in relation to environmental events change – we learn *under what conditions* to emit behaviors. We learn what to do, and when to do it. What develops are new relationships between behavior and environment, not merely the behaviors themselves. As we develop, the events and objects in our environment take on new functions.

For example, if you give a set of keys to a one year-old child, she is likely to place them in her mouth to explore them. Although you could put the keys in your mouth too, it is unlikely that you would behave the same way in relation to the keys. For you, the functions of the keys would be tied to the doors they open, the cars they start, or in some contexts, to their usefulness in prying open the lid of the jar. Not only is your behavior more complex, but it is more complex in relationship to the things and events in your environment.

Progressive Changes

Development is progressive in the sense that it is cumulative. That is, development is built upon what has come before. At conception specialized cells from the organism's mother and father combine to produce a new, single-celled organism with a unique genetic make-up. For the rest of its existence, changes will occur. For example, the elderly person with failing vision and hearing due to deterioration of his physical structures adapts to his environment in increasingly complex ways to compensate for the physical deterioration. Because he can no longer see or hear as clearly, he may learn new behaviors, such as squinting or asking questions, behaviors which were previously unnecessary. In short, later changes are built upon what has already occurred.

Note that "progressive" does not necessarily imply a higher level of functioning. With deterioration of biological capabilities, changes may result in diminished behavioral capabilities. Nevertheless, such changes are "progressive" in the sense that they are built upon earlier developments.

Changes Occur Across the Life Span

Developmental psychologists are interested in progressive changes over time. Child psychologists are interested in a relatively short span of time. Some study only infants, others study larger spans of childhood. A relatively recent trend among developmental psychologists is a life span approach. This "womb to tomb" approach enables us to get a broader overview of the entirety of human development.

The Continuum of Scientific Disciplines

There are many methods we can use to obtain knowledge of the phenomena of interest to us. Since the development of the scientific method during the Renaissance, science has been one of the most efficient ways of enabling us to understand our world. In this book we are approaching the study of child development from the perspective of the natural sciences. Just as physics, chemistry, and biology have been able to reveal basic laws and principles about the dynamical systems that concern them, we feel that a natural science approach is the best approach to understanding development.

In order to understand the unique position of developmental psychology, it is helpful to place it in the context of other sciences. In fact, it is possible to place various sciences along a continuum based on the complexity of the dynamical systems that are their focus. At one end of the continuum we examine dynamical systems involving interactions of subatomic particles. At the other end we view dynamical systems at the aggregate level of culture and society. We will start with the science that addresses the most elemental level, physics.

PHYSICS. Physicists study the physical building blocks of the universe. At its most basic level, physics is the study of electrons, protons, neutrinos, quarks, and other basic building blocks of atoms and subatomic particles, which are themselves the basic building blocks of all things, living and inert, in our universe.

CHEMISTRY. Unique combinations of protons and electrons yield unique elements. The periodic chart of elements depicts the particular combinations which result in each of the 108 known elements. Each has properties that are **quantitatively** as well as **qualitatively** unique. For example, hydrogen can be distinguished *quantitatively* from iron in terms of the quantity of electrons each possesses. Chemists study these unique properties. Furthermore, they are also interested in how chemical elements combine to produce substances with properties that emerge which are qualitatively different from their individual elements. Hydrogen and iron can also be easily distinguished based on their unique qualities – one is a gas and the other a solid.

Neale and Liebert (1980) suggested an example of how the properties of chemical compounds are lost when they are reduced to their components. Chlorine (Cl) is a gaseous element which, if inhaled, will produce severe burns, even death. Sodium (Na) is a very unstable metal which, when immersed in water, will burn vigorously. You would not make contact with either of these elements without taking precautionary measures. Yet when sodium and chlorine are combined, the resulting compound, table salt (NaCl), is something we ingest practically everyday. The resulting compound is not only essential to our health (in small amounts), but also makes life a little more palatable. The compound that emerges from the two elements has properties which cannot be understood by reducing it to the smallest basic elements studied by physics. The phenomena studied by chemistry are at a higher level and, if reduced to a more basic level of analysis, lose their unique (or emergent) properties.

BIOLOGY. Biology differs from chemistry in that it focuses on the unique combination of organic molecules which when combined produce whole living organisms and their component systems. Notice that on this continuum there are transitions between the scientific disciplines where those working at the lower level science are interested in phenomena of the next higher one. Organic chemistry is such a discipline. Notice too that some people working in this area are primarily chemists interested in the chemical compounds of living creatures, and some are principally biologists whose first interest is in the study of living organisms, and only secondarily in their chemical make-up.

What is next on our continuum?

PSYCHOLOGY. Many textbooks define psychology as the science of behavior. However, this definition is incomplete. Psychologists are not simply interested in an individual's behavior – i.e., what she does – but in the relationship of that behavior to the environment in which it occurs. For example, if a parent complains to a psychologist that her daughter is noncompliant, the psychologist needs information about the child's social environment before deciding what treatment (if any) is needed. In one environment (e.g., a physically abusive home), noncompliance may be a sign of psychological health, while in another environment, a sign of a clinical disorder. This suggests a more complete definition. Psychology is the scientific study of the interactions between the behavior of individuals and the events in their environment (Bijou & Baer, 1978)

SOCIOLOGY. Sociology is concerned with the unique characteristics of groups, not the individuals that make them up. Consequently, sociologists study the causes and effects of variables such as ethnic or racial groups, socioeconomic class, and gangs. These are analyzed as group variables, not individual ones.

ANTHROPOLOGY. As the last science on our continuum, the phenomena studied by anthropology are the most complex. Anthropology is interested in the unique phenomena emerging at the level of cultures. While cultures are composed of individuals, the effects brought about by the culture transcend the analysis of the individual. Thus, while individuals may be best understood by using psychological principles, such as reinforcement and socialization, cultural differences may need a unique set of anthropological principles to be understood. For example, cultures vary greatly in terms of the sexual stereotypes they promote, and it may be necessary to understand the values of a culture to understand the gender related behaviors that emerge in it.

A Metaphor for Development

The universe consists of many systems. As our look at the continuum of scientific disciplines illustrates, these systems may be analyzed at different levels of complexity. For example, human behavior may be analyzed at the level of the person in the environment, or at a lower level, the action of the person's biological systems. We may even analyze behavior at yet lower (that is, simpler) levels, such as the action of chemical neurotransmitters, or even the person's electrons or neutrons. At all these levels, we are analyzing systems – the interactions between parts. It is important to keep in mind that all levels of these systems are present simultaneously. That is, while we are looking at a person interacting with the environment, there are also biological, chemical and physical (lower level systems) and social and cultural events (higher level systems) taking place. We normally choose to view or analyze at one level of system at a time. Psychologists choose to look at the behavior-environment systems, biologists, biological systems, and so on.

An important point to remember is that all levels exist simultaneously. Which level you choose for your analysis depends on what level you find most appropriate to your perspective. Let me provide metaphor. There is a famous painting by the nineteenth century French painter, George Seurat, called *A Sunday Afternoon on the Island of La Grande Jatte*. It is a huge canvas, filling an entire wall. If you were to analyze it for an art appreciation class, what would you say about it? Your analysis would depend on your perspective. If you stood close to the painting you could see

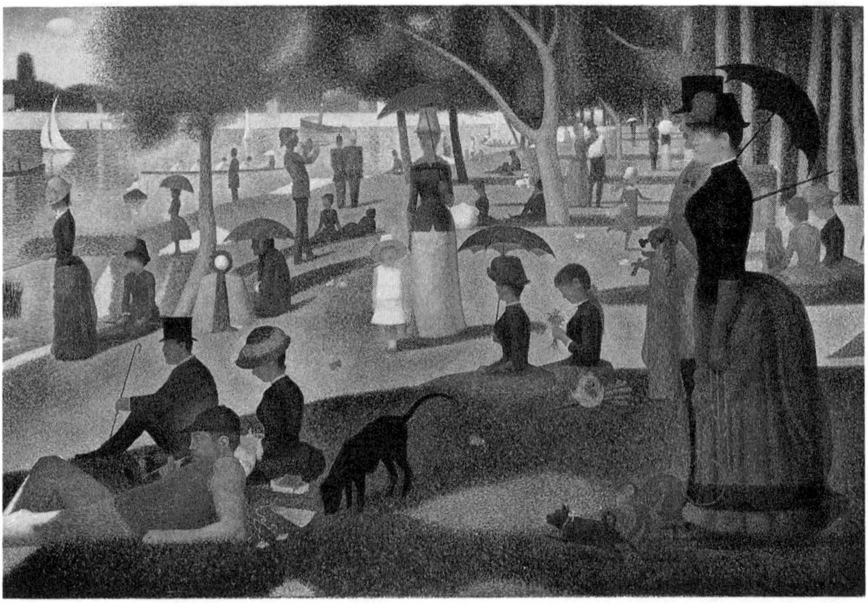

Georges Seurat, French, 1859-1891, A Sunday on La Grande Jatte - 1884, oil on canvas, 1884-86, 207.5 x 308 cm, Helen Birch Bartlett Memorial Collection, 1926.224 photograph © 1994, The Art Institue of Chicago. All Rights Reserved.

the thousands of individual colored dots on the white canvas. At this level the dots are just arrays of colors, not making any sense, but you would be able to talk about the artist's technique. You could talk about the basic processes that made up the school of painting founded by Seurat, pointillism.

Now, as you step back from the painting, the dots begin to emerge into organized shapes and forms. You see people, a dog, a tree. You could analyze how the bold use of colors makes up the forms, and you could talk about how the forms look, or how they are different from real people. Maybe you could compare the forms to those painted by Manet, Monet, or Van Gogh?

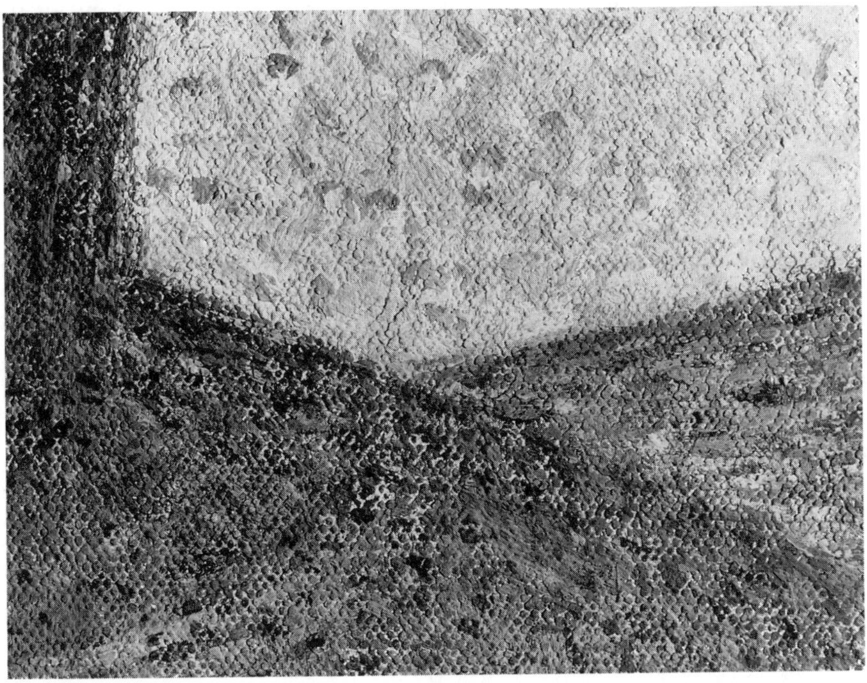

Georges Seurat, French, 1859-1891, A Sunday on La Grande Jatte - 1884, oil on canvas, 1884-86, 207.5 x 308 cm, Helen Birch Bartlett Memorial Collection, 1926.224 Detail C: close-up of back of skirt of seated women with umbrella. Photograph © 1994, The Art Institue of Chicago. All Rights Reserved.

Stepping back further, you begin to see how the forms relate to each other. They relate as aesthetic objects and as human beings. Their placement was carefully planned by Seurat and at this level you write about what is called "composition."

Finally you may be interested in analyzing the painting as social commentary – an afternoon at a working class leisure spot. You could analyze what the subjects are wearing and what they are doing. You could point out what the painting tells us about late nineteenth century culture.

Which level is appropriate? That depends on what is the purpose of your analysis and your perspective. Are you taking a course in "Techniques of Painting" or "Marxist Influences in Art?" Are you interested in paint or people? Depending on your perspective, one level of analysis may be more appropriate (*apropos*?) than another. Also certain paintings may be more appropriately analyzed at some levels and not others.

Note that all levels exist simultaneously. You could step back and do your social commentary or step forward and describe the processes of pointillism. Note also that one level cannot exist without the other. The characters are created out of the technique, but the technique would not exist without the figures that emerge. When you look at the big picture you do not notice the pointillistic dots, but the forms and the culture they produce would not exist without the basic points of paint. Likewise, *what* point gets painted and *where* is determined by the artist's cultural and societal values. Yet, sometimes we may be concerned with one level of analysis and a different level at another time. It is easy to miss the relationships among these four levels of painting.

Looking at a painting, we may analyze it in many ways. At its most basic level we may look at the canvas and the brushstrokes. At a much higher level, we may look at the social and cultural messages it conveys. The same principle of micro- through macro- analysis may be applied to the sciences we have looked at on our continuum. If we look at a person, we may analyze her as atomic, chemical, behavioral, societal, or cultural processes. All are present simultaneously. However, we tend to focus our analysis on one level because of the perspective we have taken from our formal training and informal experiences. When we focus our analysis at a lower level, we are engaging in what scientists call reductionism.

Reductionism and Anti-reductionism

Reductionism is the reducing of a phenomenon to a lower level of analysis. For example, in psychology reductionism occurs when one attempts to explain behavior in terms of physiological (i.e., biological) mechanisms, rather than in terms of the behavior of the whole organism interacting with its environment (i.e., psychological). Reductionism may be worthwhile when it is effective in producing an explanation. However, it is important to point out that it may be more useful to explain a particular phenomenon at the higher level of analysis. For instance, while NaCl may be reduced to its atomic components, you may lose the essential nature of the unique chemical compound that we know as table salt. In a similar fashion, when behavior is reduced to the physiological processes that accompany the behavior (*e.g.*, the firing of neurons), you may lose the essential psychological aspects of behavior. Just as sodium and chlorine ingested separately do not taste like salt, neuron firings do not capture the essence of person/environment interactions.

Let us provide you with an example of how different disciplines might approach a common problem of human behavior: stress induced hypertension or high blood pressure. Physicians and psychologists might both treat this disorder. Physicians, as applied biologists, might take a particularly biological approach to treatment, perhaps stressing medication to reduce blood pressure and control heart rate. Medication might be prescribed to reduce tension as well. Thus, the focus of intervention would be on the biological organs and processes. Psychologists, on the other hand, are more apt to reduce the number of stressors or try to change the person's reactions to the stressors in the environment, rather than reduce the physiological reaction to stress. Thus, psychologists would be more likely to teach coping skills and stress reduction techniques, such as progressive relaxation training and systematic desensitization, so as to change the way the person interacts with his environment. The focus would not be on changing the body's reaction to stress, but rather to change the person's reaction to the stress-inducing situations in the environment. Choosing between the two would require a cost/benefit analysis of both treatment approaches.

In recent years there has been a blurring of these disciplinary borders. The fields of holistic health and behavioral medicine incorporate many psychological principles into the treatment of human disorders. Likewise, advances in biologically based treatments have influenced the practice of psychology. Yet, it is important to understand that there are phenomena which may be best understood at a particular level of analysis and that reductionism is not always productive. The study of psychological phenomena may be most appropriately studied at the level of the whole organism's interactions with its environment rather than attempting to reduce it to the actions of biological, chemical, or atomic systems.

Dynamical Systems and Developmental Psychology

What is Developmental Psychology?

Developmental psychology is the study of the progressive changes in the relationships between an organism and its environment over the life-span of the organism. Psychologists are concerned with two parallel processes, ***developmental phylogenesis*** and ***developmental ontogenesis*** (Sheppard & Willoughby, 1975)[1].

Developmental Phylogenesis

Phylogenesis is the study of behavioral changes *within* a species over phylogenic (or evolutionary) time. Psychologists who study the evolution of behavior *across* species are called *comparative psychologists* and their field of study is called ***comparative psychology***. Comparative psychologists study, for example, the similarities and differences in perceptual, motor, and social behaviors of organisms across the phylogenic scale from, say, mitochondria to man.

Developmental Ontogenesis

Ontogenesis is the study of changes in individuals over their lifetimes. Most developmental psychologists study developmental ontogenesis. Developmental psychologists may differ with respect to the part of the life-span they study, or with respect to the approaches they take to the study of ontogenesis.

Box 1

Of Antennas and Organisms - A Metaphor

Let me provide you with a metaphor about phylogenic and ontogenic contingencies. Most people do not pay much attention to the antenna for their TV set. However, unless you have cable, your ability to receive your favorite shows is dependent on an optimally functioning antenna. I did not really notice what kind of antenna I had until a fierce wind tied mine into knots. Once I needed a new antenna I started doing some consumer research on what was best, and I also began to notice the differences and similarities of antennae on rooftops wherever I went. I began to think of why these differences and similarities existed and that led me to this metaphor:

Imagine that you are a visitor from space and you arrived in the ole US. of A. on Super Bowl Sunday. You go in search of the inhabitants. There are no people in sight (they are all inside watching their super heroes on the tube) so you might mistake some inanimate object as one of the inhabitants. You might mistake all the rooftop antennae as living inhabitants (After all, you come from the very far out planet, Anorexia), especially since they occasionally move (as their human masters adjust their antenna rotor controls).

As you travel the countryside you make two observations in your flight log. First you notice that the physical make-up of the creatures changes as you travel from area to area. In some areas the creatures are very simple, having short vertical bodies with one or perhaps two horizontal limbs. They also tend to live very close together. In other parts of the countryside they tend to be much taller, larger in size, have many appendages, and may come in many different shapes. But the individuals in a given area resemble each other to a remarkable degree. They also live farther apart from each other, or at least in smaller groups.

Your second observation is with respect to the behavior of the antennae. They roost on the rooftops like great metallic birds, occasionally turning. In a few areas there is much orienting around the central body part. In other areas, there is no movement. The entire population roosts like an enormous flock of metallic birds perched with their body parts permanently oriented toward some great eternal sun.

How do these observations relate to our discussion of phylogenic and ontogenic contingencies? First, because of general environmental conditions concerning signal strength and characteristics of television waves, owners have selected certain types of antennae over others. In areas where the signals are strong almost any form of antennae will work as well as another, and simplicity usually means a lower price. (I grew up near New York City where the signals were so strong, you could almost pick up "Leave It To Beaver" via the fillings in your teeth). Homeowners farther and farther from the signal source select equipment with greater and greater size and complexity in order to optimize their reception. Thus various species occupy various environmental niches. In the development of organisms, those which are optimally adapted to their environments are selected by these environments and survive to reproduce. They successfully compete with other organisms in that environment. These are Sheppard & Willoughby's (1975) phylogenic contingencies for selecting the characteristics of the species over evolutionary time. We call these phylogenic contingencies, ***natural selection***.

In areas where signals emanate from various directions the antennae move as a consequence of the particular environmental events (program signals) that are in effect at a given time. Thus their moment-to-moment behavior is fine tuned in accord with the specific contingencies in effect. These are Sheppard & Willoughby's ontogenic contingencies for selecting behaviors within the lifetime of the individual. We call the effects of these ontogenic contingencies learning.

Notice that in this metaphor, the effects of the phylogenic and ontogenic contingencies interact so that responding to ontogenic contingencies (*i.e.*, in our metaphor, movement of the antenna) is facilitated by those produced by the phylogenic contingencies (*i.e.*, the ability to move is determined by whether a rotor has been selected). In the development of living organisms the influence of phylogenic and ontogenic contingencies are inseparable. The manner of interaction is

Phylogenic Contingencies and Ontogenic Contingencies

Renewed interest in the genetic determination of behavior has led developmental psychologists to examine the relationship between biological and environmental determinants of behavior. One way to view this issue is in terms of the ways in which genetic and environmental factors affect the development of individuals.

Sheppard & Willoughby (1975) contrasted phylogenic and ontogenic ***contingencies***. A contingency is an **if-then** relationship. ***Phylogenic contingencies*** are the forces which shape the development of species over evolutionary time. For example, in the Arctic, **if** a bear is born with white fur – **then** it is more likely to escape detection by predators, find food, and most importantly, have off-spring than a bear with brown fur. For brown bears in the Arctic, the reverse is the case. Thus over time genes responsible for white-furry bears will predominate in the gene pool. The environmental forces which determine the physical and behavioral characteristics of species operate through the process of ***natural selection***. In natural selection, physical and behavioral characteristics which better fit the demands of the environment are possessed by an organism that is better adapted to survive and produce offspring. Over time, the effect of phylogenic contingencies is that those characteristics which result in better adaptation are the ones which will be present in the genes of the organisms.

Ontogenic contingencies are the forces which shape the behavioral development of the individuals over their lifespans. These **if-then** contingencies work through the processes of development we will study here. For example, **if** a bear comes upon a new body of water and catches a fish, **then** it is more likely to return to the same body of water to fish again. Notice the change occurred within the lifetime of the individual. In short, the bear has **learned** because of the ontogenic contingencies. This is generally the case with ontogenic contingencies.

Learning may be viewed as a parallel process to natural selection. While the latter applies to the adaptation of species characteristics over evolutionary time, learning applies to the adaptation of behaviors of a single individual to the environment over a life span. Both involve adaptations. In each case the relevant contingencies produce characteristics which allow the organism to function more successfully in its environment.

Developmental Ontogenesis and Dynamical Systems

Developmental ontogenesis (or simply, development) is the topic of this book. The view taken here is that development can be best understood as a process involving dynamical systems. The characteristics that human development shares with other dynamical systems include the following:

1. Development involves the relationship between elements, specifically the person and the environment.
2. In development, the relationship between these elements is constantly changing.
3. The effects of the elements upon each other is reciprocal. That is, not only does the environment affect the person, but the person affects the environment.
4. Development is characterized by a large number of factors (called initial conditions) acting simultaneously.
5. Development is nonlinear. The trajectory of development is not a smooth straight line progression. There may be sudden changes in the rate or form of development (called phase shifts). These phase shifts may be what developmental psychologists call "stages of development" (Thelen & Ulrich, 1992).

6. Development is emergent. The result of person/environment interactions is not simply changes in the number of cells or behaviors. Instead, new patterns of behavior emerge. The organized patterns, called "strange attractors" by dynamical systems theorists, are not just simple additions of elements, but newly organized patterns.

Levels of Analysis of Developmental Dynamical Systems

Just as it is appropriate to view science as existing simultaneously at different levels of systems, to be analyzed at different levels along our continuum, so too, it is appropriate to analyze the process of development into different levels of systems. Modern developmental theory (e.g., Bronfenbrenner & Crouter, 1983) views the child as part of many systems. For example the child may be viewed as a contributor to the dynamics of the family in which she lives or the school she attends. This systems approach is very compatible with our definition of development that emphasizes the progressive changes in interactions (i.e., transactions) between the person and the environment.

Yet the question remains: at what level of systems shall we focus when we look at development? How can stimuli and responses relate to the important context of culture and society? Horowitz (1987) suggests the answer lies in viewing the process of development as occurring simultaneously at different levels of systems. We may choose to look at one level of systems for our analysis or move among them for a more comprehensive understanding of the phenomena.

Horowitz uses the metaphor of a series of nested boxes to depict the relationship between four levels of systems. We have chosen the levels of Seurat's painting to represent the different levels of systems. At the center is system Level I. At this level we analyze development into its basic processes and components. We will be working at Level I when we look at the principles of genetics and learning. For example, meiosis in genetics and reinforcement in learning are processes viewed at Level I. In the painting metaphor, this is at the level of the dots on the canvas. As we move up to system Level II we look at larger chunks of development. At this level of analysis there emerge from the Level I processes new units to be analyzed. The basic units are organized and reorganized. These would include stages of development or characteristic behaviors such as intelligence, personality, creativity, or their facets. While we can still analyze them using the Level I processes, some of their unique qualities would disappear. In the painting, the emergence of figures from the dots would be a Level II analysis.

At Level III we view processes as transactions. "Motherese," the simplified talk used by mothers to their infants is a Level III phenomenon. It develops because the mother's talk is shaped by the slowly changing nature of the child's behavior towards mother and vice versa. Analyzing the relationship of the figures to each other in the painting is equivalent to viewing the painting at a Level III analysis.

Finally, analyzing at the systems Level IV involves looking at the effects of society and culture on the child. These involve higher order transactions, not merely transactions between the child and another. Culture and society are pervasive and form the largest context for development. In the painting metaphor, Level IV would include the societal and cultural implications of the art.

Development is occurring at all levels simultaneously. It is we who must analyze at one level of system at a time. Recalling Horowitz's nested boxes, these levels involve a system within a system within a system within a system. The power of this metaphor is in understanding *that* development can be analyzed at these different levels. All levels are equally important to an understanding of development. As you move to the higher levels you increase the breadth of your understanding of development. As you move to the lower levels you become more precise.

Let us look at sex role development. What causes it? We can explain it at Level IV by looking at the sex role stereotypes in our culture and society. We can add more to our understanding by moving to a Level III analysis involving the transactions between parents and the child. At this level we may use concepts like "modeling" and "direct tuition" to explain how sex roles develop. (But note we move back to Level IV to describe *what* the parents model and train.)

At Level II we may describe girls as having an expressive sex role and boys as having an instrumental one (or we may find androgyny). These are labels for the organized classes of behaviors that emerge out of, and are different from, the environment-behavior processes we talk about at Level I.

Yet all these levels of talking about development are occurring simultaneously. We telescope back and forth along these levels of systems to understand development more fully. In this book we will begin our analysis at Level I, Horowitz's innermost box, looking at basic principles of the organism and environment interactions. We end at Level IV viewing the unique contributions of society and culture.

Dynamical Systems, Behavior Analysis, and Development

Behavior Analysis is a field of psychology. It is concerned with the environmental influences that determine behavior. It has identified powerful laws of behavioral change which have been viewed mostly from Level I as Basic Processes. Behavior analysts (e.g., Marr, 1992; Hoyert, 1992; Nevin, 1992) have begun to incorporate dynamical systems principles into their theory and a principles. In this book, we attempt to integrate these basic processes with the principles of a dynamical systems approach to better explain the developmental process. We feel that our knowledge of phenomena that better fit Levels II, III, and IV, may be more fully understood by combining dynamical systems principles with behavior analytic ones.

For example, while behavioral mechanisms, such as reinforcement may underlie the development of sex roles, the sex roles themselves may best be understood as an organized pattern of behaviors (Level II) that emerges from the basic processes. In turn, we may better understand which sex roles emerge by understanding the functions of society and culture in shaping the roles.

We now move to the field of Developmental Psychology as practiced by its professionals. We begin with a look at the specialties within the field.

What Do Developmental Psychologists Study?

Developmental Psychologists may focus on a specific part of the life span. Some specialize in child psychology. Others may limit their interests to an even smaller segment, such as infancy. A relatively recent trend is the study of the full life-span. Those interested in this "womb-to-tomb" approach are called ***life-span developmental psychologists*** and may refer to their field as ***human development***. Those with more limited interests may call their field ***child development*** and refer to themselves as ***child psychologists***. Others focusing on the opposite end of the human life span are called ***gerontologists***.

Developmental Psychologists as Researchers

Most developmental psychologists serve as researchers and teachers at colleges and universities. They received their Ph.D.'s at research oriented universities and continue studying the processes of development. Some researchers are interested in basic issues about how development occurs. They may study perception or cognition with little regard to the immediate impact of their findings for practical problems of development. Others focus their research on applied problems related to development such as parent training or learning disabilities. Increasingly, however, this distinction between basic and applied research is fading (Whitehurst, 1986).

The traditional perspective on development taken by most researchers is characterized by a ***naturalistic*** approach. This approach has focused on the observation and description of development in its natural surroundings. For example, the researcher may describe the sequence of language development, or the development of reaching in infants. The naturalistic approach has some distinct advantages. Foremost is that this approach is very likely to describe how development occurs in real life rather than in the laboratory. To the extent the researcher *describes* rather than *interprets*, the approach yields good descriptions of what actually occurs. The primary weakness of the naturalistic approach is that its lack of control over variables make the determination of causal variables impossible. For example, because so many things (e.g., objects to describe, parents' words, the child's increasing linguistic ability, etc.) are occurring simultaneously in language development, it may be impossible to "tease out" which variables are responsible for change. Sometimes we want to know **why** things happen, not just **what happens**.

Beginning in the early 1960s there was an increasing emphasis on determining cause-effect relationships in developmental research through the use of the ***experimental method***. By bringing children into the well controlled environment of a laboratory room, or by creating special laboratory schools, researchers could control extraneous variables and determine the variables at work in the process of development. The strength of this approach was the discovery of causal variables in development, but there was a price to pay in the possible loss of accuracy in describing what happens in the real world. For example, if it is determined under controlled conditions that reinforcement of infant vocalizations by social stimuli increases the vocalizations (c. f., Rheingold, Gewirtz, & Ross, 1959), one may legitimately ask: is this how it happens in the natural environment?

In recent years the trend in developmental research has been away from over reliance on any single research approach. Criticisms of each approach have led to greater awareness of the limitations and benefits of each. New advances in statistical analysis, particularly multivariate analysis, and structural modeling procedures, and advances in single-subject designs have enhanced the ability of naturalistic researchers to ask cause-and-effect questions. Likewise, sensitivity to issues of artificiality has improved the quality of experimental research.

Today, developmental psychologists are more likely to advance their science through the use of a strategy involving a ***confluence of research methodologies*** (Nelson-Wicks & Israel, 1986). Such a strategy may follow a logical progression (although each research question may have its own requirements). A logical sequence of steps in answering a research question might involve: 1) naturalistic observation to identify the existence of the problem and potential causal variables in the real world, 2) bringing the phenomena under control in a laboratory environment to identify the processes involved, 3) returning to the real world to verify that the processes found in the laboratory function in the outside world. As we approach the dawn of the twenty first century, the promise of developmental research is more exciting than ever before.

Applied Developmental Psychologists

One reason for the excitement in developmental psychology is that basic research is producing more and more direct applications. Developmental psychologists may be involved in the prevention of developmentally based problems as well as the treatment of problems once they become clinically significant. Examples of this preventative approach spawned from basic developmental research abound, and in each chapter we will examine examples ranging from the prevention of mental retardation to the prevention of child abuse in families. Applied developmental psychologists may pursue their interests as members of university faculties, or in hospitals and other agencies in the community. ***Behavioral pediatrics*** is a recent field in which specially trained psychologists in medical settings may work on preventing developmental problems. The burgeoning field of ***behavioral gerontology*** includes researchers and applied psychologists interested in issues involving the aging process and the elderly. With the increasing number of people living to advanced age, new problems face developmental psychologists. Coupled with new interest in basic research on aging, this is an exciting new field.

Child Clinical Psychologists

These psychologists are engaged in treating existing problems of the child. Traditionally, they may be trained as clinical psychologists with additional training in developmental psychology and child treatment rather than in developmental psychology programs with an emphasis on research. They may receive their training in a clinical program approved by the American Psychological Association and include an internship in treating child cases. They may differ from other applied developmental psychologists in that their training may emphasize treating problems which already exist at levels which are significantly severe enough to result in the child's referral for treatment. While child clinical psychologists may address relatively common problems of normal development, such as discipline problems or bedwetting, they are also likely to target problems which are considered abnormal, such as autism, hyperactivity, or phobias.

Strong Developmental Questions

The above distinctions are arbitrary ones. Most developmental psychologists are engaged in a wide range of endeavors, both basic and applied. What distinguishes them from others who are interested in children is their interest in what Horowitz (1987) calls ***strong developmental questions***. Strong developmental questions are those which ask about the causal processes involved in the progressive changes we see in the individual over time. This means that the developmental psychologist is not interested in merely describing phenomena existing in children or in the aged, but rather in explaining how these phenomena came about. The rest of this book focuses on questions regarding the processes of development in a number of areas germane to the development of the whole person and how the person adapts to the environment. In the next chapter, we look at a newly emerging approach to development, dynamical systems.

Footnotes

[1]Sheppard & Willoughby use the terms *phylogenetic* and *ontogenetic*. Either usage is technically correct. We choose ***phylogenic*** and ***ontogenic*** so as not to suggest genetic inheritance with both terms.

Chapter 2

Modern Developmental Theory

The Importance of Theories

We use theories to organize our thinking. They help to bring some coherence to the many individual observations we make about our world. Theories do not stop at organizing observations; they also attempt to explain the observation in terms of cause and effect. Finally, theories often provide avenues for new knowledge by suggesting further research questions.

Two Theories – An Example

Let us look at some individual observations about the behavior of children learning language. Children enter the world unable to speak or understand a language. However, by the age of five they can understand and generate an unlimited number of grammatical utterances. Most of what they say is grammatical. Furthermore, much of what they say and understand is novel.

These are the observations. Now let us consider two theories which help organize and explain these observations about language acquisition. The first theory we shall call "The Miracle Theory." It states that the human brain contains an innate device which enables this transition from no language to fluency in a few years. The role of the environment is minimized.

We shall call the second theory "The Impossible Theory." It states that language is learned as a consequence of millions of parent-child interactions. Language develops in the same manner as other behaviors – through imitation and reinforcement. Here the role of genetic inheritance is minimized.

How would we go about choosing between these two theories? If we can teach language to an animal with a brain much less sophisticated than humans – a parrot, for example – this would lead us to reject The Miracle Theory. Similarly, if the evidence showed that imitation could only produce mimicry and not novel grammatical utterances, this would lead us to reject The Impossible Theory.[1]

As the two proposed theories just discussed suggest, specific theories of developmental psychology are frequently examples of overarching general theories or ***worldviews.*** Worldviews dominate the questions that psychologists ask and the answers they propose about their subject matter. One worldview might be that nearly everything is caused by heredity and that children are already preprogrammed for development at birth. Another worldview might be that nothing is inherited and that children are born as blank slates (or Locke's *tabula rasa*). These dominating world views bias our interpretation of data. In other words, scientists, including psychologists, tend to interpret data in ways consistent with their worldviews. Thus, many scientists conclude that we determine the very nature of what we study not by some absolute standard of truth, but by the general views of the world that we have. This ***relativistic*** view of science suggests that our conclusions, and even the basic observations we make, are colored by the scientist's own views. Thus, science is not perfect, but is influenced by the imperfect human beings who conduct it.

How Theories Differ

There are a multitude of developmental theories. If development were easy to understand, there would be fewer theories. Yet, due to the complexity of human development, we have many theories from which to choose. Some theories take a very broad view of development, but may be very scanty in details. Others may be very limited in scope, focusing on a narrow part of development, such as language comprehension, or short term memory, but give much detail on this narrow topic.

Developmental theories differ on many dimensions. We will describe three of these: structure versus function, description versus explanation, and nature versus nurture.

An Analogy

Let us say that your non-technologically oriented friend just bought a personal computer and comes to you for help. He asks you an apparently simple question: "Do you know about computers?" The answer is not that simple because "knowing about computers" has at least two distinct meanings. The first sense of knowing about computers is knowledge about what computer scientists call their "architecture." This involves knowing about the parts of the computer and how they work in relationship to each other. Thus, you may know about the differences between the Intel 8088, 80286, 80386, 80486, and pentium central processing units and the various advantages they may have in speed and processing capabilities. You may *know* the advantages of 8-bit vs. 16-bit vs. 32 bit chips. You may *know* the differences between dynamic and static RAM, between RAM and ROM, and endless lists of other possibilities. You may be able to predict that certain components will function well together and give you distinct advantages over other arrangements. You *know* about the structure of computers. You know of *what* computers are made. Your knowledge is a ***structural*** knowledge.

On the other hand, you may know a great deal about computers without knowing anything about what is inside them. You may be able to sit at the machine and get it to perform an endless number of tasks, from balancing the budget to writing a term paper with it. You "know how it works" in the sense that you know how it *functions*. You *know* the right sequence of keys to hit to perform a task. You may *know* the computer's language and be able to write programs to do whatever task you require. And while certain components may speed up operations, you do not need to know which CPU is inside in order to make it perform. You know *how* computers work or function. Your knowledge is a ***functional*** knowledge.

Structure versus Function

In both cases the answer to the question is "Yes, I know about computers." Yet the sense in which we know about them is different. In the first sense we have a ***structural*** knowledge, and in the second, a ***functional*** knowledge. Similarly, our knowledge of human development can be either structural or functional. For example, by studying language acquisition in a child we may know about the changes in grammatical structure from single words through complex sentences. Or, we may know how child/parent activities function to produce the changes. Both approaches are valid though different ways to understand human development.

Theories in developmental psychology which have a *structural* focus may emphasize the neurophysiological structures that are believed to underlie behavior. Some structural theories may also emphasize inferred structures called ***hypothetical constructs*** – such as intelligence or memory storage (Zimmerman & Whitehurst, 1979). From this viewpoint, input to the organism and the organism's responses are of interest because they provide a basis for inferring the structures that underlie them. Returning to the computer analogy, you could systematically enter certain sequences of keystrokes and see what consistently appears on the video display of the computer and from this infer that the computer has a certain CPU or is running a particular structured language.

In human behavior, *functional* explanations focus on the relationships between what happens to the organism (i.e., stimuli) and the behavior of the organism (i.e., response). We are generally unconcerned with known or hypothesized internal structures, such as short term memory or cognitive schemata. Instead. the emphasis is on identifying what events lead to what outcomes and how. From this view, it is not useful to infer hypothetical cognitive "schemata" if one is interested in determining that certain specific experiences lead to certain specific intelligent behaviors.

Both structural and functional approaches can provide complete and adequate explanations. They focus on different aspects of development. A psychologist may dislike a particular theory because she favors structural explanations while the theory is providing a functional one (or vice-versa). For example, to someone who wants to know what cognitive structures have changed during development, a theory that emphasizes environmental reinforcement of behavior will be rejected as inadequate.

Description Versus Explanation

Description and ***explanation*** are two goals of science. Unfortunately, we often confuse the two. Description means to "delineate" or "give an account of." It is one of the earliest goals of any science. In the early days of a science it is important to describe adequately the characteristics and nature of the phenomena studied. This was also true in the early days of developmental psychology. The first scientific studies of children were ***baby biographies***. In these journals, scientists and educators described the changes in their own children as they grew. Some early biographers of the nineteenth century, such as the German educator, Tiedeman, and the Swiss, Pestalozzi (1746-1827), made significant contributions to the early description of child development by chronicling the development of their own children. One such biographer, Charles Darwin (1809-1882), provided the field with scientific credibility by lending his scientific stature to the study of his own child.

In developmental psychology it is important to give an accurate account of the characteristics of children and adults at various stages, especially the behaviors that they perform, and the sequences in which they appear. Those who focus on the development of hypothetical structures miss some of the observable phenomena that are of importance in development. Therefore, careful description is a necessary activity of developmental psychology, as it is of any science. However, as sciences mature and we become aware of what it is that we are studying, the goal often switches to an attempt at explaining the phenomena.

Explanation is another of the basic goals of sciences. But what constitutes an explanation? To *explain*, in this context, means "to make clear a cause or reason." For most scientists explanation is important because it allows prediction and control.

Prediction

When there is a consistent relationship between two factors across changes in the individual factors we say these two factors are ***correlated.*** For example, there is a positive correlation between the amount of story-book reading done by parents and their children's later reading performance; that is, the more time parents devote to story-book reading, the higher their child's reading scores. Therefore, given the amount of time a parent reads to the child, we can predict, with some accuracy, how well she will perform on reading tests in school.

However, even though both factors are correlated, this does not imply that one factor *caused* the other. We cannot conclude that story-book reading by parents *causes* the level of reading achievement in their children. It may be that children who have good reading (or pre-reading) skills encourage their parents to read to them. In short, correlation does not imply causation.

Control

How then can we determine if there is a cause-effect relationship? Researchers conduct experiments in which they investigate whether changes in one variable control[2] changes in the other variable. For example, we could take a sample of 100 children and randomly assign 50 to the Experimental Group and 50 to the Control Group. Both groups will be matched on their pre-experiment reading test scores so that there is not initial difference between the groups. Both groups will be treated exactly alike by the researchers, except that the parents of the Experimental Group will be trained to read storybooks to their children and the Control Group's parents will not. After training, the children will be tested on standardized tests of reading achievement.

Assume that the researchers obtain the following results:

Group	Ave. Reading Score
Experimental	79
Control	55

Notice that the Experimental Group did much better, on average, than the Control Group. From these results we can tentatively conclude that providing increased story-book reading to children *causes* improved reading scores by their children.

We now conclude a tentative cause-effect relationship because, by manipulating the variable of parental reading in the two groups, we controlled the level of reading in the children. We now may be more confident that parental reading *causes* increased reading skills in their children, rather than some other causal relationship. In practice, prediction and control of a phenomenon constitutes an adequate explanation in science.

Developmental psychologists try to establish how hereditary and environmental conditions cause the development of progressive changes in behavior. It is not enough to merely *describe* the ongoing changes in an individual's behavior; as scientists we also want to *explain* the cause of the changes. A description merely depicts the status of things, while an explanation establishes cause and effect relationships between the behavioral phenomena and the hereditary and environmental events that cause them.

Circular and True Explanations

Unfortunately, descriptions sometime masquerade as explanations. Indeed, there are many cases in psychology where descriptions pose as explanations. I remember a psychologist telling her students that preschoolers "can't keep still and listen to long stories because they have short attention spans." On the surface it seems that the concept of "short attention span" explains why children fuss and look away if you fail to present new things every few seconds. But think about that sentence . . . it seems to be an explanation due to the word "because." However, "short attention span" is not an acceptable explanation. Rather, it is a ***circular explanation***.

Let us look at this alleged explanation. Why do preschoolers look away after a brief period? Because they have a short attention span. How do you know they have a short attention span?. . . Because they look away after a brief period! This argument takes us in circles. A "short attention span" is merely a summary description of the behavior of children who don't keep still and look away after a brief period. Thus, what the psychologist was really saying was that preschoolers "can't keep still and listen to long stories because they can't keep still and listen."

Alan Ross (1978) relates how descriptions often parade as explanations in the area of learning disabilities. One of the most common specific learning disabilities is ***dyslexia.*** We use the label dyslexia for children who, for no apparent reason (e.g., mental retardation, blindness), are significantly behind grade level in reading. Many psychologists and educators explain that the child can't read because he has dyslexia. However, you probably see what they should say. . .that dyslexia is a summary description, not an explanation. It describes children who, for no conspicuous reason, cannot read at grade level. As Alan Ross has said "Dyslexia is a way to say in Greek that your child can't read" (Ross, 1978,).

Thus, a word of caution. If someone uses the word "because" they are not necessarily providing a true explanation – it may be a circular one. Think about prediction and control. If it is a true explanation, then you should be able to both predict and control behavior. The word "because" precedes an answer to the question "why?". Ross (1982) suggests that the question to be answered in an explanation is not "why" did the behavior occur, but "under what conditions does the behavior occur."

Nature versus Nurture

Another basic issue pertaining to theories of development is the nature-nurture controversy. This issue addresses the question of which is more important, one's heredity (i.e., nature) or one's environment (i.e., nurture). This debate has raged from our earliest times and involves political and ethical as well as scientific questions.

Modern day developmental psychologists have renounced this question for presupposing that heredity and environment can function separately. Sheppard & Willoughby (1975) have called the nature/nuture issue "a false dichotomy;" meaning that it is wrong to divide the process of development into two separate parts. In a well known paper, Anastasi (1958) observed that the real question is not "***how much*** " is heredity and "how much" is environment, but: "***How*** " do heredity and environment work to produce development? Reflecting this view, it is common for present-day developmentalists to respond to the question of "How much" with the answer "It's 100% heredity . . .and 100% environment."

The reason nature/nurture is a false dichotomy is that, from the moment of conception, both genetic inheritance and interactions with the environment are important causal factors in the individual's development. No genetic material can become an organism without interacting with its unique environment and vice-versa. To analyze the contribution of one without the other is meaningless. It would be like asking "which is more important, the road or the car?", "the earth or the air?"

Judging Developmental Theories - Nine Criteria

There are many theories in developmental psychology. Each developmental theory has its followers. Each has stood the test of time. How shall we judge them? What makes one theory better than another? R. Murray Thomas (1985) presented nine criteria to use in evaluating developmental theories. However, before presenting these criteria, we must issue one warning: while most developmental psychologists would likely agree on these criteria, the simple act of selecting the criteria biases our evaluation of theories in a particular direction. These criteria emphasize an academic-scientific view whereas some other criteria might emphasize aesthetic or emotive ones. With this caveat, let us look at the criteria.

1) **Accuracy:** A theory is better if it accurately reflects the facts of the real world of children. Theories based on observation of real children are better than those based on theorists' hypotheses of how children behave.
2) **Clarity:** A theory is better if it is stated in a way that is clearly understandable to anyone who is reasonably competent. "Reasonably competent" means that any intelligent person with some knowledge of development should be able to understand the theory. Confusing, needlessly difficult theories are less desirable.
3) **Predictability:** A theory is better if it not only explains why *past* events occur, but also accurately predicts *future* events. The more *specific* the predictions, the better. It is easy to offer an explanation of events after they happen. We do this all the time with the stock market, or after an upset in football. It is also easy to make generalizations. For example, it is safe to predict that children will get larger as they get older. It is much more difficult to make specific predictions about individuals, but theories are better if they can.
4) **Practicality:** A theory is better if it offers practical guidance in solving daily problems of child rearing. Some theories are interesting abstractions, but are not very applicable to education, child care, or child welfare. Impractical theories are of limited interest to the real world of children. Good theories are practical ones.
5) **Internal Consistency:** A theory is better if it is internally consistent. It is easy to create a theory by changing the meaning of its parts to make it fit new situations. It is much harder, but the theory is better, if terms and concepts are powerful enough that they can be used consistently throughout. Let us look at a simple example of a theory that is *not* internally consistent. A physiologically based theory might explain reading reversals (e.g., reading b as d, "was" as "saw") as the result of neurological "mis-wiring" which causes the child to see some letters as mirror images of themselves. However, the explanation offered for the b-d reversal is inconsistent with any that could be offered to explain a large number of other perceptual-motor behaviors. For example, the child who reverses b-d can easily reach for a doorknob in the correct place in order to leave the classroom. If he is truly seeing the world as a mirror image of itself, he should reach for doorknobs in the wrong place. A theory which is internally consistent would provide the same explanation for letter reversals *and* grasping doorknobs. The theory just discussed cannot; the explanation offered for reversals must be changed in order to fit the observations.

6) **Parsimony:** Whereas it is easier to construct a theory that has a new principle to explain each phenomenon, a theory is better if it is founded on as few unproven assumptions as possible, and requires simple mechanisms to explain all the phenomena it encompasses. Good theories are "elegant." A few powerful concepts explain much. Behavioral theory is considered parsimonious because a few simple principles, such a reinforcement or shaping, are used to explain a great deal. The laws of nature seem to be parsimonious, in that there is a small number of powerful laws that explain many things. Developmental theories should be parsimonious too.
7) **Testable:** A theory is better if it is falsifiable or disprovable. Theories which invoke mainly mentalistic, unobservable mechanisms are untestable. Like the existence of ghosts, the existence of hypothetical mechanisms cannot be tested. Few scientists believe in ghosts because assertions about their existence are untestable and so cannot be disconfirmed or confirmed. Likewise, a theory of development that is untestable is a poor one.
8) **Productivity:** A theory is better if it stimulates the creation of new research techniques and the discovery of new knowledge. By stimulating new research, good theories provide the database for their revision and improvement.
9) **Self-Satisfying:** A good theory is self-satisfying to us in that it explains development in a way that we feel makes good sense We already have basic beliefs about children and development before we study any theory. We find theories more satisfying if they are consistent with such preexisting beliefs.

A Dynamical Systems Approach

When we looked at the nature-nurture controversy, we saw the importance of viewing development as the inseparable interaction of the child and its environment. Interactions involving both phylogenic and ontogenic factors determine development. The product of these interactions themselves interact. For example, a mother responds to her baby's babbling – the latter being the result of mainly phylogenic interactions – by using "baby talk." Because of the mother's baby talk, the babbling changes to real words – the result of ontogenic interactions. Furthermore, the words the child uses changes the mother's baby talk to more advanced language. This constant, two-way change in interactions is what characterizes transactions.

A ***transaction*** has occurred when the result of previous reciprocal interactions determine current interactions. The analysis of development into ever-changing, inseparable and interlocking systems is called the ***dynamical systems approach***. Notice that the product of the initial interactions have been reorganized and the existing person and environment conditions are different from the original ones. When mothers interact with their children, the behavior of the mother changes the child's behavior. In turn, the child's behavior changes what the mother does. In sum the mother-child system is reorganized as a function of the earlier, reciprocal interactions.

Contrast this with a static system in which the influences on the system fail to change the relationship of the parts of the system. As an example of a static system, consider the relationship between a crowbar (a lever) and the movement of a rock. By applying force to the end of the crowbar, the rock is dislodged. What makes this a static system is that the change in the rock's position does not influence the lever. The crowbar still works as before.

The outcome of development at any point in time is the result of complex interactions and resultant reorganization of dynamical systems. Alan Ross (Ross, 1982) suggested that behavior is a function of the reciprocal interaction of four factors:

1) Genetic-Constitutional Make-up.
2) History of Interactions.
3) Current Physiological Conditions.
4) Current Environmental Conditions.

One's ***Genetic-Constitutional Make-up*** is inherited at conception. This includes gross physiological characteristics such as gender, physique, race, as well as all the subtle physiological characteristics we inherit. Right from conception these inherited characteristics interact with the environment. For example, it is a common experience that females and males are raised differently by parents. How they react to the differential treatment is partly due to biological sex differences (e.g., the "sex gene" – see Chapter 3). As a result, girls and boys assume different sex roles.

The innumerable interactions one has had with the environment comprises one's history of interactions. This history determines in part, how one is likely to behave at any given moment. Kantor (1959) called this history of interactions the reactional biography. It may also be called one's learning history. These past interactions affect the interactions taking place now. For example, a child who has been punished in the past for saying a "dirty word" in his parents' presence, is now unlikely to repeat that word in their presence. Note that a history of interaction is dynamic, and not static. It is a work-in-progress which we only "take a snapshot of" for the purpose of our analysis.

The third source of influence is the organism's ***current physiological conditions.*** This is the physiological environment inside the skin. Whether you are sick or well, tired or rested, hungry or fed, contributes to determining how you behave in interaction with the other determinants. Thus, the child in our example with the newly emerging verbal skills, is more likely to say "I'm hungry" if he hasn't eaten breakfast than the child with the same genetic and interactional history, who has eaten breakfast.

Current ***environmental conditions*** affect our behavior. These include all the lights, sounds, smells, and other properties of events around us. They also include events inside our skin that act as cognitive stimuli to affect our behavior. Because of all the environmental cues present, the hungry child is more likely to ask for something to eat in the kitchen than in the garage.

This analysis of the factors necessary to understand development is, however, incomplete. We must add a fifth, behavioral dynamics, to Ross's four factors.

5) Behavior Dynamics.

Behavior/environment relationships are in a constant state of flux, influenced by changes in the relationships as they occur. While progressive, the effects of conditions are not simply additive. That is, developmental outcomes are not just the sums of genetics, history, and current conditions. The ways in which factors interact are complex. They follow principles which are characteristic of entities in change, called ***behavior dynamics*** (Galbicka, 1992; Marr, 1992). The complexity of these interactions means that simple changes can produce complex results. Small changes in conditions may produce dramatic outcomes; qualitatively new developments may emerge. The dynamical principles which must be considered are outlined next. Notice the complexities of the interactions that develop. We are not simply the result of our biological destiny, nor are we machines without a biological and psychological history. We are the result of progressive changes in the interactions between our behavior and the events in our environments.

Principles of Dynamical Systems

The dynamical principles of development are the functions which produce the structures of development. Chief among these dynamical principles are: multiple determination, equifinality, nonlinearity, emergent properties, phase shifts, coalescent organization, selectionism – organization by consequences, behavioral attractors, and developmental trajectories.

Multiple Determination

Behaviors result from many determinants (variable influences). That is, even the simplest behavior is the function of the combination of many factors. Likewise, complex human behavior may emerge from the flowing together of simple, but multiple conditions.

Equifinality

It is easy to see that a combination of different factors can produce different developmental outcomes given unique genetic, historical, or environmental conditions. This is the reason "there is no one exactly like you." Yet, it is interesting that we can reach similar developmental outcomes by different combinations of interactions. Thus two individuals who score 70 on an IQ test may have gotten there at the result of different transactions between genetics, histories, physiological, and psychological conditions. One may have had a potentially devastating genetic problem, such as Down's Syndrome, but through a history of supportive conditions, functions near a normal IQ range. Another may have inherited a "normal" set of genes, but through a less facilitative environment reached the same score. This

Figure 2.1
An Example of Equifinality

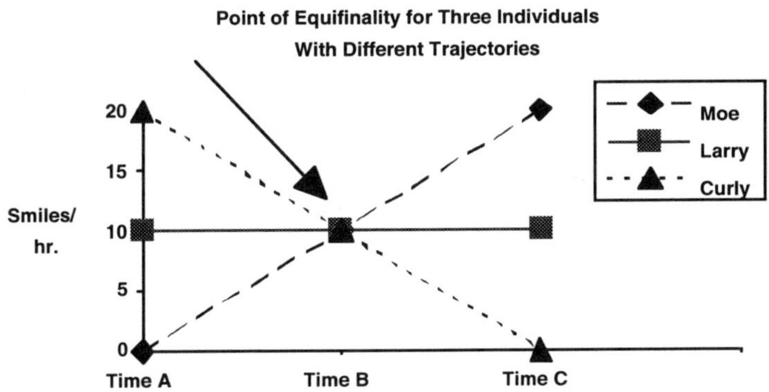

concept is called "***equifinality***" and refers to situations where similar outcomes are the result of different interactions.

The term "equifinality" is misleading. It connotes that we have reached an equal and "final" endpoint in development. Yet development is a continual process and it is only the observer who makes it into a "still photograph", freezing it in time. So these are not true endpoints, but merely points along developmental paths. While different interactions may produce similar characteristics at these points, continuation along the different trajectories of development may mean different, rather than "equal" outcomes later.

The figure 2.1 illustrates this point. It shows hypothetical data on changes in rates of smiling for three children. They start out very differently, at Time A. However, when they are measured later, at Time B, their rates are exactly the same. If we viewed development at this point, we could say this illustrates equifinality. The individuals reached the same endpoint following different paths of distinct combinations of phylogenic and ontogenic factors. Yet, development is not arrested by our measurement. It continues and we may find that at Time C the rate of smiling of the three are no longer equal. Therefore, equifinality is a useful concept, but one whose "finality" should not be taken literally.

Nonlinearity and Models of Development

In our illustration of the smiles per hour (sph) of Moe, Larry, and Curly, one common way to look at development is that it occurs on a unidirectional, straight path. That is something happens at point A (for example, you inherit the genetic predisposition to smile), there will be a particular outcome at point B (e.g., happy, grumpy). This is called a ***linear model*** because it assumes development proceeds in a straight line (i.e., in one direction.) An additional meaning of linear is that the output is proportional to the input. For example, if you are carrying a number of bricks in the back of a pick-up truck, doubling the number of bricks doubles the amount of weight you are carrying. For years, developmental psychologists used this linear model (in both senses of the term). Most statistical procedures, such as linear regression, still follow it. Figure 2.2 provides a graphical representation of a linear model.

Figure 2.2
A Simple Linear Model

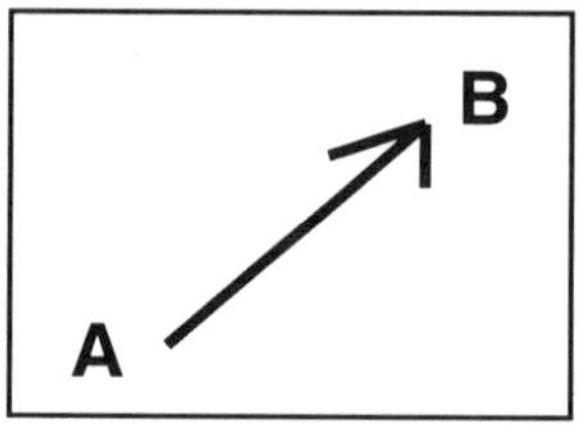

As developmental psychology became more sophisticated, psychologists saw the limitations of the linear model and turned to an ***interactional model*** (See Figure 2.3). This model is nonlinear in the sense that the causal relationships are bi-directional. This suggests that event A modifies event B, and that, in turn B modifies A. The interaction is reciprocal, involving mutual action (Baltes & Reese, 1977). Consider an interactional approach to our example involving smiling. A smiling baby increases smiling in the mother. Considered separately, a smiling mother increases smiling in her baby.

Figure 2.3
An Interactional Model

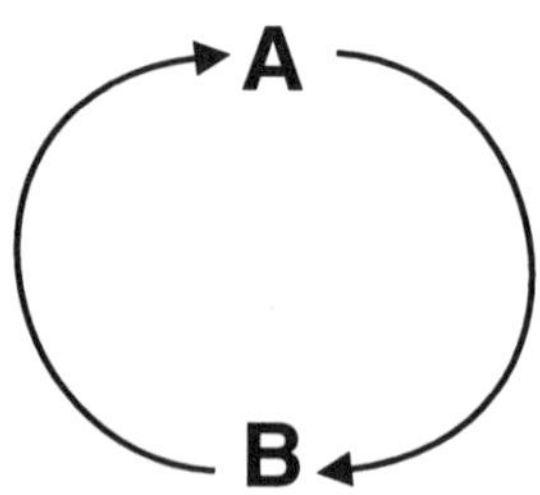

A ***nonlinear*** model emphasizes the reorganizing effects of bi-directional interactions. In a nonlinear model (Figure 2.4), not only does A affect B and B affect A, but the change A produces in B modifies the affect that B has on A, which in turn changes the effect A has on B. At first this produces a *quantitative* changes, as shown

Figure 2.4
An Nonlinear Model

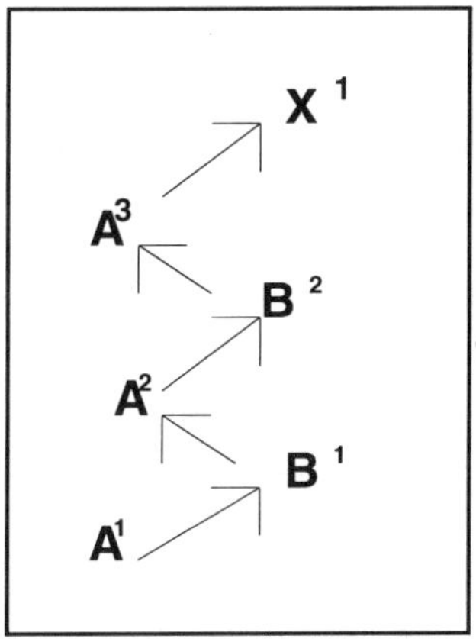

in Figure 2.4 by changes in the superscripts assigned A and B. A smiling baby (A^1) increases smiling in her mother (B^1). This increased maternal smiling (B^1) in turn may increase still further the baby's smiling (A^2). At this point the increased smiling of the baby (A^2) has further effects on mother's behavior (B^2). However, now, the high rate of baby smiling may cause mom's smiling to be replaced by an emergent behavior, laughing. As indicated by the notation, (X^1), laughing is *qualitatively*, not just quantitatively different from the behavior which came before.

Note the dynamical changes occurring in these interactions. Clearly the history of child-parent interactions (i.e., the preceding events) affects current interactions between them. The interactions have been reorganized in that the earlier system of smiling/smiling has become a system of smiling/laughing. This is the essence of the dynamical systems approach.

Remember that, beyond bi-directionality, a nonlinear model connotes disproportionality. Consider again the example of the smiling baby and her mother. Initially, small increases in the baby's smiling may cause rather large, disproportional increases in the mother's smiling. However, additional increases in the baby's smiling may lead to no changes in the mother's level of smiling. Still further increases in the baby's smiling may lead to a drastic, disproportional decrease in the mother's smiling – when her smiles are replaced by laughter.

Emergent Properties

Development is a continuous process. From conception to death, the changes in person/environment relationships are based on what has come before. Yet, as the nonlinear model suggests, not all changes are simple incremental additions to the person's repertoire. Instead, there may be sudden, abrupt change, as when a baby progresses from crawling to walking. Walking is based on what has come before, the crawling, but it is not just a faster or stronger form of walking. Walking is qualitatively different. While based on earlier forms, walking has emergent properties that are not just linear extensions of crawling.

Emergent means that the characteristic suddenly appears. An emergent characteristic, or behavior, does not resemble the origins from which it arose, but has unique properties, including a unique form or function.

While small, incremental changes may occur, at times, change is more dramatic and irregular. We describe these sudden changes in dynamical terms as ***phase shifts***. More traditional developmentists have used the term, stages.

Phase Shifts and Developmental Stages

The continuous nature of development does not mean that it proceeds at the same pace at all times. Rather than just changes in the number of behaviors, development may also involve changes in the form of behaviors. Thus development involves not only quantitative changes in behavior/environment relationships, but also qualitative changes, as well.

In the development of language, for example, we see some quantitative changes in babbling. At first the child's babbling includes all the sounds that appear in all human languages. Then, around six months of age, the number of sounds unique to the child's parents' language increases while the sounds not present in the parents' language decrease and disappear. This is a quantitative change.

However, other aspects of language show changes in the quality of the behavior/environment relationships. At around nine months of age, the child begins to use their own babbling sounds to stand for things, just as we use words to stand for things. Developmental psychologists have used the term vocables for the sounds that that child has coined. Developmental psychologists characterize the shift from babbling to vocables as a change from one "stage" to the next "stage." In the same sense, the emergence of true words constitutes a new "stage" in the development of communication.

Developmentalists have used the concept of stage to describe such qualitative changes in behavior or behavior/environment relationships. Many prominent developmental theories are essentially "stage theories." That is, they suggest that the milestones of development can be understood best by viewing them as qualitatively different states of behavior. Among the most influential of these stage theories are Freud's theory detailing psychosexual stages of personality development, and Piaget's theory identifying stages of cognitive development. We will look at these theories in detail in Chapters 11 and 8.

While stages have been widely used in developmental psychology, other sciences have also had to contend with the sudden emergence of qualitatively different states. Physical objects frequently make sudden changes from one qualitative state to another. For example, as water reaches a temperature of 0 degrees Celsius (32° Fahrenheit) there is a qualitative shift to the crystalline structure we know as ice. Gleick (1988) uses the example of applying increasing force to a metal bar. At some

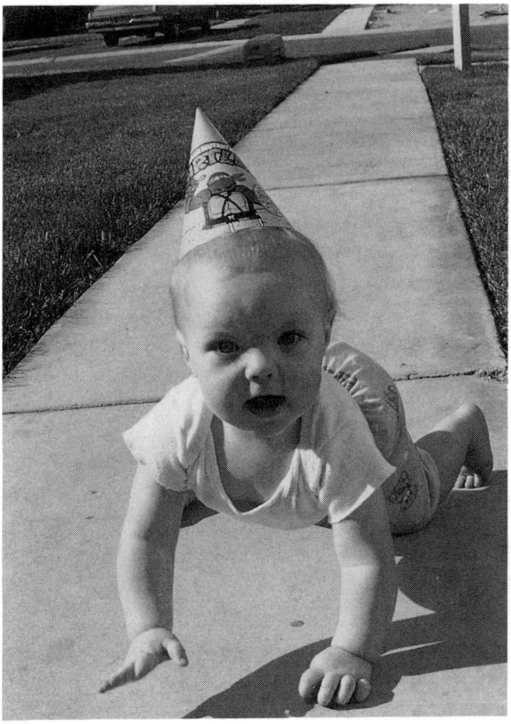

point, the bar just crumples, shifting from one state (i.e., straight) to another (bent). This sudden, qualitative change in properties is called a ***phase shift***.

Thelen and Ulrich (1991) illustrate the nonlinearity of phase shifts. They point to the sudden shift in the gait of horses from walking to trotting. With just a small increase in speed, the pattern of the horse's hoofs shifts suddenly. Trotting is not just more rapid walking; it is qualitatively different. A completely different pattern emerges from the increase in speed. The switch from walking to trotting is a phase shift.

Phase shifts have four characteristics which they share with what traditional developmental theorists describe as stages. One characteristic of phase shifts is that they are sudden. A child cannot walk at all, and then suddenly takes his first steps. A second characteristic of phase shifts is that their order is predictable. That is, we can predict that children will crawl before they walk. A third characteristic is that the new behavior is different in form from the behaviors that preceded it. The walking that emerges is quite different in appearance from crawling. A fourth characteristic is that the form and often the timing of the phase shift is predictable within a species. Thus, Piaget was able to predict a shift at about two years of age from the sensorimotor stage to the preoperational stage of cognitive development. In addition, he could predict what the differences in behavior would be in a child. However, the phase shift or "stages" don't explain the shifts in behavior, they are descriptions of it. How, then, do we explain such sudden phase shifts or "stages"? To do that we must look at the basic processes that produce phase shifts. One of the most important of these is the dynamical principle of ***coalescent organization***.

Coalescent Organization

Imagine that you can't sleep one night before a big test in Developmental Psychology. As you lie awake in your bed, thinking about child development, your attempts to try to get some sleep are thwarted by the drip...drip...drip of water from a faucet. Unable to sleep and unable to cram any more facts into your head, you get

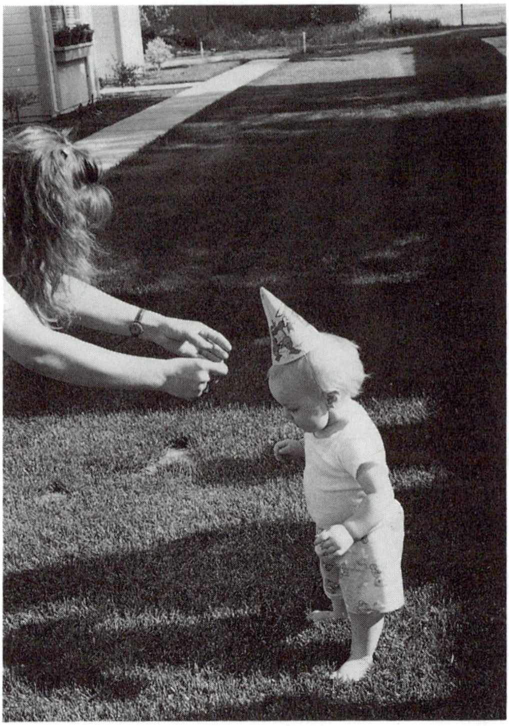

up, walk over to the faucet and are intrigued by the behavior of the water drops. You notice how the trickle of water gradually builds into a drop and how the drop produces a characteristic shape before dropping into the sink. You also notice the cadence that the sound and the pattern the drops make as they splash. You open the faucet slightly and you find that you can perturb the system and produce a completely new pattern and sound of drops. At some point the flow of water is great enough so that the faucet changes phases from dripping to running. Pleased at finding evidence of dynamical systems even in inanimate substances, you open the faucet, fall off to sleep, and visions of waterfalls fill your head.

Thelen and Ulrich (1991)[3] have pointed out that just as physical objects and biological systems develop consistent patterns of organization, so too, do psychological systems. ***Coalescent organization*** is a term for the dynamical process by which factors bring together coherent patterns of behavior. Patterns of behavior emerge because many factors, including genetics, physical structure, previous experiences, environmental conditions, and the task at hand, constrain all possible forms of behavior into the pattern that emerges. For example, the physical structure of most human infants limit the possible forms of locomotion. That is, given our phylogenically selected physique, with a large, heavy body, relatively weak arms, but long and strong legs, we are unlikely to fly. Instead, given a species typical environment shaped by and including gravity, we are most likely to develop bipedal walking. Bipedal walking emerges from the coming together of conditions.[4] Given these conditions, behavior is organized into a particular pattern. Since all humans share common species typical genetic, historical, and environmental conditions, many universal behaviors emerge. On the other hand, because of variability between individuals in the same genetic, historical, and environmental conditions, the behavior of individuals differ.

An important property of coalescent organization is that the form of the response is assembled by the particular task at hand (Thelen, Kelso, and Fogel 1987.) That is, the form of the response is organized by its function or consequences. In behavioral terms, this is called a ***response class***. A segment on *60 Minutes* several years ago illustrates this point. This segment featured a woman, Bonnie Consuelo, who was born without hands and arms. What made this segment newsworthy and fascinating was, despite the challenges that this severe birth defect presented, this woman was able to perform the functions of everyday life, including selecting fruits and vegetables at the supermarket, cleaning house, and driving a car...all with her feet! You can imagine the shock on Mike Wallace's face as he was driven around town by someone using her feet.

A second characteristic of coalescent organization is that, while the unique form of the behavior is the result of the coming together of its organismic and environmental elements, the form cannot be predicted from any of its single elements. Again, consider that walking depends on earlier behaviors and changes in neurological, muscular, and skeletal systems, further, the pattern of walking that emerges cannot be predicted from any of these elements. That is, walking is not just faster crawling or use of bigger muscles. The coming together, or coalescence of all elements produce the emergent behavior we call walking.

Remembering the principle of multiple determinants, some factors disproportionately affect outcome. Horowitz (1987) calls these elements which have the power to disproportionately affect the system "***leading parts.***" A mother in a nuclear family is a leading part for much of what develops in that family. For example, a small increase in praise from the mother may disproportionately increase room cleaning by the child. Another example of a leading part in development is the disproportionate effect the emergence of walking has on social behavior. Likewise, the attainment of muscle and bone maturation is a leading part in the development of walking (Thelen & Ulrich, 1991). These conditions which play a disproportional determining role in development have also been called ***control parameters*** (Thelen & Ulrich, 1991). That is, they are the conditions that control the development of emergent behaviors.

Rosales and Baer (Rosales & Baer, 1994, Baer & Rosales, 1994) introduced the concept of ***developmental cusps*** to describe changes in person/environment interactions which enable multiple new interactions. That is, a developmental cusp is a change, such as walking which, because it has occurred, enables the explosive development of many new interactions, such as social behaviors, exploratory behaviors, and a host of others. Baer and Rosales (1994) liken a developmental cusp to a node of a tree branch. As with the tree, a developmental cusp develops from earlier branches, and like a node, it leads to many later branches, none of which are predetermined nor precisely predictable. The explosion of multiple branches of development that are made more probable by a cusp is consistent with the dynamical principle of nonlinearity.

Selectionism – Organization by Contingencies

Bonny Consuelo's behaviors may be unique, but such adaptations to the task are hardly unusual. You are probably aware of how persons who cannot see with their eyes develop other sensory abilities, such as hearing or touching, to a much higher level than most. Such ***over-compensation*** is not rare.

This example of over-compensation illustrates the importance of the task for organizing behavior. Behavior is functional. That is, it produces an outcome. Surely, most of us would be unable to pick up a cherry or grapefruit with our feet and bring it to our nose to smell the fruit. However, we perform the same function with our arms and hands; behavior which has the same function, but a different form. Given the phylogenically selected characteristics of these limbs, it is much more probable that reaching and fetching will be done by human hands, not feet. But what if your hands are full and you drop a ball that is rolling into the street, or you are Rambo, with your hands tied behind your back, but a sharp object is on the floor in front of you? In both cases, you could use your toes as fingers, your feet as hands.

The coalescence of the behavior depends on the results obtained, that is, on the contingencies. Just as the contingencies of natural selection determine the form of the species that emerges, so to do the contingencies in the environment organize the form of the behavior that emerges. In Bonnie Consuelo's case, the complex grasping movement of the feet was assembled by the contingency of being able to pick up a piece of fruit so that it could be placed in a bag. For most of us, the hand is more likely to produce the same outcome and we develop grasping with our hands that are shaped by the contingencies. The results of these functions are the dynamic structures of development, namely, behavioral attractor states.

Thelen (1994) demonstrated how contingencies underlie the development of behavior. She focused on the spontaneous kicking of 3-month-olds, which, under normal environmental contingencies is random and uncoordinated. Thus, uncoordinated, spontaneous kicking is the norm for 3-month-olds. However, by attaching a string to a soft elastic cuff around the infants' ankles, and attaching this string to a mobile, a new contingency was put into effect: kick and the mobile moves. Furthermore, Thelen investigated the effects of connecting both ankles together with the cuff versus only one.

What she found was that all infants increased their kicking when the consequence was that kicking moved the mobile. Thus, kicking was no longer random when the contingency was in effect. Moreover, when the legs were cuffed together, coordinated movements of both legs occurred at an age where such movements are not normally observed. That is, the environmental consequences provided in this study assemble coordinated leg movements. However, the coordinated behavior was not strong enough to maintain under normal conditions, and when the cuffs were removed, the coordinated movements disappeared.

Variability in Behavior

As we shall see in detail in Chapter 7, selection of behavior depends on variability of behavior. That is, just as in natural selection, where mutation-produced variability in structures is necessary for selection to occur, so too in learning must variability (in this case behavioral) occur for contingencies to select new behaviors.

Alan Neuringer (1994) has emphasized the importance of variation in behavior for basic learning processes. Recently, Robert Siegler (1994) has recognized the importance of variability in cognitive behaviors for cognitive development to occur. He point out that a common view of cognitive development is that it develops in stages. Most people view the behavior within stages as constant. That is, when a child is at a stage of development, all their behavior is consistent with this stage. Siegler's point is that variability is "pervasive". Variability, rather than consistency, is the norm. Variablity not only occurs across different, but related tasks, but may be seen within an individual solving the same problem twice, or even within a single trial. Let us say that the child has to decide which glass (e.g., a tall, thin one versus a short, broad one) has more juice in it. One time the child may pick up each glass and look at it on all sides. Another time, the child may pick up both glasses to see which weighs more. One of these strategies may be better at getting the child more juice to drink and will become the more likely strategy due to the different consequences of the two strategies. Even in cognitive development, variability in behavior is necessary for selection by consequences.

Behavioral Attractor States

Behaviors which emerge may have consistent forms or topographies. Thelen and Ulrich (1991) have used the terms ***dynamic attractor, attractor state***, or simply, ***attractor***, for the consistent pattern that emerges as the result of coalescent organization. Thus, crawling, walking, babbling, and other functional response classes, having a specific form and assembled by the task at hand (that is, having a specific function) are attractors.

The term attractor may suggest that it is the behavior itself that attracts. In other words, the attractor assembles the components into the emergent behavior. However, the term attractor is a description of the emergent behavior. The attractor is the pattern that is assembled by the coalescence of conditions brought together by the task at hand. For example the whirlpool pattern that emerges when water goes down a drain is an attractor. It is assembled by the coalescence of conditions, such as the amount of water, shape of the sink, size of the drain, gravity, and the location of the sink (While the whirlpool rotates in a clockwise direction in the Northern hemisphere, it spins counterclockwise in the Southern hemisphere). The whirlpool emerges from the coalescence of factors; the whirlpool does not organize the factors into itself.

Thelen and Ulrich (1991) characterize attractors as "soft assemblies." This means that the patterns of behavior which emerge are rather fragile and easily disrupted by changes in the conditions which assembled them. Thus attractors are dynamic. For example, consider your own experience in learning a skill that has a particular form to it, such as a tennis swing. Given certain conditions that exist while you are taking a lesson (such as balls being hit by a machine at you at a particular speed, height, and position, and a teacher who is telling you to "keep your wrist flat"), your swing "really comes together." A nice pattern has emerged in your swing. The swing has become an attractor, it functions very well at returning the ball.

However, what if the conditions change? What if the speed increases, or the teacher now says "Keep your elbow in?" It is likely that your nice, effective pattern will be disrupted, or perturbed. Even a slight change in conditions may throw off the swing considerably. Sometimes such perturbations in attractors provide the basis for variability that will be selected by the environment, and a new attractor, better suited to the current conditions, will emerge. Thus, after a short period where your swing has "gone to pot" a new, better swing will emerge.

Developmental Trajectories

Thelen and Ulrich (1991) characterize development as a "dynamic, multilevel, non-stationary process" (page 27). Many levels of systems are involved. Because of the transactions between the person and environment, the influences of each on the other are dynamic and constantly changing. As a dynamic process, development is often viewed as a pathway or ***trajectory***. From a dynamical systems view this means that transacting behavior/environment systems can be seen as tracing a path through time and space.

In simplest terms, the path, or ***trajectory*** of behavior can follow one of three patterns. Behavior can remain stable, it can continue on the same linear or curvilinear trajectory, or, it can exhibit sudden phase shifts.

Given consistency in the conditions determining behavior, behavior is likely to remain stable. That is, with no changes in organismic or environmental conditions, there should be no changes in person/environment interactions.

However, even in the absence of changes in conditions, behavior may continue on its dynamic trajectory. That is, behavior/environment relations which are moving in a particular direction, at a particular rate, may continue on that trajectory. This is the principle of ***developmental momentum*** (Nevin, 1994). Unless conditions change to disturb the person from this path of development, the tendency of the organism is to continue to develop on this path. Conditions that can perturb this developmental trajectory can include genetic-constitutional ones (such as changes in neurological, skeletal, and muscular structure), history of interactions, and environmental conditions, especially control parameters. Some of these changes will be a function of the changes in the organism/environment relations that result from previous transactions.

Finally, as conditions change, behavior/environment relations change. Thus, when transactions produce changes in conditions, trajectories of development change too. Behavior developing along a particular path may be perturbed and a new trajectory may emerge. Thus, discontinuities or non-linearities of development (i.e., phase shifts) may result from the ongoing processes of dynamic transactions (Thelen & Ulrich, 1991). In summary, development is dynamical in two ways. First, *developmental outcome*, while cumulative and progressive, is essentially nonlinear. Second, the *factors determining development* are multiple and non-additive.

A Model for Development

In Horowitz's (1987) view, developmental outcomes are products of the transactions between the organism and environment. In her view, the organism provides the structures of development, while the environment provides the functions. The result is a constant transaction between the structures of the organism, such as arms, limbs, and brain, and the functions of the environment; the contingencies that shape development. Therefore, not only is the organism changed by the environment, but the changed organism affects what the environmental influences will be.[5]

Figure 2.5

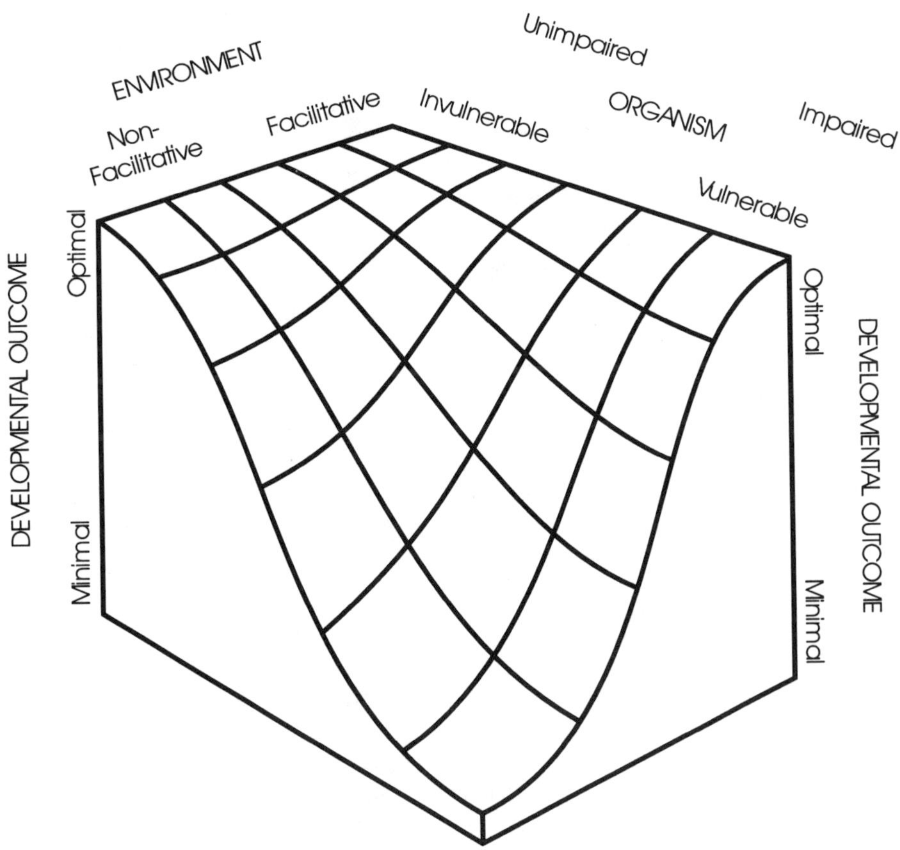

Horowitz's model of developmental outcomes

Horowitz's Organism/Environment Model

Horowitz (1987) termed her view of development a "structural/behavioral" model, but her organism/environment dimensions fit our "structural/functional" definitions. Horowitz represented the developmental outcomes of these organism/environment transactions through the figure above. In this figure, the structures of the organism form one base of the cube (the organismic dimension) and the functions of the environment form the other base (the environmental dimension.) The location on the surface of the figure that results from the interactions of these two factors is the level of developmental outcome.

Organismic Characteristics

Organisms are living beings. What is important from a psychological perspective is that they do things, that is, they behave. At any given time the organism has certain characteristics consisting of a genetic make-up, physiological structure and ***repertoire of behaviors***. These organismic characteristics are the result of the transactions that have occurred up to this point. Thus these characteristics are the result of the organism's genetic make-up and interactional history. Horowitz sees these characteristics of the organism as running along two dimensions, Vulnerable–Invulnerable, and Impaired–Unimpaired.

Vulnerable – Invulnerable

At a given time, the organism's characteristics can be categorized as running on a continuum from vulnerable to invulnerable. This dimension concerns the relative resiliency in the face of an aversive environment. Thus the same threatening environment could have a large effect on a highly vulnerable child, but have no effect on an invulnerable child. "Crack babies," by virtue of prenatal exposure to crack cocaine, have many characteristics that make them vulnerable to aversive environments. These characteristics may include hypersensitivity to stimuli (e.g., noises seem louder) or distractibility (e.g. noises take them off task). These organismic variables make them less resilient to aversive conditions. For example, an infant who is hypersensitive to noises is likely to cry more thus increasing its chances of being abused by a parent (Vasta, 1982).

Unimpaired – Impaired

This dimension pertains to the physiological integrity of the child. For example, a child may be impaired in the sense that she suffers from Down's syndrome, with its neurological defects. On the other end of the continuum, the child would be considered unimpaired if she had no physiological defects. Again, a particular environment will have one effect on a severely impaired child, and a different effect on an unimpaired one. For example, an infant prenatally exposed to crack cocaine may be born with a small head and brain (microencephalic). This child will be considered impaired and his interactions with the environment will be less optimal than the unimpaired infant in the same environment.

Types of Behavior

Psychologists study behavior. Behavior is what an organism does. Behavior includes events both outside and inside the skin. Examples of external behaviors include running and talking out loud. Examples of private behaviors include thinking, feeling, and physiological events. While non observable behavior may lead to problems for the scientist (e.g., they cannot be objectively observed by two people), internal behaviors such as thinking or physiological arousal play important roles in development.

Horowitz (1987) distinguishes between three categories of behavior: Universal I, Universal II, and Non-Universal behaviors. These can be placed on a continuum based on the relative influence of the environment (e.g., learning) on their development. Along this continuum, learning's influence varies from playing a minor to the major role in development (Horowitz, 1987).

Universal I Behaviors (UI)

These behaviors are universal in the sense that all members of the species are "hard-wired" to exhibit them. Examples of UI behaviors include reflexes and perceptual capabilities (e.g., sensitivity to the part of the color spectrum to which humans are sensitive). They are "hard wired" in the sense that they are part of the physiological nature of the species, having been selected over millions of years by evolutionary pressures. Some members of the species had genes for structures that produce behaviors that enabled them to compete more successfully in their environments than those not possessing such behaviors. They survived to pass these genes on to their offspring. This process is ongoing today.

Universal I behaviors are like arms and legs in that they will be a part of the make-up of all members of that species. Yet, like those physical characteristics, UI's require a ***species typical environment*** for the behaviors to appear. Just as you need a species typical environment that includes certain nutrients and exercise for arms and legs to develop, Universal I Behaviors require the stimulation of a normal environment. Just as with arms and legs, individual genetics and environments may influence the subtleties of Universal I behaviors but their basic forms are inherited as part of the species. These behaviors are so strongly determined, that only massive deprivation or injury will prevent them from occurring. Learning plays "a" role, in the sense that experience is necessary for development of the characteristics.

The category of UI behaviors appears to be restricted mostly to simple, yet vitally important behaviors. To reiterate, Horowitz (1987) suggests that this category includes most reflexes and elementary perceptual and autonomic responses. For example, the ability to perceive only a specific part of the visual spectrum (Horowitz, 1987) or perceiving language sounds as phonemes are UI behaviors. Thus innate capacities to respond to the environment fall into this category. Often they may be the essential building blocks from which most other behavior emerge. In Chapter 4 we will look in more detail at these when we look at the behaviors of the newborn.

Universal II Behaviors (UII)

Many behaviors, such as walking or talking are universal behaviors in that nearly all members of the species do them. Yet, they differ from the Type I Universals in several key ways. First, while "hard-wired", they are less "hard-wired" than UIs in the sense that they are inherited as behavioral *capabilities.* With UIs the behavior/environment relationships are there, with UIIs the potential for their development is there. Second, they exhibit more variability in form and quality than do UIs. While nearly everyone walks and talks, the quality of how they do varies enormously (Take Little Eva . . .She walks, she talks, she craaawls on her belly like a reptile.) Third, the *level* of development of these behaviors attained by individuals differs. Fourth, UII behaviors typically take a longer time to develop. Finally, environmental factors exert a greater influence on Universal II compared to UI behaviors. This means learning plays a larger role in the development of UIIs.

What do these facts imply? First, although all humans share the same UII behaviors, the specific levels, forms, and qualities of each of these behaviors will vary from person to person. Second, the paths of development of UII behaviors will be longer, reflecting a greater influence of the environment than was true with UI behaviors. Horowitz (1987) views the development of Universal II behaviors as "a conspiracy between the nature of the organism and the nature of the environment. As we shall see in Chapter 3, genetics clearly plays a role (see genotype/environment interactions). Yet , the influence of the environment is also strong. Thus, nearly all children inherit a basic physiology which allows them to learn language. But the language skills they develop differ widely, depending not only on individual genetic make-up, but also their unique environments.

Non-Universal Behaviors (NU)

Horowitz (1987) defines Non-Universal (NU) behaviors as those "that are the result of learning opportunities determined by cultural values and variations in functional environments." Thus what makes each of us so different from others is the role of cultural and socially determined environments transacting with our genetic make-up and interactional histories. Note transactions are still crucial here. Unlike UI behaviors where the environment constrains the influence of the genes, with Non-Universals, the genetic make-up constrains the role of the environment. Thus, no matter how facilitative the environment, our genetically based body structure will not allow us to flap our arms and fly. We must develop very different behaviors to accomplish that task.

Functions: The Environment

The characteristic action of the environment has just one dimension: ***Facilitative-Nonfacilitative.***

Facilitative means that, with respect to the behaviors involved, the characteristics of the environment are optimal. Thus, given a particular set of organismic characteristics, a facilitative environment will maximize outcomes while a nonfacilitative environment will minimize outcomes. For example, "crack babies" are often exposed to nonfacilitative environments in which nutritional, social, and educational deficits work to minimize developmental outcomes. Such babies may have parents who provide inadequate nutrition, poor socialization experiences, and fail to provide an adequate language environment (e.g., are less likely to read to their children).

Developmental Outcomes: Minimal–Optimal

The developmental outcome of a particular characteristic, such as intelligence, language, or social skills, is dependent on the transactions between organismic and environmental factors. We see how the dynamic transaction of factors fits here. Genetic-constitutional make-up and the history of interactions are organismic factors. Current physiological conditions and current environmental conditions are environmental factors. Their dynamical transactions produce developmental outcomes.

Horowitz has represented this in the model shown in Figure 2-5. Notice the organismic characteristics lie on one base of the figure and the environmental characteristics on the other side. The height of the intersection of the two is the extent of developmental outcome. Thus, we have a model that enables us to see the potential outcomes of interactions of various values of the organism and the environment. We can use this to see that a given organismic characteristic (e.g., Down's Syndrome) could have different developmental outcomes (e.g., IQ) depending on the facilitativeness of the environment. We also can see how equifinality can occur, where two different sets of organismic and environmental characteristics could produce the same developmental outcome.

This model is neither detailed nor specific. The details have to be filled in by research. Still, it is a very powerful tool for generating understanding of development because it can be applied to any area of development to give an overview of the type of transactions that are possible. It may guide us in doing research to identify the specific organismic and environmental factors in development.

Box 2.1

Chaos – An Emergent Theory

The problems facing the scientist in predicting human development is not that different from those facing the scientist attempting to predict the weather. Both involve large, ever-changing, dynamical systems. Both involve a seemingly infinite number of initial conditions from which we must select those on which to base our predictions. Both seem to involve rapid, random, and apparently unpredictable changes. It was from the science of weather prediction, meteorology, that arose a new science, Chaos science (Gleick, 1988). Some of these new ideas may be relevant to the science of developmental psychology as well (Barton, 1994). Let us look at some of the principles of chaos science and their relevance to development.

Chaotic Systems. In predicting the path of a hurricane, or even the flow of a molecule of water down a stream, simple linear models are of limited use. Up to a point our predictions are reasonably accurate, but once past this point a predictable event tumbles into seeming randomness – chaos. In nature it seems chaotic behavior is inherent in large systems – we can predict that systems will reach a point in which they are unpredictable. The laws of Newtonian physics are powerful and useful – they have produced a technology that has sent man to the moon and discovered cures to diseases – yet there are points at which predictions based on linear models fail. These failures to predict do not invalidate the Newtonian principles, but they do call for elaboration of them. The same may be seen as true for current developmental predictions. We may make some predictions about children in general with a fairly high probability of accuracy. Yet, our linear models may be insufficient to predict individual development in detail. Chaos may be inherent in the system of human development too.

Nonlinearity. This may be demonstrated by your opening of a bag of potato chips. You start to tear the top, but nothing happens. You apply more force. Still nothing happens. Finally, you reach a point where the bag suddenly ruptures, dumping chips all over you and on the floor. This is a case of nonlinearity. Rather than tearing gradually and tearing faster as you increase the force, the bag does not tear at all and then suffers complete failure. A phase shift has occurred in wihc the bag went from one state (closed) to a qualitatively different one (empty). Development may be like this. Experiences may have no observable effect and then suddenly a new behavior may appear as if out of nowhere. The child suddenly gets up and walks and never again needs to crawl. The effects of past experiences is crucial, but the importance of each experience is not simply additive. Traditional developmental theory based on linear models would fail to see the major role played by discrete, minor events in the development of behavior during childhood.

Horowitz's leading parts may be an example of the nonlinearity of development. Remember, leading parts are experiences or influences in development that seem to have a disproportionately large effect compared with other conditions. For example, early mother language interaction with the infant may influence later language development more than would be predicted from a simple count of interactions. Or, having one good friend might insulate the child from the effects on divorce more than would be predicted from the child's overall popularity. Linear regression models might miss the unusual significance of these influences. Chaos science suggests that such leading parts may be more characteristic of development than originally thought.

Horowitz's leading parts concept may also reflect the chaos science principle of sensitivity to initial conditions. If you start two identical balls rolling down a plane, where they stop will be influenced to a significant extent by where they started. That is, by the initial conditions. Development clearly is influenced by initial conditions, including genetic make-up and early interactional history. These may function as leading parts.

Another issue raised by chaos science is how we measure things. The yards, feet, meters, or miles we use to measure the coastline of California are arbitrary. The length of the coastline will be different if we use a tape measure that is accurate to one foot or one-one thousandth of an inch. Likewise our measures of intelligence and social development are arbitrary and affect our findings. Within behavior analysis there is a debate between those pursuing a microanalysis of behavior and those taking a more molar approach. Chaos science may help lead us to better understanding of the relationship between various measures of development and behavior.

In sum, Chaos science is new and has created an impact among scientists. It may serve to improve, rather than replace current scientific principles. It is too soon to tell whether it will yield principles that lead to better prediction and control than current theories. Still it has led scientists in all fields to question their current theories and find ways to improve upon them. Behavior analysts have incorporated its principles into their science (See Galbicka, 1992; Marr, 1992; Hoyert, 1992; Nevin, 1992). It may be useful to the science of developmental psychology, too (Barton, 1994).

Footnotes

[1]The terms "Miracle Theory" and "Impossible Theory" have been applied frequently in the past to describe the psycholinguistic and behavioral theories of language acquisition respectively. The theories will be considered in some detail in Chapter 8.

[2]Notice that the word "control" in this context does not mean the same thing as in the expression "Control Group." The former refers to causing changes in a variable to occur. The latter refers to a group which provides the comparison for the experimental group.

[3]The term "coalescent organization is used in this text because it more clearly connotes that it is a coming together of factors. "Self-organization carries the connotation of the organism (the self) doing something to bring the factors together. Thelen and Ulrich (1991) noted this concern.

[4]Paul Andronis and his colleagues (Andronis, 1983; Andronis, Goldiamond, & Layng, 1983) have used the term ***contingency adduction*** for a complex skill which is assembled from component parts by reinforcement contingencies.

[5]For an earlier treatment of this model see Bijou & Baer, 1961; 1978.

Chapter 3

Behavior Genetics

Controversy – The Role of Genetics in Development

In Chapter 2 we saw that the nature-nurture controversy was one of the most basic and oldest in developmental psychology. In recent years a consensus has emerged that we cannot separate the influence of heredity and environment in development.

An Interactional View

The view that heredity and environment each contribute to development is known as the ***interactional view***. Furthermore, the role of heredity and environment appears to be more complex than a simple interaction. The mutual or reciprocal modification of effects of one on the other that result from simple interactions is called a ***transaction***. Transactions are characteristic of dynamical systems, including developmental systems.

What factors transact in human development? To recap, Ross (1982) identified four sources of influence that transact to produce development:

1) Genetics (constitutional make-up).
2) Previous interactions (transactional history).
3) Current physiological conditions.
4) Current environmental conditions.

Genetics - constitutional make-up

This is your genetic inheritance. For practical purposes, it is fixed at the moment of conception, when you receive half your genetic code from your mother and half from your father. At conception, this single cell (called the *zygote*) begins to multiply. As each new cell emerges it contains the same genetic code as the original. That same exact genetic make-up is duplicated in the nucleus of every cell in your body. This source of influence is the subject of this chapter.

Transactional History[1]

Development is a continuous process of change. Once a change has occurred (due to learning or maturation), the organism is different. The individual is the product of its previous interactions. Horowitz (1987) points out that once learning occurs its influence shifts from the environmental to the organismic dimension.

That is, when learning is occurring, it is determined by the environment. Once learning has occurred, the history of interactions are part of the organism's history and will render the person more or less vulnerable to ongoing environmental influences.

Who we are now is determined by what went before. The longer we are on a particular path of development, the more difficult it is to divert us from that path. This is due to the cumulative effects of our interactional histories.

Current Physiological Conditions

We are also affected by the current physiological conditions inside our skin. So lack of key elements (e.g., nutrients, stimulation), diseases, and other conditions will prevent growth of the developing organism. On the other hand, good nutrition and freedom from disease or injury will promote desirable development.

Current Environmental Conditions

Right from the moment of conception, interaction is present. The plight of the zygote is dependent on what Horowitz (1987) calls the ***functional environmental surround***. This is the part of the environment that comes into contact and affects the child. The functional environmental surround for the zygote is initially one of the fallopian tubes, where fertilization occurs. From the start, the quality of the environment interacts with the genetic make-up of the child. For example, a blocked fallopian tube would stop development entirely, while a healthy prenatal environment contributes positively to development.

In addition, many similar functional aspects of the current environment affect our behavior outside the womb. They are the changes in light, sound, touch, and social conditions influencing behavior. Most importantly, they are the events inside and outside the skin which produce learning. Inside the skin, thoughts are stimuli for other thoughts or external actions. Outside the skin, events signal and strengthen our actions.

Dynamical Transactions

The interplay between these factors is significant in a dynamical systems approach. Each individual will be unique due to the unique ways in which genetic, historical, and environmental factors act on each other. Two children could be raised in apparently similar, depressed environments. A parent may be absent, nutrition may be substandard, social and educational opportunities may be lacking. One child may become a high school dropout, get arrested for a violent crime, and die before the age of 21. The other may become good at sports, go to college, and become a lawyer. One becomes a casualty because of the environment, the other a success, seemingly in spite of the environment. How can the environment produce such opposite effects?

The answer is that the effects of any of these factors is not simple. Development is a continuing series of complex transactions between all four factors producing unique coalescent reorganization of behaviors. Prediction may not be made from only one factor. Prediction of developmental outcomes is difficult because of the ever-changing, dynamic transactions between all factors.

Predictions made on the basis of group generalizations are not likely to predict individual development. Because each individual has a unique set of initial organismic and environmental conditions which are critical, group generalizations are only likely to yield crude probabilities about individual development.

Behavior Genetics – The Structures

To understand these complex transactions, it is necessary to start at the beginning. At the beginning is conception, a process which virtually guarantees hereditary uniqueness. To understand how we start our existence unlike anyone who ever lived requires some basic knowledge of the genetic code.

DNA – Secrets of the Genetic Code

An absolute wonder of development is the genetic code. A simple but enormously powerful set of universal mechanisms is responsible, in large measure, for producing all living things in their infinite variety. You share the same genetic building blocks as all living things, including your distant relatives, the trees! (Sagan, 1980).

A molecule of DNA exists as the well-known double helix. Each strand of this spiral staircase consists of sequences of nucleotides. There are only four distinct ***chemical bases*** in a DNA molecule. These four and only these four determine the genetic make-up the DNA of all living things. How can this be? How can only four simple bases be responsible for all our inherited attributes and the genetic uniqueness of living things?

The answer is that while the elements of the genetic code are extremely simple, the sequences of these elements are infinitely long and complex. The genetic code has a small alphabet but an enormous vocabulary. The alphabet consists only of the letter A, C, G, and T. These stand for Adenine, Cytosine, Guanine, and Thymine. These are bases or amino acids, and there are only four of them in DNA. Yet, the genetic code has a dictionary of traits that may be thousands of letters long. Each unique word, or sequence of bases, may produce a unique characteristic. Thus AACAGAT may mean blue eyes while CACCAGT could mean brown. Furthermore, not only is the sequence of the letters significant, but the position of the words in the sentences is crucial as well. Just as the positioning of the words in "The dog bit the man" and "The man bit the dog" is crucial, the positioning of the sequences of bases at different locations is decisive. These locations that determine physical or behavioral characteristics are called genes and the sequences of bases determining the form of the gene are called alleles.

Genes are therefore locations on strands of DNA called chromosomes. There may be 20,000 or so of these locations (i.e., genes) that determine characteristics on each chromosome. Each species has a unique number of chromosomes. Humans have 23 pair of chromosomes or a total of 46 chromosomes in the nucleus of each cell. Thus each cell of your body may contain nearly a million genes! (46 chromo-

Figure 3.1
Locations on a Chromosome = a Gene

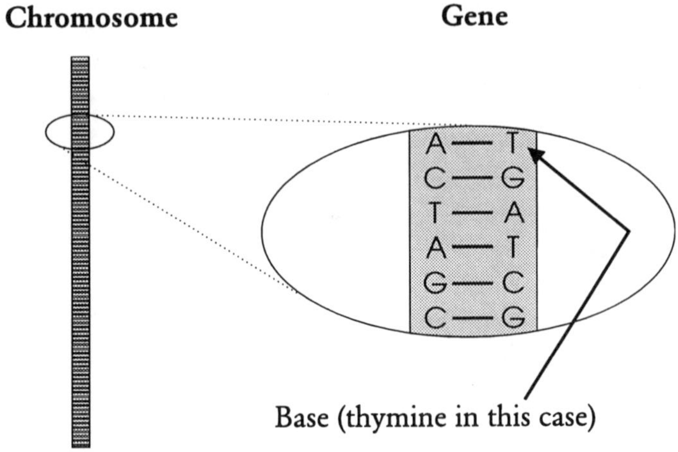

The number of possible sequences of bases is infinite. Therefore the variability of characteristics among organisms, even within the human species, is infinite. Sagan (1980) pointed out that there are combinations for putting together humans that have not yet evolved.

How does every body cell of an individual come to contain exactly the same genetic code? Your genetic make-up is established at conception in the single cell, the zygote, which is the fertilized ovum. At that point cellular development proceeds by the process called mitosis. In mitosis, a cell divides into two new cells (ironically, multiplication by division!) and the chromosomes are duplicated so that each new cell has exactly the same genetic code as the original cell and all others.

Figure 3-2 shows how mitosis produces two identical chromosomes, shown at the gene level. Because of the enormous complexity underlying your genetic code, how can the critical sequence of bases in all the hundreds of thousands of genes be duplicated exactly? The answer to this lies in the double helix of the DNA's structure. In the early stage of cell synthesis, the DNA double helix unzips. This leaves two half strands of DNA, each with one of the bases in its exact position in the sequence. Thus, we now have two half-complete DNA replicas of the original molecule. Now remember, each base can only be paired with another single base, its compliment (i.e., Adenine can only pair with Thymine and Cytosine only with Guanine.) In the latter part of constructing new molecules, an enzyme binds the complimentary base onto its existing partner up and down the molecule. The result is that the original double helix yields two new double helixes that are the mirror image of each other. For every new cell that your body produces the enormous complexity of the genetic code is duplicated exactly.

Does the process ever result in a mistake? Occasionally, the wrong base is attached and the enzyme that "proofreads" the combinations does not correct this. The resulting proofreading error produces what is called a ***mutation***.

Where do the particular combinations that make-up our genes come from? They come from our parents of course. One of the great evolutionary breakthroughs was the natural selection of ***biparental reproduction***. With two parents an organism receives half its genetic make-up from its mother and half from its father. Thus the offspring is genetically different from either parent, insuring variability within the species.

If each cell contained all 46 chromosomes from each parent, the resulting zygote of the offspring would contain 92, and the next generation 184 and so on. Much too many to fit into our tiny cell nuclei. Fortunately, specialized ***sex cells*** or ***gametes*** are involved in biparental reproduction. Gametes, the female's ***ovum***(or egg) and male's ***sperm***, are produced by the process called ***meiosis***. Meiosis involves several stages, but the essential part of the process is an alignment of the individual chromosomes into pairs. The individual chromosomes touch, then separate again. Next, one from each chromosome pair moves into one of two resulting ***daughter cells***. Consequently meiosis produces two "daughter cells" (or two "son" cells for sperm?), each of which has 23 single chromosomes, or one half the parent's genetic make-up. Therefore, at conception, the union of the 23 **single** chromosomes in the ovum and 23 single

Figure 3.2
Replicating chromosomes through mitosis.

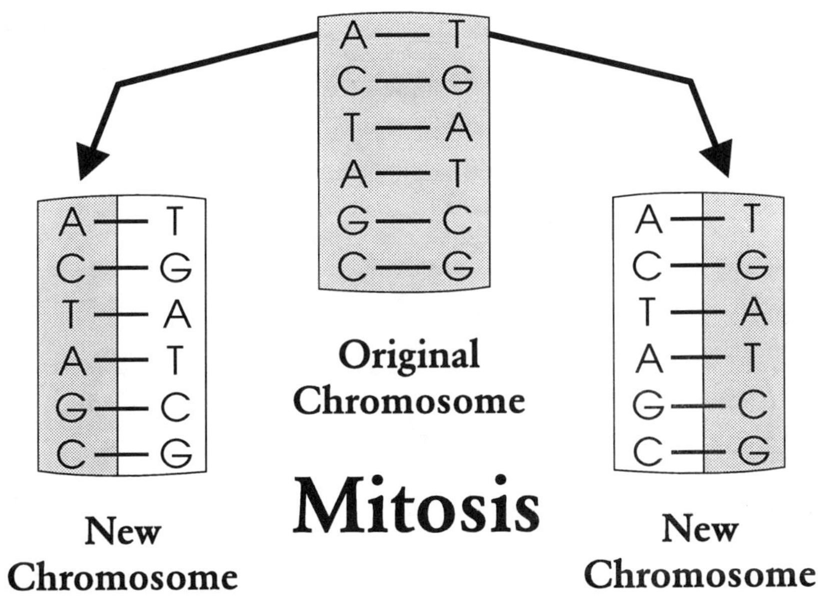

chromosomes in the sperm yield the full complement of 46 (23 **pairs**) chromosomes of the new zygote. These 46 will be the basis for all the individual's genetic code as development now proceeds to duplicate these through mitosis.

Genetic Variability

Biparental variability, mediated by meiosis, ensures that each offspring will be different from either parent. While some similar characteristics will be inherited, the result is variability in the species. Why is variability important?

It is important for the survival of the species. Natural selection dictates the survival of the fittest. Those who are better adapted to the environmental conditions will survive to carry on reproduction. Since environments are continually changing (*e.g.*, global warming/global cooling) species that are unable to adapt may become extinct. The dinosaur extinction is a case where extreme environmental changes outpaced the species ability to adapt.

There are three main factors that ensure genetic variability in species. The first two, ***random assortment*** and ***crossing-over,*** occur during meiosis in the production of the gametes. The third, ***mutations*** are random (*i.e.*, erroneous) changes in the DNA sequence and occur during mitosis or meiosis.

Random Assortment

Recall that during meiosis the chromosomes sort themselves into 23 pairs. When the two daughter cells are formed, one of each pair is "shuffled" into one or the other cells. However, which one of the pairs winds up in which daughter cells is entirely by chance. This "random assortment" occurs for each of the 23 pairs. Hence the probability of any particular combination (such as 1a, 2b, 3a, ...23b) is 2^{23}. This calculates as 2 x 2 x 2 x...2 (a total of 23 times). When combined with the same random assortment from the other parent, this equals 64,000,000,000, or 64 trillion possible combinations from the same mother and father. Thus the likelihood of your receiving a particular genetic combination from one parent is one in 64 trillion! That is more than all the people who have ever lived!! So, it is highly probable that you

Figure 3.3
Crossing Over - Chromosome segments switch

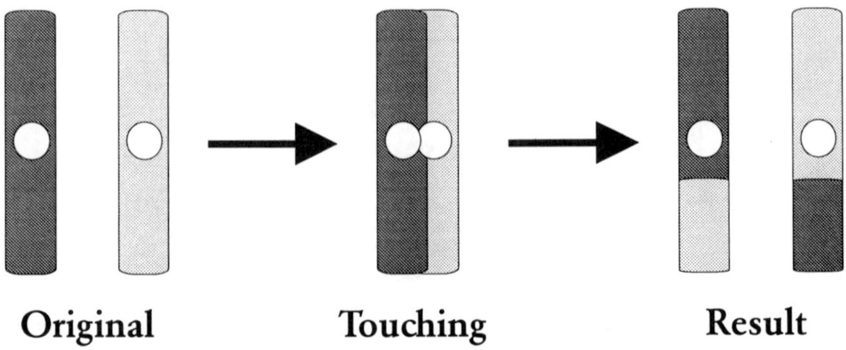

will inherit a unique genetic mixture from each parent. Furthermore, one cannot calculate which of the two combinations will ultimately be the one that contributes to the zygote. Every time a sperm is produced a new assortment of chromosomes occurs.

Crossing-Over

If the odds for genetic variability were not already enormous, then crossing-over makes them even more astronomical. Crossing-over involves the actual exchange of parts of genetic material, as segments of one chromosome in a pair changes places with segments of its compliment. The chromosomes pair-up and touch along their lengths during meiosis. At this point parts of the chromosomes (containing many genes) may trade places. When they unzip we have two chromosomes that are unlike

Figure 3.4
A mutation produces a different sequence on the right.

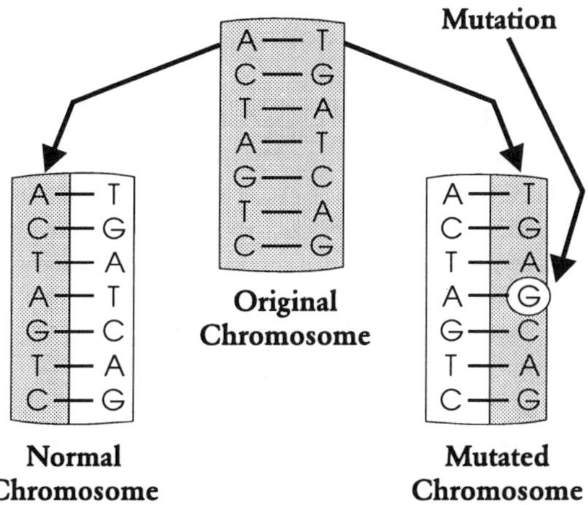

the originals, being composed of parts from both compliments. Thus new combinations of genes appear on these chromosomes produced by crossing over. This process is random and unpredictable. When it occurs, it increases the variability in offspring since it produces chromosomes that have different values of genes. The locations on the chromosomes are the same as the originals, but the sequences are different.

Mutations

Mutations, which are proofreading errors that result in a new sequence of DNA bases, are the third process producing variability. If an error is made during chromosome replication, a new sequence of bases is the result. Most of these mutations are "nonsense words" in the genetic vocabulary and are irrelevant for development. Figure 3-3 shows a mutation. Normally adenine (A) only combines with thymine (T). Through a "proofreading" error, guanine (G) has been inserted instead. When this is duplicated, the new chromosome has a segment that reads TGAGCAG instead of the original TGATCAG. If duplicates of this mutated chromosome become a zygote, this new genetic code is transmitted.

Many mutations are genetically "nonsensical" and cause significant imperfections or malfunctions in development. Most are lethal. A few of these new combinations produce characteristics that enable the organism to better adapt to its environment. These are "naturally selected" and are passed on to offspring. This is how new genes evolve.

Alleles - Dominant & Recessive

Biparental inheritance would be irrelevant if the values of each gene at equivalent locations on each pair had the same strength. That is not so and these differences are the real power behind biparental inheritance. Each alternative form or value (that is the sequence of DNA bases) of a gene is called an ***allele***. (Actually, an allele can mean either the different forms of genes or merely refer to the gene on one chromosome, even if the other is the same form). In a simple example, the alleles for eye color include blue and brown. Since we inherit 23 chromosomes from each parent, and since each gene is a location on these chromosomes, at each pair's location there are two alleles, one from either parent. Both the alleles for each gene can be the same value (***homozygous)*** or they can be different (***heterozygous***). The terms "homozygous" and "heterozygous" refer to the values (or sequences) of alleles at the level of actual genetic makeup, or ***genotype***. An individual with two alleles for blue eyes would have a genotype that is "homozygous, blbl." A person with one allele for blue and one for brown would by "heterozygous, blbr." These genotypes represent their actual genetic make-up. But what of their actual eye color?

When we deal with the actual expression of a genetic trait we mean the ***phenotype***. The genotype/environment interaction determines the phenotype. Some phenotypes, such as eye color, are so strongly influenced by the genotype that environment has little influence. Phenotypes that are deeply entrenched along a path of development from which it is difficult to deviate are said to be canalized. Other phenotypes, especially many psychological characteristics such as intelligence, are more obviously the result of the genotype interacting with a far more influential environment.

Is Development Only Canalized by Genes?

Until recently, developmental psychologists defined canalization as the restriction of development to a single pathway by the action of genes. This genotype-only view of canalization was the result of the influence of Waddington (1957), a geneticist. Thus the view common among developmentalists was that if a developed characteristic was difficult to influence by changing the environment, the canalization meant that the characteristic was genetically determined.

Recently, Gottlieb (1991) has suggested that the environment can also cause development to be restricted. That is canalization can also be due to the long time effects of the environment. This ***experiential canalization*** suggests that behavior can be organized by the action of environment-gene transaction, not just genes. For example, an individual's scores on an intelligence test may be difficult to change much. One may assume that this is because IQ is strongly determined by genes. That is, that it is genetically canalized. However, an IQ score is a sample of complex human behavior. Many of these behaviors may be difficult to influence because of the long-term person/environment interactions that have occurred over a lifetime. Gottlieb's point is that behaviors do become canalized, but canalization may be the result of environmental as well as genetic factors. This latter view is consistent with a dynamical systems approach.

Let us return to eye color to see how the genotype determines the phenotype. With homozygous genotypes (*e.g.,* blbl or brbr) the relationship is simple. With a normal ***species typical environment*** the homozygous genotype will be expressed in the phenotype (blue eyes or brown eyes, respectively). Yet in heterozygous genotypes the relationship between genotype and phenotype is a bit more complex. Some alleles are relatively stronger than others and are more likely to be expressed if present in the genotype. These alleles are called ***dominant.*** Those masked by the presence of a dominant allele are called ***recessive.*** The rule is that dominant alleles are expressed in the phenotype whether they are homozygous (*e.g.*, BRBR) or heterozygous (*e.g.*, BRbl). Recessive alleles are expressed in the phenotype only when they are

Figure 3.5

How a trait skips a generation. Both mother and father have brown eyes. Baby has BLUE!!

Father (Brown Eyes) \ Mother (Brown Eyes)	BR	bl
BR	BRBR (Brown)	BRbl (Brown)
bl	blBR (Brown)	blbl (**Blue**)

homozygous (*e.g.*, blbl). Since you receive one eye color allele from each parent, it is possible for a blue-eyed child to have two brown eyed parents (each heterozygous BRbl). This is how a characteristic can "skip a generation". Figure 3-5 shows the possible outcomes associated with the matings of various genotypes producing offspring with particular phenotypes.

Sex-linked Characteristics

Certain characteristics, including red/green color blindness, hemophilia, and the dreaded MPB (Male Pattern Baldness) occur more frequently in males than in females. We call these ***sex-linked characteristics***. They occur because of the unique characteristics of the ***sex chromosomes***, the X and Y chromosomes. In the other 22 pair of chromosomes, both chromosomes are identical in length so they carry the same gene locations on each strand. On these ***autosomes***, only the value (*i.e.*, dominant or recessive) of the genes (or alleles) differ. For a person to express a recessive characteristic in the phenotype, two recessive alleles must be present. The sex chromosomes present a different case. The X chromosome is longer than and carries more genes than the Y chromosome. (The reason it is called the X chromosome is that with two of these long strands joined at the center, they look like the letter X. The short Y joined with the longer X strand makes it look like the letter Y).

Gender is determined by which of the sex chromosomes the child has. A zygote with two X's (XX) will be genetically female, while one with an X and a Y (XY) will be male. Since the ovum develops from the mother, who is XX, it always contributes an X to the child. It is the sperm from the XY father that determines the gender of the child. If it is the result of a sperm that contains the Y chromosome, the zygote will be a male. With an X, the zygote will be a female.

Because the Y chromosome of the male is lacking the sites for some genes, it means that males are more vulnerable to the influence of recessive genes. Instead of needing two recessive genes for the characteristic to appear in the phenotype, a single recessive gene on the extra arm of the X chromosome will manifest itself. This is because there will be no dominant gene to mask its effects. Because there is no gene on the Y chromosome, a male must inherit the recessive gene from his mother, a carrier who may not show the characteristic herself. Besides the simple dominant-recessive relationship, there are other possibilities in ***single gene inheritance patterns***. ***Co-dominance*** occurs where two alleles are equal in strength. Here characteristics of both are expressed in the phenotype. Blood type is an example of co-dominance (Shaffer, 1989). The alleles for Type A and Type B blood each act as dominant if heterozygous with Type O. In that case the person will have either Type A or Type B blood respectively. Yet, a child who inherits Type A from one parent and Type B from the other (AB phenotype) will have type AB blood. So co-dominance means that both characteristics appear in the phenotype.

Another interesting characteristic is ***incomplete dominance*** (Shaffer, 1989). If a person has one allele that shows incomplete dominance, only some of its characteristics will be evident. This occurs in sickle cell disease where if the person is heterozygous for sickle cell, mild symptoms appear. If the person has two sickle cell alleles, the disorder is much more severe.

We have been looking at simple, ***single gene*** inheritance patterns of the kind that Mendel used to derive his very basic laws of genetic inheritance in the 1860s. Yet it is likely that many characteristics, particularly behavioral ones, involve the influence of many genes. Such ***polygenic inheritance patterns*** are apparently very common. Yet, one must be cautious not to invoke the idea of polygenic inheritance only because a single gene cannot explain the development of a complex characteristic. It may be that the genotype/environment interaction is a better explanation for such complexity of development.

Sources of Development – The Combined Roles of Heredity and Environment

We have already looked at the mechanisms in biparental inheritance that virtually guarantee each individual will be genetically unique (save for the case of identical twins who start as a single zygote that splits after fertilization and who therefore share the same genotype). Crossing-over, random assortment, and chance fertilization of a single ovum from millions of potential sperm are responsible for this uniqueness. The zygote contains all the person's genetic potential, but how is that potential realized over a life span?

Genes signal the production of cells at particular times and sites. Thus they produce the physical being. Their effects on behavior may be significant, but indirect (Liebert & Wicks-Nelson, 1981). Plomin (1989) suggests that the effect of genes on behavior is ***multifactorial***, that is, not fitting the single gene model. Among the factors are the influence of many genes and the environment. He concludes that genetic influence on a specific behavior involves many genes, each of which has a small effect by itself. Thus human behavior is ***polygenic***. These genes may contribute to behavior by determining the physical structures (*e.g.*, the central nervous system, muscles, etc.) that interact with the environment to produce behavior.

Heritability

Heritability is a statistical concept. It is the amount of the variability across individuals, of a characteristic, (e.g., IQ), that can be attributed to genes. Generally, heritability statistics are computed from twin studies. In these studies ***concordance rates*** are calculated to establish the correlation between two persons on a measure such as IQ or personality. If two people score similarly on a measurement, such as IQ, their concordance rate is high. If their scores are dissimilar, then the concordance rate is low. Generally, comparisons are made in the concordance rate differences among groups based on the strength of their genetic similarity. This ranges from the same genetic make-up of identical twins through the random make-up of unrelated individuals.

According to Plomin (1986), individual differences in IQ are estimated to be 50% heritable (*i.e.*, 50% of the variance in scores is due to genetic make-up). Yet, if a characteristic is heritable that does not mean genes alone are responsible. Instead, behavior geneticists have identified several important sources of influence.

Sources of Influence

Formerly twin studies were viewed as comparing the effects of the same genes (identical twins) with different genes (fraternal twins, siblings, unrelated persons). They also viewed the environment as the same (reared in the same home) or different (twins separated shortly after birth and reared in separate homes). Thus they were seen as a clear test of heredity versus environment in that they were comparing the effects of same or different genes with rearing in the same or different environment.

We now see this as conceptually naive. Whereas the genetic differences were valid, the environmental ones were not as simple as first thought. Identical twins have the same genotype, but people living in the same house **do not have the same environment**. Correlations for siblings living in the same home for characteristics such as cognitive abilities (r = .40), personality (r = .20), and psychopathology (r = .10) is low (Plomin, 1988). This means that the home environment does not function to make siblings very much alike.

What then are the sources of influence on development of the phenotype? Plomin (1989) has identified three.

Genotype

The actual genetic make-up contributes to many characteristics, at least indirectly. This is measured by genetic analysis techniques such as karyotyping.

Shared Environmental Influences

The facets of the environment that affect all persons equally are called ***shared environmental effects***. Certainly living in the same household restricts the range of environmental influences. Children growing up in middle-class America share similar environments. Their shared environmental influences are different from those in other cultures. Living in the same household focuses the environmental influences even more. Psychologists believed that living in the same household meant only shared environmental influences were at work. Yet, the small correlations for siblings in the same household shows that is not true. In fact, Plomin and Daniels (1987) reported that correlations for unrelated children adopted into the same family are low. Plomin (1988) concludes that shared environmental influences have near zero effect on most characteristics studied. If these effects are relatively unimportant, what aspects of the environment are influential?

Nonshared Environmental Influences

Even if two people live in the same household they have different environments. Because no two things can occupy the same space, no two organisms can have the same environment. While their physical environments may appear similar, their ***functional environments*** may be very different. The unique effects the environment has on the individual are called ***nonshared environmental effects***. Dunn and Plomin (1990) have argued that nonshared environmental factors appear to have the major influence on an individual's behavioral development.

Rowe and Plomin (1981) provide a way to calculate the approximate strength of nonshared environmental effects. They argue that by taking the correlation for identical twins living together (i.e., same genetics **and shared environmental influences**) and subtracting it from 1.00 (the correlation if all effects were included) the result is what is due to nonshared environmental influences. A hypothetical illustration follows: Suppose the correlation for the IQ scores of identical twins is .70. The nonshared environmental influence would be .30 (1.00-.70).

To recap, we have three identified sources of influence, genotype, shared environmental, and nonshared environmental. There is a fourth factor which influences our estimates of heritability . . .***measurement error***.

Measurement Error

We measure human characteristics in calculating concordance rates and correlations. To measure intelligence we use IQ tests. To measure personality we use various personality tests. Sometimes we measure behavior directly (*e.g.*, the mean length of utterance is a common direct measure of language development). Many of our measures are standardized samples of behavior called tests. In every case we make a certain amount of error in our measures, just as there is often error in measuring the dimensions of a window or the amount of flour that goes into a recipe. The more reliable our measurement, the less error it contains.

We also commit errors in our measurement of human characteristics. While tests are constructed to be reliable and limit the measurement error, no test is close to achieving 100% reliability or validity. Additionally, reliability on many tests may be acceptable for the overall measurement of groups of individuals, but may be quite poor in measuring single individuals. Even our ability to measure genotype in identical twins may contain some error. While improved measurement techniques such as karyotyping has reduced much of this type of error which happened in earlier studies, researchers still make mistakes. In the early days of twin studies the techniques were so poor that twins, thought to be identical, turned out to be fraternal (*cf.*, McGraw, 1935).

In sum, there are four factors determining the correlations between nature and nurture: genotype, shared environmental influences, nonshared environmental influences, and measurement error. These are factors relating to the *"how much?"* question. Let us turn to the question of *"how?"*.

How Do Genes and Environment Interact?

Since genotype is fixed at conception, it makes sense to view the genotype as setting the limits on development. That is, the development cannot exceed the range (up or down) set by the genotype. Within this range of potential or ***range of reaction*** (Gottesman, 1963) shared, and especially *nonshared* environmental influences determine the ultimate influence of the genotype on the phenotype.

However, this restricted range of reaction view has been challenged. Gottlieb (1991) has pointed out that there are no preexisting, fixed limits within which the environment reacts. He suggests instead that we view the role of genotype as establishing a ***norm of reaction*** as suggested by Platt and Sanislow, (1988). That is, certain genotypes make potential limits more probable than others, but do not determine limits of development by themselves. Rather, because of the constant dynamical interaction of multiple factors, including genetic, neurological, and environmental ones, prediction of a specific developmental outcome is unlikely to be very accurate.

Different genotypes have different ranges of reaction. Some characteristics, particularly physical ones like eye color, have small ranges of reaction and so the environment has little influence. These characteristics with strong genetic limits and small ranges are said to be highly canalized. Universal I behaviors show strong genetic canalization and small ranges of reaction. Given a ***normal species typical environment,*** there will be little variability in Universal I behaviors that is due to environmental effects.

Other behaviors have hypothetically much broader ranges of reaction and are less canalized. The environment has more effect on their ultimate expression in the phenotype. Universal II behaviors and especially Non-Universal behaviors have increasingly wider ranges of reaction. Shared and nonshared environmental effects are potent.

Note that these concepts apply *not only across* different characteristics of a given individual, but *also* across individuals for a specific characteristic. For example, two individuals may have different ranges of reaction for their IQ. It is estimated that the average range of reaction for IQ under current environmental conditions is about 20 to 25 points (Zigler & Seitz, 1982). Yet this may vary from genotype to genotype, that is, from person to person. The range of reaction for an individual with a genotype for ***Down's syndrome*** may be more restricted than one without the condition.

The ***rubber band hypothesis*** is a metaphor to help understand the role of the environment with various genotypes. Genotypes are depicted as different types of rubber bands, some short and thick, some long and thin. Some may be stretched more (have wider ranges of reaction) than others. In this metaphor, it is the environment that stretches the range of rubber band. The ultimate expansion of the rubber band is the interaction between the genotype and the environment. Horowitz's environmental dimension reveals another facet of this metaphor. The environment may run from non-facilitative to facilitative. In the metaphor, a facilitative environment would exert more stretch on the rubber band.

Genotype/Environment Interactions

Earlier we suggested that genes do their work indirectly. How might a genotype indirectly produce behavior in the child? One place to look is at ***genotype/ environment effects*** (Scarr & McCartney, 1983). In these effects, genotypes interact with the environment producing behavior in one of three ways: passively, evocatively, or actively.

Passive Genotype /Environment Effects

Parents may provide an environment that is compatible with the child's genotype. These environmental events facilitate the development of the phenotype. For example, parents may enjoy reading to a child. A child with a genotype for hearing will benefit from this. In other words, in an environment containing parents who read to her, a child's genotype causes her to read, while a child with a genotype for hearing impairment will not so benefit.

Evocative Genotype /Environment Effects

Some genetically determined characteristics of the child (*e.g.*, small size) may evoke different responses (e.g., protectiveness, gentleness) from the parents or others in the social environment. A large baby might evoke independence or roughhouse play from the parent. In turn, this child will develop more independence, vigorous activity, and exploration due to the parenting styles his genotype evoked.

Active Genotype /Environment Effects.

People with certain genotypes may actively select certain environments. Scarr and McCartney (1983) call this seeking out of compatible or stimulating environments **"niche picking"** or "niche building." A person with a high IQ may pick a very different environment than one with a low IQ.

Scarr & McCartney (1983) suggest a developmental sequence for these effects. They suggest that passive genotype - environment effects are most frequent in the early years as the parents provide much of the child's functional environment. These become less important and the active genotype/environment effects dominate as older children and adults select their own environments. The dramatic changes brought about with the appearance of crawling and walking illustrate a change to active effects. They see the evocative effects occurring over the life-span as the environment reacts with the person's characteristics.

A Behavioral View – The Organism as Host

Scarr and McCartney (1983) show how genotypes can influence the course of environmental transactions. Transactions, particularly of the evocative and active type, could explain the correlations for identical twins even when they are reared apart. It suggests that they have genetically based characteristics that evoke or select certain interactions from the environment. Over time these interactions serve to maintain similarities in environments rather than leading to vastly changing environments over developmental time. But are genes the only basis for producing consistency in behavior over time? Are our personalities caused by genes?

Donald Baer (1976) suggest that it is environment/behavior interactions that cause consistency in behavior over time. In his view, not only are characteristic behaviors reinforced by our environments, but we also emit behaviors that select a consistent environment. Reinforcement of characteristic behavior is more likely in certain "person typical" environments.

We emit behaviors that keep the environment consistent and more reinforcing. We have the same friends, go to the same places, and do the same things because these are likely to be reinforced. If we wind up in a drastically different environment, our repertoire of behaviors does not work. We act like "a fish out of water." We may find that we are a "different person" at home and at school.

While emphasizing the learning rather than the genetic aspect, Baer's view shares many parallels to genotype/environment effects. We may instead view these as ***person/environment transactions.***

Passive person/environment effects

The person has acquired characteristics which enable her to respond to events in the environment. The role of the environment is to evoke and reinforce certain behaviors that the person has acquired. If the behavior is not in the repertoire the behavior will disappear (extinguish) or be "shaped" (see Chapter 7) into behavior that will be reinforced.

Evocative person/environment effects

The behavioral repertoire evokes certain events in the environment. These events bring consistency to the environment based on the characteristics of organism. The way you dress affects what your environment is like. A soldier's uniform affects how others responds to him/her. Likewise a person may speak a different way "on the street" or in a college class because the styles evoke different reactions from different environments.

Active person/environment effects

We call friends, go to familiar places, select certain things to read or watch. In each case we select a certain environment. These environments strengthen behaviors already in our repertoires. So, in Baer's view the consistency in our characteristics is due to consistency in our environments.

A Dynamical Systems Approach

Returning to our transactional view, both heredity and environment produce changes. Our behaviors react to, evoke, and actively select our environments. These behaviors are the result of our genes, our history, and our current environment. The coalescence of these factors means that highly consistent physical and behavioral characteristics emerge, in what we view as canalization. Plomin and his associates (Plomin, Reiss, Hethrington, & Howe, 1994) have found that environmental factors, such as the mother's positive and negative behavior directed at the child, are, in part, a result of the child's genetic characteristics. Their findings suggests that characteristics of the child determine to some extent the reactions of the environment towards her. So, even nonshared environmental effects may be the result of a long interactional history involving organismic and environmental characteristics in a complex, nonlinear fashion.

In recent years the pendulum that is our dominant world view has swung toward the *nature* side of the controversy. We expect to find, and as a result, therefore do find, increased evidence for genetic determinants of behavior. Like the pessimist, we now find development to be half genetic where formerly it was half environmental. We have begun to take an increasingly simple genetic view of development.

Robert Plomin, one of our most respected behavior geneticists, has offered some wise words of caution (Plomin, 1989):

> ...genetic effects on behavior are polygenic and probabilistic, not single gene and deterministic. The characteristics in the pea plant that Mendel studied and a few diseases such as Huntington's disease and sickle-cell anemia are due to single genes that have their effects regardless of the environment or the genetic background of the individual. The complexity of behaviors studied by psychologists makes it unlikely that such a deterministic model and the reductionistic approach that it suggests will pay off. There is no firm evidence for a single-gene effect that accounts for a detectable amount of variation for any complex behavior . . . Behavioral genetic research clearly demonstrates that nature and nurture are important in human development. (pg. 110)

Footnote

[1]At this point we prefer to use the term "transactional history" since we are talking about reciprocal interaction.

Chapter 4

Prenatal Development

Conception

The moment of conception fixes your genetic make-up and sets into motion the complex interactions between the person and environment that will continue for roughly eighty years. From that moment, a single cell, the zygote, barely visible to the human eye and vulnerable, begins to adapt to its environment. Within nine lunar months it will have increased in size two hundred billion times. It will emerge from its highly specialized environment capable of surviving in the world of human beings. Let us look at this process.

The menstrual cycle lasts an average of 28 days. Approximately halfway through the cycle, one of many eggs or ovum is released by one of two ovaries. If the ovum is not fertilized, it will eventually break down and be sloughed off along with other mucus membrane material and blood.

However, if a sperm were to penetrate the cell wall of an ovum moving in the fallopian tube, fertilization takes place. Which ovum will be fertilized by only one of the hundreds of thousands of sperm is determined at random. Once one sperm fertilizes the ovum the cell's membrane protects it from any further penetration. With 23 chromosomes from the mother and 23 from the father, the child's genotype is now fixed. Only mutations can now change this code.

The Periods of Prenatal Development

Psychologists divide the prenatal period (conception to birth) into three periods. These are the periods of the ovum, embryo, and fetus. Each period has a distinct end that serves as the beginning of the next period.

Period of the Ovum-Germinal Period

The establishment of the fertilized ovum, now called the ***zygote*** marks the beginning of the period of the ovum or germinal period. It lasts approximately from day 2 to day 14. The name "germinal" period comes from the word "germ", meaning "the rudiment of a living organism" (Random House, 1973).

Indeed, the rudiments of what is to become the child begin here. As the zygote moves through the fallopian tube, it begins the process of mitosis. The first cell divides, producing two identical cells. These two divide to produce a total of four. Gradually a mass of cells begins to develop.

At this early stage the cells are undifferentiated. That is, there is no difference in the cells. Not only do they have the same genetic make-up, but they look alike and function alike. At this point a cell could be moved from any one spot to any other without affecting development. This will not be so later when cells are earmarked for certain parts of the body.

A malfunction during mitosis at this early stage of development may cause a parting of the cells into two separate spheres. If these two spheres continue to multiply on their own, twins will occur. Twins of this nature originate from the same zygote and therefore have the same genetic make-up. These are referred to as ***identical, monozygotic,*** or ***paternal twins.*** In contrast, ***dizygotic twins*** are formed when at conception two unique ova are fertilized by two separate sperm. Therefore, these twins are no more similar in genetic make-up than any two siblings from the same parents.

The journey through the fallopian tube takes about three to four days. Near the end of this time the cell ***differentiation*** occurs. When this happens the entire mass of cells forms what is called the ***blastula.*** Within the blastula a group of cells develops into a hollow ball, the ***blastocyst.*** The blastocyst will develop into the organism proper. This growing inner mass of cells will develop into all of the body parts such as the heart, skin, bones, and muscles. Another group of cells forms a distinct layer surrounding the blastocyst. This outer, protective layer of the blastula, called the ***trophoblast,*** ultimately will develop into the membranes surrounding the developing child. The amnion, chorion, placenta, umbilical cord, and allantois will all develop from the trophoblast.

Figure 4.1
The Blastula and Its Parts

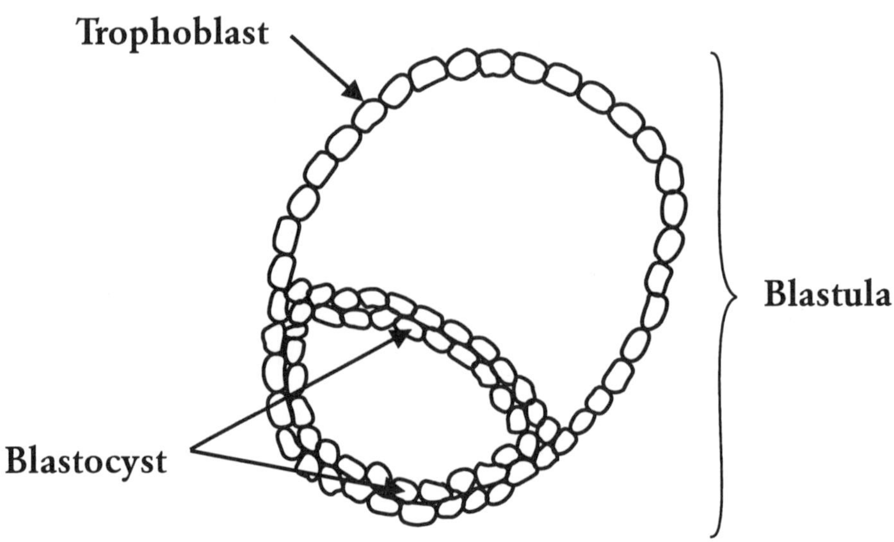

At around seven days the blastula consists of 100 - 150 cells. It floats free inside the uterus for a few days before making contact with the uterine wall. The lining of the uterus is, as part of the menstrual cycle, engorged with blood. Normally this lining sloughs off, carrying an unfertilized ovum with it during menses. But, if the blastula begins to send tendrils into the lining of the sensitized uterus, hormones inhibit the menstrual flow. It is this embedding of the blastula (more specifically, the trophoblast) that is called ***implantation***. This event, around the fourteenth day after conception, marks the end of the germinal period and the beginning of the embryonic period.

Period of the Embryo-Embryonic Period

Once implantation occurs many dramatic changes take place. This formerly free-floating blastula is now connected to the mother's body. At first hair-like blood vessels from the trophoblast burrow their way into the mother's uterus establishing a connection with the mother's blood system. During the embryonic period these tendrils will become the placenta. The outer membrane of the placenta will form the placental barrier, a semipermeable membrane. The placental barrier functions as the interface between the blood supply of the mother and that of the child. The barrier allows the child to receive nutrients and discard waste products.

Other organs that develop out of the trophoblast include the following:

The ***allantois*** becomes the ***umbilical cord***, the conduit for substances between the child and the placenta.

Figure 4.2
The Embryo and Its Environment

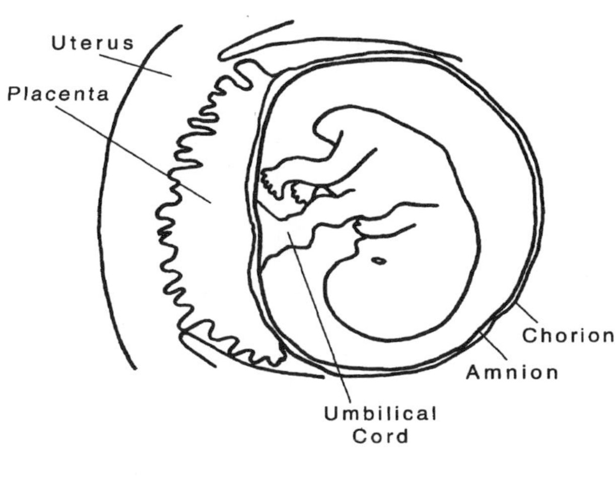

The ***chorion*** is the protective membrane that surrounds the child and amnion.

The ***yolk sac*** is the initial source of embryonic blood cells.

The ***amnion*** is an inner membrane surrounding the embryo and containing amniotic fluid.

The Three Layers of the Embryo

What was once the blastocyst is now the embryo. The next major change after implantation is the differentiation of the embryo into three distinct layers, the ***endoderm, mesoderm***, and ***ectoderm***. The individual's organs will emerge from these layers. The innermost layer is called the endoderm. During the next few weeks, the inner organs will develop into the digestive tract, respiratory system, pancreas, and liver. The middle layer is called the mesoderm and will yield the muscles and bones, as well as the circulatory system. The outer layer, which is termed the ectoderm, will turn into the skin, hair, and nails. Curiously, this outer layer is also the origin of the central nervous system. The location of the spinal cord along the back and the brain at the very top reflects the legacy of their origins in the ectoderm.

The embryonic period lasts from approximately the second through the eighth week. During this brief span all the organs of the body arise. Once all the basic structures are formed, we cease to call the organism an embryo. We now leave the embryonic period for the last prenatal stage, the period of the fetus.

The Period of the Fetus-The Fetal Period

The fetal period is by far the longest period of prenatal development. It lasts from approximately the ninth week until birth at about the 38th week. It is a period marked by growth and refinement. At the beginning of the fetal period the fetus is about 1.5" (3cm) long (Tanner, 1970). At birth the average male baby is about 20 inches (51 cm), about a fourteen-fold increase in length.

Much more than an increase in size or weight occurs during this period. Notably, all basic structures of organs that emerged during the embryonic period are refined during the fetal period. At the beginning of the period the fetus has only the most elemental forms of its organs. During the fetal period they are increasingly refined to the point that, at birth, the organ structures can support life outside the mother's body. The turning point, called the ***age of viability***, occurs around the 26th week. At this time the child's structure is sufficiently developed to sustain life outside the womb.

Principles of Prenatal Development

The prenatal period initiates the beginning of the lifelong interactions between the person and the environment. Already there are processes of development occurring that follow basic principles. Among these principles are some general laws regarding the order in which development occurs.

The Laws of Developmental Direction

The laws of developmental direction are generalizations that state the order in which characteristics emerge. The laws are not restricted to physical development or to prenatal development. They are general guidelines that seem relevant also to motor development and to early postnatal development. The three specific laws and their combined effects are as follows:

The Cephalo–Caudal Law

This means literally that development proceeds from head (cephalo) to tail (caudal). In other words, characteristics closer to the head (eyes, nose, arms) will develop before things closer to the lower part of the body (legs, toes).

The Proximo–Distal Law

This law implies that things nearer to the center of the body will develop before those that are more extreme. It suggests that the heart will develop before the hands, that the elbows will develop before the fingers (This makes intuitive sense. If you were going to make a sculpture, would you ever start with the fingers and work to the middle?).

The Gross–Fine Law

This law states that general, unrefined characteristics develop into specific, refined ones. For example, the basic unrefined characteristics of the embryo turn more specifically into the finely honed features of the newborn. At the beginning of the embryonic period hands are just nubs. At birth they are elongated, composed of many bones, and covered with skin and fingernails.

The General Law of Developmental Direction

Although these guidelines are stated as if they are three separate laws, it is essential to be aware that they are interconnected. Considered in combination, they help us predict when characteristics will emerge relative to others. Internal general features located near the head will emerge before refined parts of the lower extremities. For instance, the laws suggest that toe nails will be among the last parts to emerge. Taken together the laws suggest the importance of timing to development.

The Role of Timing in Development

The laws of developmental direction reflect the importance of timing in development. The timing of an event often determines its impact. Growth is more rapid during the prenatal period than any other stage of development. If the 200 billion-fold increase in size continued, when we reached our first birthday we would be around 476 billion feet tall. Imagine the bottles of formula this would require, or the diaper disposal problem it would create! Fortunately, growth is not always so rapid.

Figure 4-3 shows the velocity of growth in length during prenatal development and the first two postnatal years. Note, that after a slow start growth accelerates rapidly and is fastest around the fourth month. The velocity for weight follows the same pattern, except that the peak velocity is reached later, at the 34th prenatal week (Tanner, 1970).

Figure 4.3
The rate of prenatal and infant growth (birth at month 9)

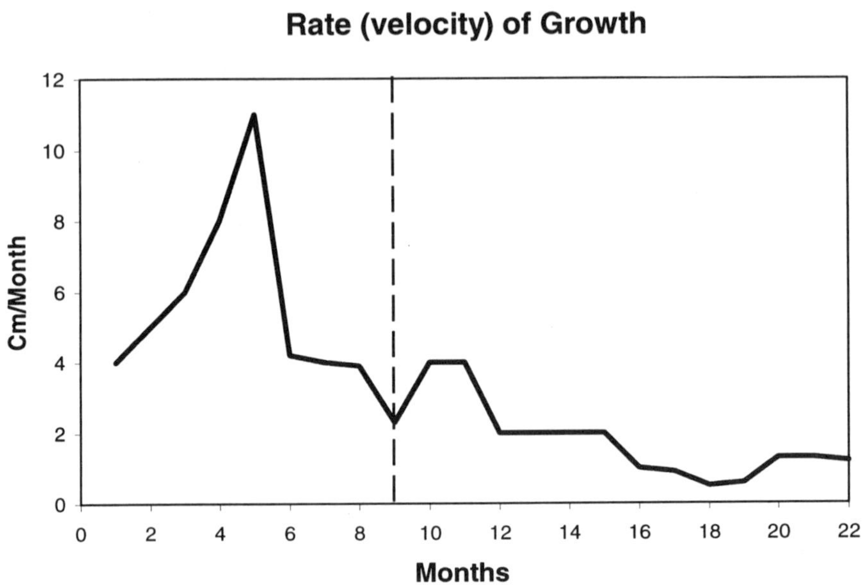

Timing and Teratogens

This rapid growth has important implications for development, particularly when things go awry. ***Teratogens*** are substances such as diseases or drugs that cause physical or psychological abnormalities. (Teratogen comes from the Greek word for monster.) ***Teratology*** is the study of birth defects (Wilson, 1973).

When growth is rapid, events that halt it will have much greater effects than when growth is slower. Many more cells will be affected in the same short time. The presence of teratogens during the germinal period may be catastrophic. Those present during the embryonic period may cripple entire organs or systems. Because basic organs are present, but not fully refined, the effects of teratogens during the last months of pregnancy may be much less severe than if teratogens are present during the embryonic period.

It is also important to remember the laws of developmental direction. Different organs will be affected by teratogens present at various times. Some teratogens, such as ***rubella*** have their most damaging effects only during the first trimester. This is during the embryonic period when the central nervous system and related organs are developing. Rubella is a mild disease for an adult, and also for a fetus. Yet, it has effects on the embryo which include blindness, hearing problems, and mental retardation. A teratogen such as this is dangerous because the mother is often

Box 4

Benifogens?

Scientists use the term **teratogen** for environmental agents which have harmful effects on the prenatally exposed child. In contrast, recent research has shown that prenatal exposure to other environmental agents may have beneficial effects. Two that are discussed below are folic acid and AZT.

Folic acid is a B vitamin that is naturally present in foods, especially dried beans green leafy vegetables, and members of the broccoli family. Folic acid is necessary for the proper formation of the neural tube through which the spinal cord runs. The absence of folic acid has been linked to spina bifida, a common birth defect. Spina bifida occurs in nearly one out of every 1,000 live births and is characterized by small or large openings in the spine so that parts of the spinal cord protrude. Because the nerves have very little protection, the spinal cord is likely to be injured or infected. This usually results in paralysis, mental retardation, other major disability, or even infant deaths from infection.

Some of the effects of spina bifida can be prevented through surgically enclosing the spinal cord. However, it may be possible to prevent spina bifida itself. It has been reported that women who take folic acid vitamin supplements in the earliest stages of pregnancy may reduce the likelihood of having a child with spina bifida (American Medical Association, 1991). It is believed that American women follow diets that are low in folic acid (Willett, 1992). Even taking a multi-vitamin may not provide enough folic acid to prevent many defects.

Because the defects are likely to occur in the embryonic period, even before women are aware that they are pregnant, the Federal Drug Administration has proposed fortifying flour and other grain products with folic acid (Williams, 1994). Recently the New York Times (Kolata, 1995) has reported that although the importance of folic acid in preventing this common birth defect is well established, the importance of supplementing the diets of females of child-bearing age is still not widely understood and attempts to alter dietary habits have been unsuccessful.

The drug AZT may be considered a "benifogen" for children of mothers infected with the AIDS virus, HIV. Originally found to slow down the development of AIDS-related symptoms in adults with the virus, AZT (or Zidovudine) has recently been found to offer protection to the prenatal child. In a study by Boyer, Dillon, Navaie, Deveikis, Keller, O'Rourke, and Bryson (1994) only one out of 26 (4%) mothers treated with AZT transmitted HIV to their children. This is in contrast to the children of the AZT group versus 15% of those receiving a placebo (Cowley, 1994). This discovery caused the researchers to abandon the placebo and administered the AZT to all participants.

Unlike the use of folic acid to prevent spinal tube defects, the use of AZT is not without controversy. In the view of many, it is one thing to add an inexpensive, natural substance (vitamin B) to food, and yet another to administer AZT. AZT is expensive, has potential side effects (Center for Disease Control and Prevention, 1994), and therefore requires that mothers be tested to determine if they are AZT positive. Ethical concerns revolving around a person's right to privacy versus the benefits of AZT therapy for the child have been raised (Bayer, 1994). However, in 1995, the U.S. Public Health Service developed guidelines which strongly urged that all pregnant women voluntarily obtain an AIDS test as early in the pregnancy as possible. The Center for Disease Control estimated that with testing and administration of AZT, among the 7,000 HIV infected women who give birth each year, at least 1,00 babies could be saved from HIV infection through the voluntary guidelines. Furthermore, the CDC believes that the $240 million spent in the U.S. on the treatment of HIV infected children could be cut in half. Ultimately, research, debate, and education will determine the use of this "benifogen".

unaware of its presence. By vaccinating all women of childbearing age *prior* to conceiving, the devastating effects of this disease could be prevented.

The Earliest Environment

The progressive interactions between the person and environment that characterize behavior start immediately at conception. Thus far we have focused mainly on the developing child. Now we must turn our attention to the highly specialized context in which the prenatal organism develops, its mother's body. The amniotic sac is the entire functional environmental surround for the child's first nine months. Over our phylogenic history the mother's body has evolved special characteristics that truly place it in the category of a species typical environment. All members of the species develop in the specialized structures of the child's protective membranes and its mother's body (test tube babies and MacDuff to the contrary).

The ovaries, oviduct, and uterus are structures that serve very specialized functions. They transact with the characteristic of the developing organism. The structures of the mother's body change as the developing child changes. Each affects the other.

These structures play very specific roles. For example, the oviduct is designed to function as a conduit to transport the blastula into the uterus. Its tiny, hair-sized tubing is unsuitable to nourish the baby to full term. Unfortunately things can go terribly wrong even in the earliest stages of the mother/child interaction and a blastula can implant in the oviduct rather than in the uterus. This ***ectopic*** (or ***tubal***) ***pregnancy*** is lethal to the developing embryo and a serious medical emergency for the mother, requiring surgical treatment. It is the much more spacious chamber of the uterus that evolved as the appropriate species typical environment for the growth and development of the embryo and fetus.

Nutrition and Development

Another important factor in growth and development is the availability of nutrients. Look again at figure 4.3. Notice the relatively slow initial growth. An important limitation for the free floating blastula is the lack of available nutrition. It can only ingest nutrients available by absorption through the cell membranes, a process called ***phagocytosis***. This is a very inefficient way to take in food (although I know several people who claim to be able to put on fat just by standing next to a dozen jelly doughnuts).

This lack of nutritional supply is part of what makes implantation in the uterus lining such a milestone. Now, with the availability of substances in the maternal blood supply, growth can accelerate. Let us look at this mother-embryo connection.

Initially the trophoblast sends its hair-like tendrils burrowing into the lining of the uterus. Eventually, some cells of the trophoblast form the placenta. It is the placenta at which occurs the exchange of nutrients from the mother and metabolic waste products from the child. These exchanges occur because the placenta is a semipermeable membrane that functions through ***osmosis***. Substances flow from a location of high concentration (e.g., nutrients in the mother's blood) to one where there is a low concentration (e.g., the child's blood).

As a semipermeable membrane, this placental barrier allows small molecules through, but it keeps large particles, especially blood cells, from crossing between the two blood systems. Thus the two blood systems are separate. This is why the mother can carry a child with different ***rh antigens*** (rh positive, rh negative) without her immune system producing antibodies against this foreign substance. Because the blood cells and their antigens are kept separate, they do not trigger an immune response.

The enormous capacity of the placenta to exchange nutrients and wastes between the two blood systems is striking. The placenta is very convoluted and filled with tiny hair-like capillaries. This gives it an immense surface area, facilitating the exchange of substances. To fully appreciate the enormity of the placenta's surface area, consider one estimate of the size of its surface area relative to the size of the child it nourishes. While the weight of the placenta is only 14% of the weight of the child at birth (Eichorn, 1970), Aherne and Dunnill (1966) estimated the following: The surface area of a newborn is about .22 square meters or about *two square feet*, while the surface area of the placenta is estimated to be 11 square meters or about *99 square feet.* This enormous surface area is present to allow nutrients to pass from the mother to the fetus. It enables the prenatal child to grow at a prodigious rate.

Another Look at Teratogens

Unfortunately, the placental barrier does not only bring nutrition in and wastes out. The mother's body is also the environmental source for many teratogens. If the substances are small enough to pass through the semipermeable membrane, the placenta transmits these as well. Vorhees and Mollnow (1987) have looked at many suspected environmental teratogens. Below is a list of environmental agents, rank ordered in terms of the strength of the evidence (strongest to weakest) concerning their detrimental effects.

1. **Agents Established as Behavioral Teratogens:** these include Fetal Alcohol Syndrome, lead poisoning, and Fetal Minamata disease caused by mercury poisoning (methyl mercury).
2. **Agents That are Probable Behavioral Teratogens:** Fetal Anticonvulsant Syndrome (caused by anticonvulsant drugs), cigarette smoking & nicotine, narcotics, PCBs, hormones, and radiation.
3. **Agents Suspected of Being Behavioral Teratogens:** Marijuana, anesthetics, antidepressants, aspirin, thalidomide, and anxiolytic drugs (e.g., diazepam and chlordiazepoxide). In addition maternal infections (including rubella and AIDS – See Box 4) and other heavy metals and industrial solvents are also suspected.

Accordingly, there are many possible detrimental environmental influences on prenatal development, all mediated by the mother. A question arises: what are the long term effects of this interaction of the child with the environment?

Dynamical Systems Model

Reproductive Risk Versus Caretaking Casualty

For years, the linear model had us focus on reproductive risk. In this view, exposure to a teratogen or other nonfacilitative conditions, such as anoxia produced a poor developmental outcome. This idea was based on assumptions and backed by faulty research findings supporting the view that some of the above teratogens and birth complications such as anoxia (i.e., lack of oxygen) carried a near 100% probability of later developmental problems. To recap the linear model, if something happened at A (e.g., mild anoxia) it caused a difficulty at B (e.g., mental retardation, learning disabilities).

Sameroff and Chandler (1975) took issue with the linear approach inherent in the term ***"reproductive risk."*** They cited improved research which showed that mild anoxia usually did not necessarily lead to long term problems for the children. They argued that long term parental caretaking over a period of years was more influential than a single early event in affecting developmental outcomes. Thus they argued for replacing the term "reproductive risk" with the ***continuum of caretaking casualty.***

A continuum emphasizes the long term and continuous nature of the caretaker's role. The idea of caretaker casualty implies the importance of the environmental dimension mediated by the caretaker. Thus, the expression "continuum of caretaker casualty" suggests that interactions between genetic, historical, and current environments are crucial. While the term "continuum" sounds linear, their thinking was transactional. Thus they found that the effects of mild anoxia gradually disappeared over a period of years, as caretakers provided a facilitative environment.

The transactional model seems particularly useful when viewing prenatal development. It will be helpful to refer again to Horowitz's model in Figure 2.6 . Genetic make-up falls on the organismic continuum, contributing to where the child falls on the impaired/unimpaired and vulnerable/invulnerable continuum. For example, a child with Down's syndrome has certain impairments which will influence physical, intellectual, and social development. Likewise, inherited characteristics, such as ear canals which retain fluid, make the child vulnerable to developing language problems since the child's hearing is affected. The prenatal environment the mother provides falls on the environmental dimension. Conditions in this environment, such as appropriate nutrition or diseases, determine the child's placement on the nonfacilitative/facilitative dimension.

It is important to note that the effects of the environment on the child become part of the organismic dimension. For example, if mother's exposure to high concentrations of alcohol (nonfacilitative environment) produce detrimental effects, the child will be more impaired on the organismic dimension. The long run effects also fall on the environmental side, with sensitive childrearing, remedial education, and other facilitative events eradicating the early nonfacilitative ones.

Getting Ready for the World

The intrauterine environment provides a mostly facilitative environment for the fetus. During the last months of development the fetus is acquiring the physical structures which will ensure survival in the outside world. At the same time, basic behavioral adaptations are taking place that will enable it to adapt to its environment. As a result, it enters the outside world ready to profit from the full range of potential learning experiences in this new functional environmental surround.

Chapter 5

The Remarkable Newborn

After some 266 days the newborn emerges from the highly protective environment of its mother's body. It has spent the time not only developing physically, but behaviorally as well. Not only has it acquired the biological structures necessary for survival, but also the ability to interact with the outside world.

Birth is an event that changes the child's environmental surround. Auditory stimuli were muffled, visual stimuli were dim or nonexistent, but birth has changed that. The newborn enters an environment filled with multiple stimuli. Is the newborn capable of sensing these? Do newborns react to the stimuli immediately, or do they first need to experience the world for a while before they can react to it? William James, the preeminent American psychologist of his day, described the newborn's world as a "booming, buzzing, mass of confusion." Today, a century later, we know that the newborn enters this new world already capable of responding to it in systematic ways. Such response capabilities set the stage for rapid learning. What are these capabilities? When do they begin? How do we assess them? These are questions to be answered about the remarkable newborn.

Birth

First, we shall call the newborn by the technical term "neonate." ***Neonate*** literally means newborn. The full-term neonate averages 20 inches (51 cm) and weighs between 6 and 9 pounds (2.7 - 4.1 kg) at birth. Hormonal changes signal the mother's body to produce changes that induce labor. On average, labor for firstborns lasts sixteen to seventeen hours (Lamb & Bornstein, 1987).

Already the neonate is brimming with the capacity to respond to the external environment. How early do these capabilities appear? Sakabe, Arayama, and Suzuki (1969) measured changes in the ***EEG*** (electroencephalograms) of fetuses in the 32nd to 38th week following conception. The study measured changes in brain waves that occurred when changes in sound were presented. These brain wave changes have two implications. First, they are indications that perceptual capabilities may already exist one month before birth. Second, they show that exposure to external stimuli is possible while the fetus is still *in utero*.

The Ability to Respond to the Environment

Sensory Capability

Two capabilities are necessary to respond to the environment. The first is the ability to detect changes in the environment. This is the sensory capability of the child. The second is the ability to behave or respond. We start by looking at the first of these, the sensory capability of the neonate.

Sensation vs. Perception

There is a sudden bright flash of light. What is it? What color it is? Is it a photo flash, an explosion, or what? What did you see? We can look at this event (the flash of light) in many ways.

Sensation

First we need to know whether it had an effect on the person. If a tree falls in the woods . . .is there a sound? This philosophical question deals with the act of sensation. ***Sensation*** is the actual stimulation of sensory receptors and their connection to neurons traveling to the sensory center in the central nervous system. Sensation is the detection of the presence of stimuli.

Humans have five basic senses: seeing (visual), hearing (auditory), smelling (olfactory), tasting (gustatory), and feeling (touch, pain, proprioceptive). Each of these senses involves a relationship between an event in the environment (i.e., stimulus) and a specific sensory receptor. Receptors are stimulus specific; only certain stimuli will fire them. Visual receptors detect changes in light; sound receptors detect changes in sound waves. Likewise, receptors tend to be located at specific sites, such as the retina of the eye, or the outer, middle, and inner ear.

The stimuli that fire the visual receptors are changes in light. Light is physical energy occurring in waves[1] of a distinctive length. Specifically, the visual spectrum for visual receptors is energy in wavelengths from 3800 to 7600 angstroms. While other organisms have receptors that can sense light in the ultraviolet or infrared parts of the spectrum, we cannot.

There are several specific types of cells that are receptors for vision. All are located in the eye. The retina, the lining of the back of the eyeball, contains these cells. Two specific visual receptors are the ***rods*** and ***cones***. Each of these is sensitive to a particular aspect of the visual stimulus, light. Cones, concentrated in the central portion of the retina called the fovea, come in different varieties. These different cones are sensitive to light of a specific wavelength, corresponding to colors. Because the fovea contains a high density of many cones, vision is most acute in this area.

Rods are cells located in the periphery of the retina and fire in response to small changes in light. Thus they are light-dark receptors, but cannot detect color. When a dim object, such as a shooting star is detected, it is because of the sensation of these rods.

Sound also takes the form of waves of energy, but sound waves are larger and travel much more slowly. They are detected by receptors in the inner ear after being enhanced by the action of the ear drum and parts of the middle ear. These organs respond to the presence of waves of energy in the auditory range. Note, although sound waves also consist of physical energy, because of the wavelength differences we do not see sounds or hear light. Nevertheless, if sound waves are slow enough (as in the deep bass of a drum) and amplified enough, we may sense them with something other than our ears. With a good stereo (or when someone is riding by with a boom-box in their car) we not only hear the sound, we feel it with the pressure sensors in our bodies.

In short, because of natural selection, we have evolved certain cells that serve the role of specialized receptors. These receptors are sensitive to particular events in our environment. Thus, for purely physical reasons, some parts of our environmental surround will be sensed and others not. We will now turn to another reason why some stimuli affect our behavior and others do not.

Perception

Perception is the organized response to a stimulus. Perception requires sensation, but entails more. The firing of a cone by a stimulus is sensation, but an awareness of blue in our "mind's eye," or responding to that sensation with the word "blue," or pushing a key, or feeling an emotion is perception. Perception involves an integrated response to a stimulus. It is an integration of a sensation with the activation of appropriate response systems. A question arises: is our perception of "blue" innate or acquired?

Nativism versus Empiricism

In the field of perception, the nature/nurture controversy becomes the nativism versus empiricism controversy. ***Nativism*** proposes that perception is innate, that it is hard-wired, and present at birth. In contrast, ***empiricism*** states that we acquire perception through experience. As in the nature/nurture controversy, there is probably no way to make a clear determination of which is true.

Our physiology provides us with some hard-wired Universal I behaviors. Among these are basic sensory responses to stimuli. We detect light versus dark, horizontal versus vertical lines, and other innate perceptual responses. In addition, we have apparently hard-wired responses to stimuli called ***reflexes***. Some reflexes may be complex enough that we consider the response of the child as demonstrating that she is perceiving the stimulus, not merely sensing it.

For example, in a series of experiments, Meltzoff and Moore (1977, 1983) have reported that within hours of birth, neonates imitate the gestures of adults. The authors (Meltzoff & Moore, 1984, p. 155) stated that . . ."our working hypothesis is that human newborns have an innate ability to appreciate equivalencies between their acts and the acts they see." This "appreciation of equivalencies" is perception inferred from the neonate's organized imitative response. Seeing a newborn stick out its tongue after an adult does, or opening its mouth after an adult does, leads us to the conclusion that the child *perceives* the adult behavior as something to be imitated.

How Do We Know the Sensory/Perceptual Capabilities of the Infant?

As James's famous quotation implies, we underestimated the newborns sensory/perceptual capabilities. We did this because of the difficulty in assessing these capabilities. To assess the visual acuity of adults we present them with an eye chart and ask them to tell us what line they can read. We use a similar procedure to assess auditory perception. Yet how do you ask newborns what they can see or hear? The difficulty in posing the question meant we had little data on infant sensory capabilities.

This dilemma was solved by Robert Fantz, a psychologist at Case Western Reserve University in Cleveland. Fantz (1958, 1961) devised a simple procedure to test visual acuity. Like many breakthroughs, his method, called the ***visual preference method***, was simple. Yet it was so powerful in its conceptualization that it led to the development of many other methods and revolutionized the field.

Methods of Perceptual Research

Let us look again at how adults are tested. You give them a line of letters and ask them to tell you what letters they see. You stop when they can no longer give you a response that correlates with the stimulus. Or, you change the pitch of a sound and you ask them to tell you if they hear it. In both cases, you present them with a change in stimulus (e.g., letters, pitch) and then you see if there is a correlated change in behavior (e.g., "f," "e," or "yes, I hear it.").

Fantz recognized that this relationship between a change in the stimulus and a change in behavior was common to all measures of perception. His problem was to identify a neonatal response that was reliably related to visual perception. Again the solution was simple . . . looking itself was correlated with perception. If a change in what the child was looking at followed a change in the stimulus, it could be concluded that the child could detect or see the change.

Fantz realized that if the child spent more time looking at one stimulus over another that this *preference* indicated that the child could tell one stimulus from the other. Admittedly, in some cases the child would show no preference, even though he could perceive one as different from the other, as, say, a circle from a square or a coke or pepsi. Such a lack of a preference would not allow us to attribute the lack to perception or motivation. However, if the child does show a reliable preference, looking longer at one stimulus than the other, then it means he can tell one from the other. That is, he can perceive a difference.

To use this preference method Fantz created a visual chamber. The child could be placed on its back inside the chamber. Lying in an infant seat, the infant would be facing the top of the chamber. On this "ceiling" Fantz could place two pictures that were his stimuli. By carefully lighting the chamber, an image of what the child was looking at was reflected on the cornea of the child's eye and could be seen by an observer looking through a peep hole in the top of the chamber. By carefully recording the amount of time each stimulus was reflected in the child's eye, the observer would have the total duration that the child looked at each stimulus.

If the amount of time were equal for both stimuli (after reversing the location of the square and circle to prevent a "side bias"), this could mean one of two things: either (1) the child could not tell one stimulus from the other or (2) that the child could see a difference but did not prefer one over the other. Therefore, finding equal durations would be inconclusive regarding visual capability.

However, an infant who spent more time looking at one stimulus over the other, showed not only a preference, but the ability to perceive a difference in the stimuli. By varying the stimuli and the amount of detail, researchers could use this preference method to determine visual acuity, color perception, and other characteristics of vision.

To measure visual acuity, Fantz chose a neutral gray square for one stimulus. The other stimulus was a box containing lines of specified thickness. These repetitive black-white patterns are called ***gratings***. Varying the thickness of the lines would be like varying the size of the letters for adults. As long as the infant perceived the lines as lines, their complexity attracted the infant's gaze. But, as the lines became thinner, they became fuzzy. A lack of preference for the lined stimulus over the gray one meant the infant could no longer distinguish between the two stimuli and perceived

Figure 5.1
Stimuli for Testing Visual Acuity with the Preference Method

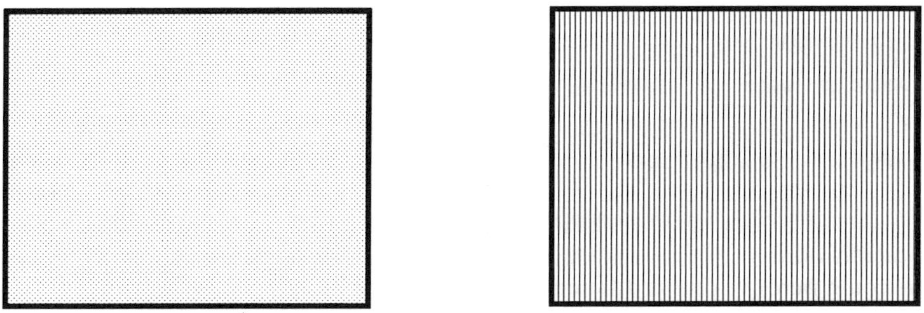

these lines to be the same as the gray stimulus. (You can try this yourself by propping up figure 5.1 on one side of the room and looking at it as you back away. There will be a point where you can't distinguish between the two squares – they will both appear uniformly gray.) By comparing the thinness of the lines that produced this infant response with those that adults see, an estimate of infant acuity could be made.

Fantz's preference method broke the conceptual logjam that had prevented researchers from designing methods to test infant perceptual capabilities. Within a few years other researchers developed methods that have enabled us to know much more about how the infant perceives its world. Some of these methods are described below.

Visual Cliff

The question of whether depth perception is innate or develops due to experience prompted Walk and Gibson (1961) to develop the ***visual cliff*** apparatus (Walk & Gibson, 1961). The visual cliff is a large glass covered table with a "shallow end" and "deep end". The shallow end has a checkerboard pattern of black and white squares immediately under the glass. The deep end has the same pattern placed on the ground, a few feet below the glass. The infant is placed on a board between the two ends and is enticed by its mother to crawl to her, either over the shallow or the deep end.

Walk and Gibson (1961) showed that children at six months avoid crawling on the deep end, indicating they perceive the "depth" of the deep end, despite the feel of the glass sheet. However, you probably can see why this method cannot answer the nativism - empiricism question. You need a child who can crawl (about 6 months of age) to use the cliff. Later Campos and his colleagues (Campos, Langer, & Krowtiz, 1970) tested non-crawlers using the visual cliff by lowering them onto the deep side and measuring their heart rate. They found children (as young as two months of age showed a change in heart rate (a *decrease)*. This meant children could detect the depth from visual cues, as a decrease in heart rate is taken as a measure of attention. About a month after learning to crawl, the same procedure produces an *increase* in heart rate. This is associated with fear responses and suggests perception of depth is possible prior to crawling, but that fear of falling is acquired with the experience that comes with crawling.

Habituation-Dishabituation

In this procedure the researchers record a consistent, ongoing response such as a newborn's sucking response to a nipple. (This can be done systematically by using a high-tech nipple: one with a micro switch attached to a recording device.) Now the researcher introduces a sound such as the phoneme "ba," The sucking stops as the child orients to the sound. If you continue the "ba" sound the sucking will resume. This is ***habituation*** (See Chapter 6) and involves adaptation to a repeated stimulus (e.g., "ba"). Now change the stimulus slightly, from "ba" to "pa." If the neonate stops sucking again, then it perceives the difference between these two auditory stimuli. This reversal of a habituated response is dishabituation. This is the procedure used by Eimas (1971) and his colleagues at Brown University to show that infants as young as six hours could discriminate "ba" from "pa". Among the most frequently used responses in the habituation-dishabituation procedure, besides sucking, is heart rate (Miller, 1987).

Operant Conditioning Procedures

Many procedures used to assess neonatal perceptual capabilities involve operant conditioning (See Chapter 7). The basic process involves reinforcing the child for differentially responding to stimuli, that is the infant is reinforced for making one response (e.g., turning head to the right) for one stimulus and a second response (turning head left) for another stimulus. If she now turns her head in the appropriate direction when presented with a given stimulus, perception of this stimulus is inferred. Stimuli may be presented one at a time or simultaneously. Among the responses used by researchers include head turning (e.g., Siqueland, 1968; Engen, Lipsitt, & Kaye, 1963), sucking a nipple at a high (or low) rate (e.g., DeCasper, & Fifer, 1980), or kicking a mobile (e.g., Rovee-Collier, Griesler, & Earley, 1985).

Reinforcers for the neonate have included the mother's voice (e.g., DeCasper & Fifer, 1980; Barrett-Goldfarb & Whitehurst, 1973), milk (e.g., Siqueland, 1968), visual stimulation (e.g., Rovee-Collier, Griesler, & Earley, 1985), and even a recording of the intrauterine heartbeat (DeCasper, & Sigafoos, 1983).

Thus, there are a wide range of stimuli, responses, and reinforcers that may be employed with young infants. Taken together, the use of various operant conditioning procedures has been very effective for studying a wide range of infant perceptual capabilities.

Box 5

Sound Localization – A Developmental Problem.

It is pitch dark. You hear a ticking sound. Tick...tick...tick. Where is that watch? You listen and turn your head a bit and then you quickly walk over and pick up the watch you never saw. We have found a solution to a very common problem. The problem is called "***sound localization.***"

Bower (1977) presents an interesting illustration of the interaction of biological maturational structures and learning in the problem of sound localization. Biology is important. Our biological make-up includes a ***binaural*** hearing system. That is, we have two ears, one on either side of the head. In the case of sound localization, it is true that two ears are better than one. Since the sound has to travel through your head to get to the opposite ear, when a sound emanates from your left, the sound wave hits your left ear microseconds before it reaches your right one. The difference is called the ***interaural time difference.*** The differences are maximal when the sound is 90 degrees to the side. As the sound travels directly in front or to the rear of you, the delay differences disappear. In fact, we have difficulty knowing if something is directly in front or directly to the rear of us because there is no time discrepancy to use as a cue. Although a matter of microseconds, this difference is sufficient enough for adults to readily identify the source of the sound.

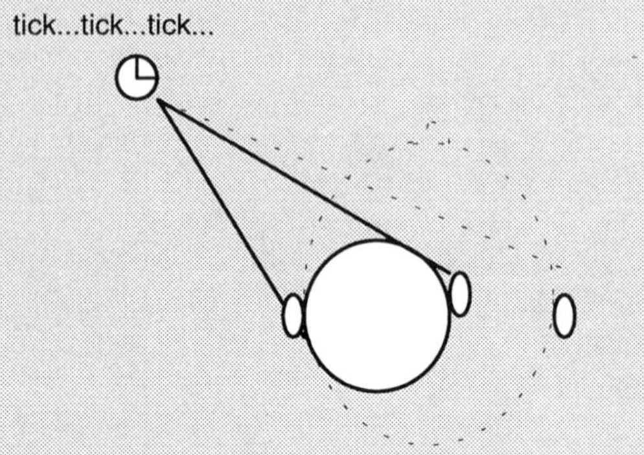

Is such localization ability hard-wired (Universal I)? Ashmead, DeFord, Whalen, and Odom (1991) presented some data relevant to this issue. They found that the precision of the infant's sound localization abilities does increase dramatically during the first year. However, the increase is not as great as the increase in our ability to detect interaural time differences. At 10 weeks there must be a difference of at least 170 microseconds for the neonate to detect the difference. By 80 weeks, a much smaller difference (63 microsec) is detectable (adults can detect differences as small as 20 microsec). So, our abilities to detect differences improve significantly during a few short months.

Why should our localization ability lag behind our sensitivity to sound differences? Bower suggested that it is because of physical changes occurring over the first year. During the first year, head size increases from 60% of adult size to nearly 85% . To make his point, consider the above illustration of changes in head size. Notice that as the head size increases, the distance, and therefore, the time it takes for the sound to reach the right ear increases too. The interaural time difference is greater. This means we have to constantly recalibrate these interaural timed differences to the position of a sound to accommodate changes in head size, if we are to successfully localize a sound. Are we able to do this? Such recalibrations require transactions between the child and her experiences. It requires learning the relationship between a sound and its visual location. This is a skill made more difficult by the constant change of head size that changes the interaural time difference for something in the same place.

Since nearly all humans learn to localize sounds it is a universal behavior. Because it requires a longer period of development and requires learning experiences we classify it as a Universal II behavior.

These are a few of the many methods and variations used by developmental psychologists to determine the perceptual capabilities of young infants. Now we turn to an overview of what these capabilities are.

Sensory Abilities

Visual Abilities

Acuity. The acuity of the newborn is not as good as that of the normal adult, but during the first six months acuity improves by three- to fourfold (Dobson & Teller, 1978). It is possible that the poorer vision occurs because the neonate does not use the fovea, which contains the largest concentration of cones, for focusing.

Color Perception. Regarding sensitivity to different stimuli on the visual spectrum, one- and 3-month-old infants have about the same range of sensitivity to colors as adults (Powers, Schneck, & Teller, 1981). Furthermore, based on habituation data produced by Bornstein (1981), Anslin (1987) concluded that by four months, infants group wavelengths into the same categories that adults do.

Auditory Capabilities

Studies by Sakabe, et al. (1969) using EEG and Grimwade, Walker, Bartlett, Gordon, & Wood (1971) using heartbeat indicate that the auditory system is already functioning prior to birth. In addition to detecting sounds within the normal adult range, auditory discrimination may develop surprisingly early.

Perceptual Abilities as Universal I Behaviors

Basic perceptual abilities fit Horowitz's (1987) definition of Universal I behaviors. They are hard-wired responses to stimuli which all normal human infants possess at birth. They are the result of the interaction of genetic and prenatal environmental variables. Most importantly, they enable us to learn from our environment even before the moment of birth.

A study by DeCasper and Spence (1986) provides an example of just how early learning may occur. Mothers in the experimental group were instructed to read a specific Dr. Seuss story aloud during the eighth month of pregnancy. A control group was not given a specific story. During the first few days after birth their infants were tested using the conditioning procedure. The Dr. Seuss story was used as a reinforcer. Infants from the experimental group mothers sucked faster to hear the Dr. Seuss story than to hear another story. The control group children did not.

Reflexes as Universal I Behaviors

We also enter this world with certain behaviors (or responses) that are made to certain events (or stimuli). We call these behaviors ***reflexes.*** They too are Universal I behaviors. All normal newborns possess these reflexes. These relationships between certain stimuli and certain responses are part of our genetic make-up. Table 5.1 lists the reflexes of the neonate.

Psychologists believe that natural selection has produced these reflexes that are common to our species. They reason that it is adaptive for the infant to possess these from birth. The alternative would be that we would have to learn these behaviors. This is a sobering thought -- imagine a mother needing to teach her newborn to suck or to swallow to keep it alive. Fortunately, our inborn nature provides these functions for us.

Note that a reflex is not just the behavior. It is a relationship between an environmental event (the stimulus) and a behavior (the response). Since this behavior is unlearned (or unconditioned) we may look at it as an ***unconditioned response.*** Since the stimulus that causes it is also an unlearned relationship, we may call it an ***unconditioned stimulus.*** To recap, a reflex is a relationship between an unconditioned stimulus and an unconditioned response. Because the stimulus draws out or brings forth the reflexive response, we say the stimulus "elicits" the response.

Table 5.1 (from Bijou & Baer, 1965) gives an extensive list of the range of neonatal reflexes.

Table 5.1

Neonatal Reflexes

Eyelid Responses -
opening–correlated with other activity
closing–touching the eye, lid, lashes, forehead, nose, cheeks, mucous membrane of the nose, sound, strong odors, bitter tastes, strong light, correlated with crying and sneezing
Pupillary Responses -
dilation to weak light
constriction to strong light
widen to strong stimulation of the skin
Ocular Responses -
pursuit–follows stimulus
saccadic (fast lateral motions of very small sweep, maintaining constantly wavering image on retina; stabilization of image produces fading of image in adults)
nystagmus–cold (20 degrees C.), rotation of body
coordinated compensatory eye movements–correlated with infant's own head movements, or with sharp jerks of head by the investigator
unspecific movements, random
Face and Mouth Responses -
opening–touch stimuli around mouth
closing–touch stimuli around mouth
sucking (tongue and jaw motions)–tactile and taste stimuli; hunger (?)

Table 5.1 (Continued)

grimacing, twisting of face and mouth–bitter, salt, sour tastes, pricking of nose
yawning
tongue pushing–bitter, salt, sour tastes rejected
licking
lip pursing–touch about mouth
sneezing–smells of ammonia
coughing
gagging–tongue stimulation, bitter tastes
swallowing
hiccoughing
vomiting

Head Responses -

rooting (or search)–tactile stimulation of the side of the mouth elicits turn in that direction.
dorsal (drawing back of head) nose-holding, strong odors, bright light ventral–less
turning–tactile stimuli to face or nose, touch on cheek, bright light away, weak light toward; turning of rest of body producing similar turn of head
head shudder–bitter tastes
head balancing–within few days

Hand and arm Responses -

radius reflex
scapulo-humeral reflex
handcloses–tactile stimulation to fingers or palm
flexion (withdrawal)–sharp tap or pinprick to hand
face rubbing–tickling stimuli to face, irritation of mucous membrane of nose, strong odors
random movements
startle (outward flinging of hands and arms)–sudden strong stimulation

Trunk Responses -

back arching–nose pinching, being held upside down, crying, and stimulus producing dorsal head response
twisting–trunk twists in same direction as head is rotated by the investigator. If chest held, pelvis twists in opposite direction of head, squirming, in effect
abdominal reflex

Sexual Responses -

raising of testes–tactile stimulation of inner thigh, erection of penis (?)

Picture 5.1
J. B. Watson demonstrates the rooting reflex (top) and the Babinski reflex (bottom) with an infant (circa 1920)

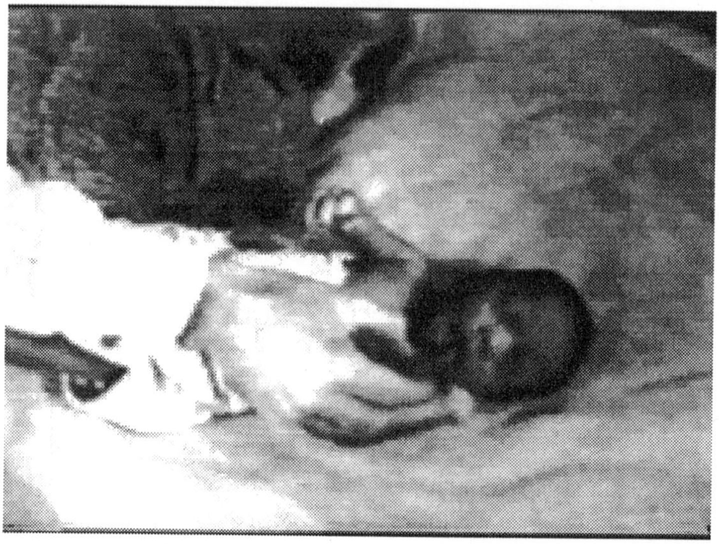

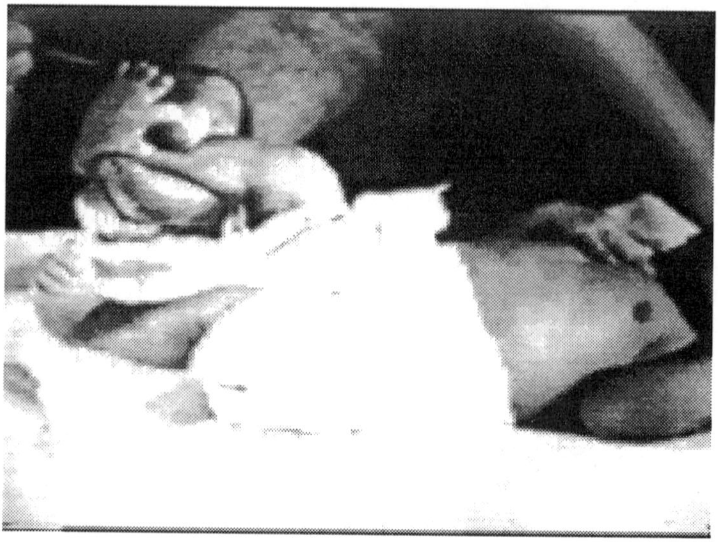

Table 5.1 (Continued)

Foot and Leg Responses -

plantar–pressing on the sole of the foot elicts a curling in of the toes

Babinski–gently stroking the sole of the foot elicts a fanning back of the toes

Table 5.1 (Continued)

knee–jerk reflex

Achilles tendon reflex

flexion of leg–needle prick to foot or leg, pushing head down towards chest

extension of leg–gentle push sometimes strong enough to support baby's weight

kicking– free foot kicks at other when other is restrained, leg is pinched

inside knee–kicking with both legs usually alternating ; correlates with crying

stepping– when held upright, feet touching surface

Coordinated Responses -

resting, sleeping position–legs flexed, upper arms straight out from shoulders, forearms flexed to lie parallel with head, fists closed

opisthodomic position–back arch dorsally, head to heals (more extreme form of head rearing)

back bone reflex–concave bending of side of body which is tickled stroked; leg on stroke side extends, contralateral leg flexes

lifting head and rump–if held horizontally in the air, when head is raised, rump rises too

"fencing"–when head is turned, faced arm extends, other flexes faced leg extends other flexes

"springing"–if held upright, inclined slightly forward, arms extend and legs are flexed

stretching–back arches, head arches back, leg extend, arms extend over head

startle responses–head thrown back, arms thrown apart from body, fingers extend and fan out, legs extend, crying in extreme cases, sudden loud noises, falling, sudden touches, sudden widespread change in temperature over surfaces of body, sudden blow to chest or abdomen, and also at random moments in absence of any obvious stimulus

creeping– in prone position, arms and legs drawn in under body, head lifted; feet may push against traction, and arms will move too shivering, trembling, during urination

You can see the enormous number of environment-behavior relationships, called reflexes, with which the child enters the world. They form the initial repertoire of human behavior.

How Do Reflexes Change?

The Universal I behaviors we call reflexes comprise much of the initial behaviors in the newborn's repertoire. At birth nearly all person-environment interactions are reflexive ones. While they start us on the path of developmental change, reflexes themselves are very inflexible. While humans are characterized by their ability to change in relation to their environment, reflexes are hard-wired and inflexible. They change very little over time. There are four developmental paths that reflexive behaviors may take.

1. Reflexes May Stay the Same

Many reflexes remain virtually unchanged from birth. A puff of air still elicits an eye blink reflex and a bright light elicits pupillary dilation *across the life span.*

2. Reflexes May Disappear

Many reflexes disappear over the first year of life. These include the moro, swimming, and Babinski reflexes. Let us look at these three. The moro reflex is elicited by stimulation of the balance organs in the middle ear, as occurs during a fall. The child first arches his back, next opens his arms, and then closes the arms in a grasping motion. The swimming reflex is elicited by cold water. The child holds her breath and makes basic swimming movements. The Babinski reflex is the fanning of the toes when the sole of the foot is lightly touched.

As other behaviors develop and physiological development of the brain proceeds, the cortex suppresses these sub-cortical responses and they disappear during the first year. Therefore, when you fall (e.g., in an elevator) you do not respond with a moro reflex. In fact, the reappearance of these responses is used as clinical evidence of cortical damage.

3. Reflexes May Be Elicited by New Stimuli – Respondent Conditioning

As we interact with our environment, other stimuli become associated with the stimuli that elicit reflexes. As this association continues, a new stimulus comes to elicit the response. For example, Mom regularly talks to Baby as she feeds him. The nipple elicits the sucking reflex, but soon Baby is sucking to Mom's voice, even before she gives him the nipple. This is a form of learning known as ***respondent conditioning***. It is the topic of the next chapter.

4. Reflexes May be Elaborated into New Behaviors – Operant Conditioning

Finally, behaviors elicited in the newborn may develop into behaviors that are sensitive to the changes they produce in their environment. For example, some crying may start as a reflex to pain, but it becomes crying that gets mother to pick up the child. This is what is called operant conditioning and is the topic of chapter 7.

However, not all behavior develops from reflexes. Indeed, only a small percentage of human behavior originates in this way. Most behavior appears to develop through principles of operant conditioning.

So, we are at the point that at birth we have a neonate who senses its environment and responds to it in ways that will help it survive. From this excellent start we embark on a journey involving an infinitely large number of reciprocal interactions with our environment. To understand the basic principles of this process, we must understand how learning occurs and how it relates to development.

Footnote

[1]However, light is also conceptualized as a particulate when explaining its behavior in certain contexts.

Chapter 6

Learning I: Habituation & Respondent Learning

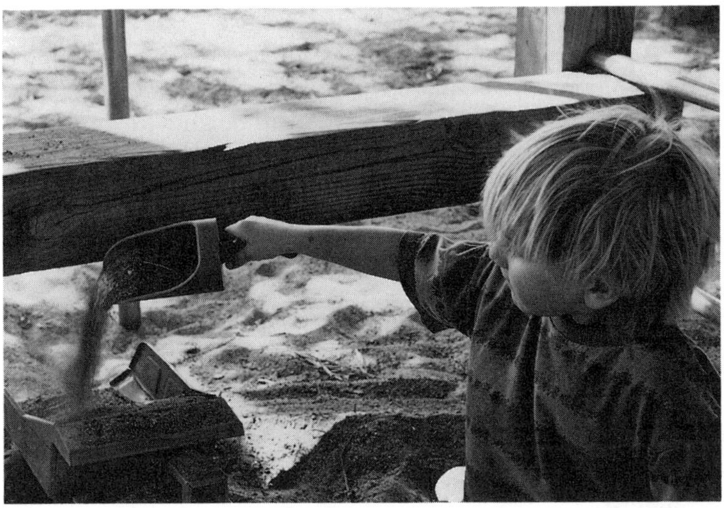

What is Learning?

Learning is a basic process in human development. It is responsible for change. **Learning** is defined as *a relatively permanent change in behavior in relation to the environment that is due to experience.* There are three parts to this definition. 1) Learning is a change in the behavior-environment relationship. Behaviors may change, but they do so in relationship to events in the environment. Our behavior changes when we learn to walk. But when we learn to read the word "cat" aloud the behavior that produces the sound does not change compared to just saying the word, but it does change in relationship to the environment (the written word cat versus a cat itself). 2) This change is *relatively permanent.* Thus changes are not merely momentary, such as with a sneeze, but lasting. When we learn to walk that change remains just as it does if we reliably read "cat." If the behavior is not relatively permanent (i.e., we say "cat" one time, but do not respond another) we have not yet learned the behavior. Why do we need the qualifier "relatively"? Sometimes behaviors disappear after we have learned them, as when we forget what a word means. The exact length of time required to demonstrate learning is vague, but researchers often explicitly define learning as a number or percentage of correct responses in a row.

The final part of the definition is that learning is due to experience with the environment. What else could produce relatively permanent changes? Physical growth or physiological changes (e.g., sickness) can change behavior. ***Maturation*** is a term to describe physical and behavioral changes that are due to biological growth. Yet one must keep in mind that the effects of biological growth may also be influenced by the environmental experiences occurring, so that maturation may also involve learning as well as physical growth.

The Evolutionary Significance of Learning

Sheppard and Willoughby (1975) stated that what separates humans from other species is the human species' remarkable ability to adapt to the environment. What would be the evolutionary importance of inheriting increased ability to learn? Unlearned behaviors are fine as long as the environment remains consistent and stable. Animals may have elaborate patterns of unlearned behavior that are elicited by particular environmental stimuli. Ethologists call these patterns ***Fixed Action Patterns*** and the stimuli that elicit them ***Innate Releasing Mechanisms.*** Indeed the stimuli are fixed and cannot vary once the automatic response is released by the species specific stimulus.

The evolutionary significance of such innate patterns is that they provide behaviors that enable members in their species normal environment to survive. Equipped with these innate releasing mechanisms, bees will signal the location and distance of honey, wolves will fight but not slash the exposed throat of its white marked victim, and the lowly freshwater stickleback fish will engage in an elaborate mating dance. But using an unlucky stickleback, we may illustrate the adaptive limits of such inflexibility.

An innate releasing mechanism for the courting dance of the male stickleback is the red belly of the female in spring, when she is ripe with eggs. The males, in whom the dance is released, build a nest and lure the female into the nest where the eggs are fertilized. This ensures the survival of the species, and presumably the best dancers are the fittest.

But woe the poor male stickleback living in a stream that falls victim to a stream filled with red Christmas tree balls (the result of a train derailment accident). The red spot is a brighter and larger stimulus, which ethologists refer to as a ***supernormal stimulus***, and is a more effective releaser of the male dancing behavior than the gravid females' spots. The poor males in this stream dance and dance into the night and to exhaustion. Alas, no little sticklebacks are born in that stream that spring and the population is threatened.

Learning is much more adaptive to the individual, and, in the long run, to the species. Species that can learn can adapt to short run changes in their environment. They may even change the environment from what they have learned. Individual humans are extremely adaptable to the environments. Over evolutionary time they have been selected on the basis of their ability to learn. As a consequence, humans exist in a wide range of environments. . . we have even walked on the moon. We do this through our ability to change with respect to the environment as no other species can.

A Parallelism Between Evolution and Learning

Recall Sheppard & Willoughby's (1975) concepts of phylogenic and ontogenic contingencies. Recall that natural selection was the process in evolution and learning was the process in individual development. We may take this parallelism further and point out that both are forms of adaptation to the environment. For natural selection the adaptation to the ecological niche works over phylogenic time. Learning is adaptation to the ecosystem of the individual over his or her lifetime.

Selectionism - Learning as a Natural Process

As noted previously, our view is that learning and natural selection are parallel processes. Learning involves the contingencies in ontogenic development while natural selection involves the contingencies in phylogenic development. Recently (Donahoe, Burgos, & Palmer, 1993; Donahoe & Palmer, 1994) it has been argued that selectionism is the basic process in ontogenic, as well as phylogenic development. That is, that learning functions as a type of natural selection too. The difference is that selection of an individual's behavior is made by contingencies that work directly on the individual during her lifetime.

Donahoe and Palmer (1994) list three requirements for selectionism to function: (1) variation, (2) selection, and (3) retention.

How Does Learning Relate to Development?

What is the difference between learning and development? Development is the overall process. It is the progressive changes in the interactions between behavior and environment. *Learning is a process* (or **the** process) that determines development.

Is Learning "A" Process or "THE" Process in Development?

For Horowitz (1987) the question is significant, but the answer is not simple. For her, the answer depends on what behaviors you are asking about. In the development of Universal I behaviors, such as basic perceptual behaviors or the production of early language sounds, learning is "a" process in development. These Universal I behaviors are hard wired in the child's physiology due to his/her genetic inheritance. Yet even with these simple behaviors, exposure to a ***species typical environment*** is necessary for the behaviors to develop. Thus the changes occur due to experience. Learning is therefore **a** process in development of Universal I behaviors.

Why is a species typical environment necessary for the development of Universal I behaviors? The selection of genes that hard-wire these species characteristic behaviors would have happened in the environment that the species normally found itself. Thus the selected behaviors would have been the product of genotype/environment interactions. Selection did not occur in an environmental void.

Still the role of heredity in these Universal I behaviors is so strong that only minimal environmental experience is necessary. For example, being exposed to the visual stimuli present in human environments is sufficient to produce basic perceptual skills. For these behaviors learning plays a role, but genetics plays the most important one.

As they become more individual and unique, behaviors show greater influence by the environment and therefore more of a role for learning. Horowitz suggests that learning plays "THE" role in the development of non-universal behaviors. Remember, these are behaviors that develop over a long period of time and show great individual variation. So for the great majority of human behaviors, learning plays THE role in development.

Figure 6.1

The Role of Learning
(Hypothetical)

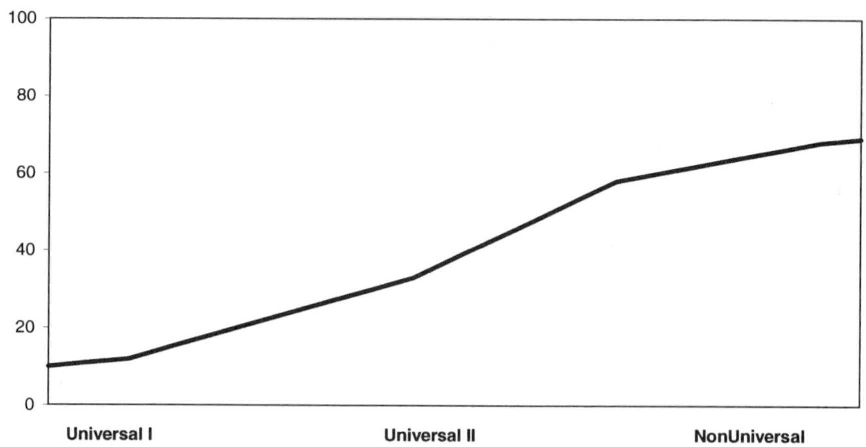

Two points must be emphasized. First, behaviors can be placed on a continuum ranging from Universal I to Non -Universal along which learning plays an increasingly significant role. Second, regardless of where you move along such a continuum, both physiology and learning play a role. The difference is in how the influences combine. We are reminded that the important question is not "How much?", but "How?". Let us look at how the environment works. Let us look at the processes of learning.

Where Does Learning Fit in Human Development?

Learning is a process in development, but where does it fit with respect to other developmental topics, such as language, cognitive, and social development? To help understand this relationship we turn again to our painting metaphor (see Chapter 1). In our metaphor, learning is the paint itself, the dots that make-up the picture. We might extend the metaphor to suggest that biology is the canvas. These are basic processes of development. We sawthem at Level I of analyzing the systems of development. The basic processes of genetics and learning underlay all development. To understand development at other levels we also need to understand these basic processes.

Learning – What Develops?

Remember our definition of development: Progressive changes in the interactions between a person and her/his environment. This definition is consistent with the role of learning in development. However we should use new terms – technical terms to describe what changes in learning. To analyze at the level of basic processes we need to be more precise about the person and the environment. Specifically, we shall be focusing on what the person does as a ***behavior*** or ***response***. Behavior and response can be used interchangeably. They are the actions or changes that individuals do. Snapping your fingers, walking, talking, whispering, and writing a letter are all behaviors. Imagining a sunset and thinking about what you will do tomorrow are also included among the actions of the individual.

Are thoughts appropriate phenomena for those studying behavior? In a word, yes. As early as 1953, Skinner (1953) wrote about the role of thoughts in a natural science. He referred to thoughts as ***private events***. That is, they are like other behaviors of an individual such as walking or talking, but unlike these public events, thoughts are observable only to the individual producing the thoughts. This may make them difficult to objectify, but they are behaviors and as such, are governed by the same basic principles that affect all behaviors. The main difference is that they occur inside the skin and are therefore private, not public.

In analyzing the environment we talk in terms of ***stimuli***. A stimulus is an environmental change or event. A flash of light, a ringing bell, the letter "A", these are all environmental events or stimuli. In looking at the environment we can identify countless stimuli. However we normally are only interested in those aspects of the environment that have a functional relationship to behavior. That is, we are most interested in those stimuli which actually have an effect on behavior.

Classifying Stimuli

We can categorize stimuli in a number of ways. A common way is to classify stimuli based on their physical characteristics. This is a structural approach to classifying stimuli. The classes are based on what the stimuli look like and not what they do. Bijou and Baer (1978) identified four physical stimulus classes. These are:

1. Physical: objects and natural phenomena - e.g., tools, furniture, plants, trees, etc.
2. Chemical: gases that have an effect at a distance – e.g., the aroma of roast turkey, perfume, smoke; liquid solutions in contact with the skin – e.g., water, soap, etc.

3. Organismic: the organism's own biological structure – e.g., stimulation from breathing and digestive processes, proprioceptive stimulation.
4. Social: the appearance, action and interaction of people and animals.

Functional Stimulus Classes

While physical classifications are a common way to look at stimuli, in psychology it is more important to identify the ***functional stimulus classes.*** The function of a stimulus is the effect it has on behavior. We exist in a sea of stimuli. Not all stimuli have an effect on (or a function for) our behaviors. Many stimuli in the environment are outside the limits of our abilities to sense them. The dog whistle may have a function for Fido, but its pitch is too high for most people to be affected by it. A nearsighted person may not respond to a stimulus that a person with 20/20 vision would. Other functions are the result of our developmental history. If you grow up in the United States, the French word "*sortie*" may not have an effect on your behavior. (It is the word for "exit.") So, while we may analyze the environment as composed of an infinite number of stimuli, in psychology we are only concerned with what Horowitz (1987) called the ***functional environmental surround.*** That is we are concerned with those events in the environment that actually have a function for our behavior. While still large, the number of possible functional events is limited and consists of stimuli that function universally (that is, for all humans) and those that are unique to the individual.

Types of Learning

In this chapter we look at two types of learning that are specific to the Universal I behaviors that we called reflexes. We start with a simple type of learning called habituation and then turn to respondent learning.

Habituation

Consider the following story. In an attempt to discourage a pesky crow from eating her crop, Farmer Joan decided to install a loudspeaker system in her fields and broadcast at regular intervals the sound of a shotgun blast. At first, this tactic successfully scared the bird and it flew off, only to return much later when the fear subsided. However, after repeated exposures the bird failed to respond at all. Expressed in the technical language of the behavioral sciences, the bird's fear response habituated to the auditory stimulus produced by the speaker system. As generally defined (e.g., Jeffrey & Cohen, 1971; Fantino & Logan, 1979), ***habituation*** is a decrement in responding to a particular stimulus as a result of repetitive presentations of that stimulus.

Nonhuman Studies

There is an extensive history of research reporting habituation in nonhumans, including spiders (e.g., Peckham & Peckham, 1887), rats (e.g., Prosser & Hunter, 1936), and cats (e.g., Sharpless & Jasper, 1956). For example, in a recent experiment with cats, Crampton & Lucot (1991) exposed cats to a "motion sickness" stimulus, eliciting a retching response. With repeated exposure to the stimulus, there was a pronounced decrease in the incidence of retching which suggested habituation. In addition to the nonhuman studies already identified, habituation has been demonstrated in a large variety of other species including frogs, birds, earthworms, and squirrel monkeys (Catania, 1984).

Infant Studies

In an early study conducted around 1950 in the Soviet Union, Bronstein & Petrova (1967) found that non-nutritive sucking habituated to the repeated presentations of each of a variety of auditory stimuli (e.g., a whistle, a harmonica) in neonates as well as older infants. In a classic American study, Bridger (1961) reported the habituation of both accelerated heart rate and the startle response to auditory stimulation in neonates. Subsequent research demonstrated habituation in infants not only to auditory stimuli, but to visual and olfactory stimuli as well (see Jeffrey & Cohen, 1971). Further, habituation has not only been demonstrated in neonates and older infants, but with fetuses as well. For example, Madison, Madison, and Adubato (1986) applied a vibrating stimulus to the abdomens of women pregnant between twenty-eight and thirty-seven weeks. After repeated presentations, fetal movements habituated.

Defining Characteristics

The previously cited definition of habituation identified two necessary conditions: (1) there must be a decrement in responding; (2) this decrement must follow the repeated presentations of a particular stimulus. However, to distinguish habituation from related behavioral phenomena, additional necessary conditions must be met. A third necessary condition for habituation is that it only applies to those stimulus-response relations commonly called reflexes (Catania, 1984). As we saw earlier, a ***reflex*** is an automatic and unlearned relation between narrowly-defined stimulus and response classes. However, while reflexive S-R relations do not require any prior experience with the stimulus, the waning of reflexive responding that is characteristic of habituation does require that the organism experience repeated presentations of the stimulus. In short, although reflexes are unlearned, the habituation of reflexive responding is a type of learning.

A fourth necessary condition for habituation is that the decrement in responding must not be the product of other processes such as satiation or fatigue. For example, an infant's rate of drinking decreases as it becomes satiated. However, this is not a result of habituation, but a result of physiological processes accompanying ingestion of water. Unlike the infant exhibiting habituated responding, the satiated infant is not unresponsive to a particular food-related stimulus, but to food-related stimuli in general. Similarly, a response decrement which is the result of muscle fatigue is not an example of habituation. The fatigued muscle is unresponsive to all stimuli which normally elicit its contraction, not just to a particular stimulus (Fantino & Logan, 1979).

How then do you distinguish habituation from these other types of decremental responding? Jeffrey and Cohen (1971) suggested a procedure which has been widely used: present the infant with a novel stimulus from the same sensory modality as the habituated stimulus. If the infant's response returns to its earlier level, the response decrement was probably habituation; if it does not, the response decrement was probably the product of another process. For example, if you repeatedly clap your hands in the presence of an infant, her orienting response to that auditory stimulus will decrease. If you then ring a bell in the infant's presence and she orients to the sound, the response decrement following repeated hand clapping was probably habituation.

In summary, there are four necessary conditions for habituation:

1. There must be a decrement in responding.
2. This decrement must follow the repeated presentations of a particular stimulus.
3. The initial S-R relation must be a reflex.
4. The decrement in responding must not be the product of other processes such as satiation or muscle fatigue.

These four necessary conditions, taken together, constitute a sufficient condition for habituation.

Why Study Habituation?

There are two principle reasons why those interested in child development should study habituation. First, habituation is a form of learning which plays a critical role during a child's life. As William James put it, the child is exposed daily to a "buzzing, blooming confusion" of stimuli. The ability to stop responding to some stimuli while continuing to respond to others has implications for her long-term survival. For example, a nursing infant is likely to stop feeding when exposed to a loud auditory stimulus. However, after repeated presentations of this stimulus, the infant's orienting response habituates; it no longer stops feeding when it hears the sound. As Fantino & Logan (1979) expressed it, "the organism that continues to respond to an innocuous stimulus is wasting valuable time and energy engaging in uneconomical behavior."

Secondly, habituation should be understood by students of child development because of the role it frequently plays in infant studies, as we saw in Chapter 5. For example, the fact that an infant has habituated to a particular stimulus is useful as a way of determining whether the infant recognizes or remembers a stimulus. Researchers have indeed used habituation to determine whether infants recognize and/or remember particular faces. Similarly, if an infant has habituated to a stimulus and then is presented with both it and a novel stimulus, the fact that it responds only to the novel stimulus is taken as evidence that it can discriminate between the two stimuli.

Respondent Learning

Consider again the story of Farmer Joan. While she was busy trying to keep the crow from feeding in her fields, her two year old daughter Jenny conducted her own "training" program with a bird of another feather. On a number of occasions when her mother was outside, Jenny used a large spoon to strike the cage of the family's pet parakeet, Frankie. Frankie responded to these disturbances by excitedly flapping her wings in an attempt to escape. As a consequence, whenever anyone with a spoon in hand now comes within close proximity of the cage, Frankie flaps her wings in a similar fashion. Frankie has been respondently conditioned to fear spoons.

In the earlier discussion of habituation, unlearned S-R relations such as a bird's fear response to auditory stimulation were identified as reflexes. However, because this term has a number of popular meanings, it lacks the precision necessary for scientific discourse. Therefore, reflex will now be replaced with the more precise term respondent. Respondent S-R relations in humans include increased illumination eliciting pupillary constriction, a loud sound eliciting the eye blink, and a frightening stimulus eliciting an increase in heart rate. What then is respondent learning?

In a respondent S-R relation, the stimulus is termed the unconditioned stimulus (UCS) and the response (UCR), the unconditioned response. Note that conditioning is a synonym for learning. Therefore, unconditioned means "unlearned". In our example involving Frankie, the UCS is the loud noise and vibration produced by the spoon, and the UCR is the flapping of wings and other, related behaviors. Prior to Jenny's having banged the cage numerous times with the spoon, the presence of a spoon was a neutral stimulus (NS). It did not elicit the flapping of wings. However, as a result of Jenny's having paired presentations of the UCS (the noise and vibrations produced by the spoon) with presentations of the NS (the spoon), the spoon is no longer a neutral stimulus. It is now a conditioned stimulus (CS), and the response it elicits (the flapping of wings, etc.) a conditioned response (CR). Frankie has learned to respond in a new way to the presence of spoons. The relation between the presentation of a spoon and the behavior of wing flapping is a conditioned respondent relation.

Nonhuman Studies

Does the name Pavlov ring a bell? Ivan Pavlov was a Russian physiologist who received the Nobel prize for his study of the physiology of digestion. However, as notable as was that achievement, Pavlov is best remembered for his discovery of the importance of respondent learning (also known as classical or Pavlovian conditioning)[1]. During his research on the digestive processes of dogs, Pavlov noted that the dogs would begin to salivate when they saw the person who normally brought them their food. He hypothesized that the dogs had somehow associated the sight of attendant with the presence of food in their mouths. Pavlov tested this hypothesis by ringing a bell immediately before feeding the dogs. Following several bell/food pairings, Pavlov presented the sound of the bell alone. The dogs salivated. In technical terms, the presence of food in the mouth was the UCS, and salivation was the UCR. Before conducting the experiment, the bell was a NS. However, after pairings of the food presentation with the bell, the previously-neutral sound of the bell became a CS eliciting the CR (salivation).

Since Pavlov's time, there have been a large number of studies investigating respondent learning with nonhumans. For example, Harlow (Mason and Harlow,

Picture 6.2

J.B. Watson, Little Albert, Rosaline Rayner and the rat (circa 1920)

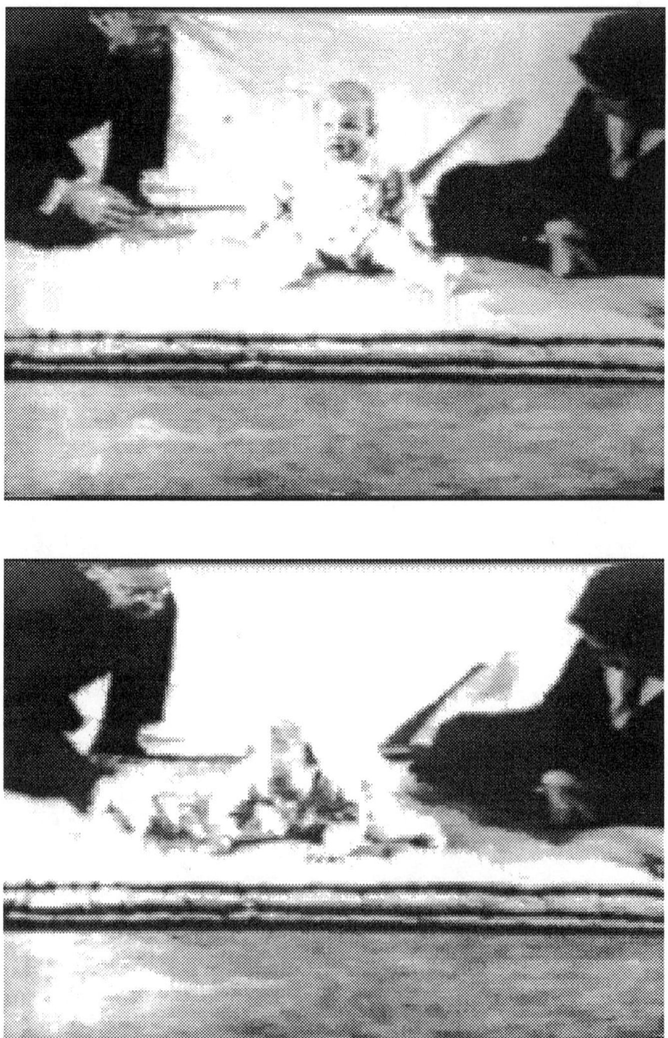

1958; Harlow, 1959) trained infant rhesus monkeys by pairing presentation of a tone (the NS) with an electric shock (the UCS). After completion of training, the presentation of the tone alone elicited movement. In an experiment with newborn albino rats, Caldwell and Werboff (1962) paired the presentation of a vibrotactile stimulus (the NS) with an electric shock (the UCS) to the forelimb. After a number of such pairings, the vibrotactile stimulus alone (now the CS) elicited movement (the CR).

Infant Studies

The case of Little Albert is the most famous respondent learning experiment involving an infant. During the initial stage of their classic experiment, Watson and Rayner (1920) presented a friendly white rat to their subject, 11-month-old Albert. Albert approached the rat and played with it. During the next stage of the experiment, a loud noise (produced by striking a metal rod with a hammer) was paired with presentations of the rat. The loud noise elicited crying. Eventually the presence of the rat alone elicited crying. Further, other similar objects (e.g., cat, fur coat, Santa Claus mask) reportedly also elicited crying (see Novak, 1990).

Additional respondent learning experiments have been conducted with fetuses (e.g., Ray, 1932; Spelt, 1948) and infants (e.g., Grunzke, 1961; Levin and Kaye, 1964; Kolata, 1987). For example, Spelt (1948) paired a loud clapper (the UCS) with vibrotactile stimulation (the NS) in an experiment with fetuses between seven and nine months of gestation. Eventually the vibrotactile stimulus became a CS, eliciting fetal movements. Lipsitt and Kaye (1963) paired presentation of a tone with the insertion of a nipple in the mouths of newborns three or four days old. Eventually the presentation of the tone alone elicited a sucking response.

Defining Characteristics

Based upon the previous discussion, three necessary conditions for respondent conditioning have been identified: first, the initial S-R relation must be an unlearned, automatic, respondent relation; second, the UCS must be paired with a NS. Third, presentations of the CS alone must elicit the response. A fourth necessary condition of respondent learning is that the response must not be the product of other processes such as sensitization. For example, presentation of the UCS alone might predispose the infant to respond to the previously-neutral stimulus. In other words, the capacity of the previously-neutral stimulus to elicit the response may not be the product of pairing the UCS with the NS; rather, it may be a product of simply presenting the UCS, thereby sensitizing the infant to many other previously-neutral stimuli. One way to distinguish respondent learning from sensitization is to utilize a control group which is presented with the UCS alone. If the previously-neutral stimulus fails to elicit the CR in the control group, but does elicit the CR in the experimental group (i.e., the group trained with UCS/NS pairings), it is likely that the experimental group exhibits respondent learning.

In summary, there are four necessary conditions for respondent learning:

1. The initial S-R relation must be an unlearned, automatic, respondent relation;
2. The UCS must be paired with a NS;
3. Presentations of the CS alone must elicit the response.
4. The response elicited by the previously-neutral stimulus must not be the product of other processes such as sensitization. Taken together, these four necessary conditions constitute a sufficient condition for respondent learning.

Generalization

When a conditioned response is established, the CR is not only elicited by the CS, but by other stimuli that are similar to the CS. For example, in the Little Albert study, Albert not only showed fear to the rat, but to a rabbit, cotton wool, and even Watson's hair. Generalization explains how new stimuli not directly present can come to elicit conditioned responses, particularly fears.

Discrimination

This is the opposite of generalization. Discrimination is demonstrated by the lack of a response to a stimulus. In Watson & Rayner's (1920) study, wooden blocks did not elicit a CR. Albert showed respondent discrimination to the blocks.

Respondent Extinction

The defining characteristic of respondent extinction is that the CS no longer elicits a CR. The CS has returned to serving as a NS. If a CS is created by the pairing of a NS with a UCS, extinction is brought about by presenting the CS without the UCS. Many CS alone presentations may be necessary to produce extinction.

One impediment to the extinction of some conditioned responses, particularly emotional ones, is that the conditioned emotional response is also accompanied by escape behavior such as running away or closing the eyes. When this behavior occurs, the child does not experience the CS without the UCS and extinction will not occur. Psychologists treating the intense fears known as phobias have developed some specialized procedures to reduce the intensity of the conditioned emotional response and to reduce escape. Two of these are systematic desensitization and counter conditioning.

In systematic desensitization, a hierarchy of stimuli is created by ranking the intensity of the fear produced by each stimulus from most to least. That is, a child with a fear of dogs may be terrified of petting a snarling pit bull and only a bit uneasy watching the Disney animated film, *Lady and the Tramp* (although *101 Dalmatians* may be a bit too intense for her). The child would be allowed to watch the film without escaping until the film elicited no emotional response at all. Extinction to this first stimulus would make successful desensitization (another term for extinction) to the next stimulus possible. Thus the child would be presented the second stimulus on his hierarchy until it could be presented without eliciting an emotional response. Successive stimuli on the hierarchy would be presented until the child's response to the last stimulus (the snarling pit bulls) is also desensitized (i.e., extinguished).

In counter conditioning, the conditioned stimulus is paired with an unconditioned stimulus which elicts a response opposite (or counter) to the conditioned response. Thus a new conditioned response is established to "counter" the original. This procedure was first reported in 1924 by Mary Cover Jones, a student of Watson. Jones reported the case of Peter who exhibited a fear of rabbits (that should be easy to remember). In her study, Jones gave Peter candy to eat and then introduced the rabbit while Peter was eating the candy. This pairing of candy and rabbit led to the rapid elimination of Peter's fear of rabbits.

Why study respondent learning?

Students of child development should study respondent learning for a number of reasons. First, like habituation, respondent learning plays a critical role in helping the child successfully adapt to her environment. Some common examples may be a child who avoids a dog that has bitten her or when a child opens her mouth in the presence of food. Both examples show the child behaving in ways which enhance her chances of surviving. These and many other adaptive responses are products of respondent learning. Second, the process of respondent learning helps explain the wide variety of emotional responses a child makes to the world. Consider a young boy who has been strongly admonished by his father for going outside without his pants. Months or years later that same boy may then blush when he discovers that his pants are unzipped (Bijou & Baer, 1978). Many instances in which we cry, become fearful, or sexually aroused can be explained in terms of respondent learning.

At this point, let us examine more closely some important aspects of respondent conditioning.

Types of Behaviors

As we have noted, a defining characteristic of respondent behavior is that it involves reflexive behaviors[2]. However, are the UCR and the CR the same response, but differing only in terms of the stimuli which elicit them? The answer is no. In most cases the CR will be at least slightly different from the UCR. For example, the arousal produced by a conditioned stimulus (e.g., a white rat) may be lower than that produced by an unconditioned stimulus (e.g., a loud noise). However, unless we are careful in our observations, the behaviors may appear identical.

What Factors Influence Respondent Acquisition?

Order of Presentation

Must the neutral stimulus precede the UCS or can the UCS come first for respondent conditioning to be successful? Is it more effective for the NS to remain on with the UCS present, or is it better that the NS end before onset of the UCS? These are some questions regarding the order of presentation of the stimuli.

First, the order of stimulus presentations seems important. The most effective conditioning occurs when onset of the NS precedes the UCS and terminates either with onset of the UCS or remains present for a time along with the UCS. This procedure is called ***delayed conditioning*** (Klein, 1987) or ***forward conditioning***. Delayed conditioning is used in the following example. A nipple on a bottle is an UCS which elicits sucking (the UCR) in an infant. This is the sucking reflex. Engen, Lipsitt, & Kaye (1963) preceded the onset of the UCS with the onset of a tone (NS). With repeated presentations, the tone alone elicited sucking demonstrating that the tone had become a CS, since it elicited a CR, the sucking to the tone.

Such anticipatory sucking can frequently be observed outside the laboratory. Since mothers often talk to their infants prior to feeding them, a mother's voice often becomes a CS, eliciting sucking even before the nipple is placed in the child's mouth.

A second type of sequence is called ***trace conditioning*** (Klein, 1987). In this procedure, the NS also precedes the UCS, but the NS is terminated before the onset of the UCS. For example, the mother would stop talking before placing the nipple in the baby's mouth. This procedure produces weaker conditioning than delayed conditioning, particularly if the gap between the end of the NS and onset of the UCS is long.

A third sequence is called ***backward conditioning*** (Klein, 1987). In this procedure, the UCS precedes the NS. In our example, this would mean that the mother would place the nipple in the infant's mouth and then begin to speak. This is the least effective of the three procedures.

The implication is that respondent conditioning is more likely to occur when a neutral stimulus precedes and remains present with the onset of an unconditioned stimulus. Is there an optimal time that the NS should precede the UCS?

NS–UCS Interval

We noted that in trace conditioning a long delay between the NS and UCS will be less effective. Indeed, it is unlikely that an association will be made between a threat (NS) and a spanking (UCS) if the spanking occurs the following day, for example. Too long, or too short a latency between NS onset and UCS onset will also inhibit the formation of a CR (Smith & Moore, 1966). One-half second seems to be optimal in adults (Kimble, 1961).

Intensity of the UCS

The intensity or magnitude of the unconditioned stimulus effects the development of a conditioned stimulus. Generally speaking, an intense UCS (e.g., loud sound, bright light) will lead to easier conditioning, within fewer trials. Highly intense stimuli may produce ***one trial conditioning***, as when a fear of an object may be produced if there is a stimulus which elicits an intense emotional response. Many phobias are the result of such brief, intense exposures.

Respondent conditioning is limited to the class of behaviors which originate as reflexes. As such, they are limited to responses which have a strong phylogenic basis. However, the simple learning which occurs in respondent conditioning extends the functioning of these responses to a wider range of ontogenic stimuli. Of special interest is the development of emotional reactions to the world around us. However, most human behavior is not limited to respondents. Instead, new behaviors are acquired in a different manner. We shall examine this important developmental process in the next chapter when we look at operant learning.

Footnotes

[1]Although the discovery of respondent type learning is generally attributed to Pavlov, some have considered an American, E. B. Twitmyer, who completed his doctoral dissertation on the knee jerk reflex (1905), to be the discoverer of the phenomenon.

[2]Recently, Turkkan (1989) has argued that Pavlovian Conditioning principles can be applied to a more extensive range of behaviors, including physiological responses, such as endocrine secretions, and changes at the level of the individual neuron synapse. Although the issues in this area are hotly debated, renewed interest in classical conditioning processes may lead to revisions in how we view this form of learning.

Chapter 7

Operant Learning

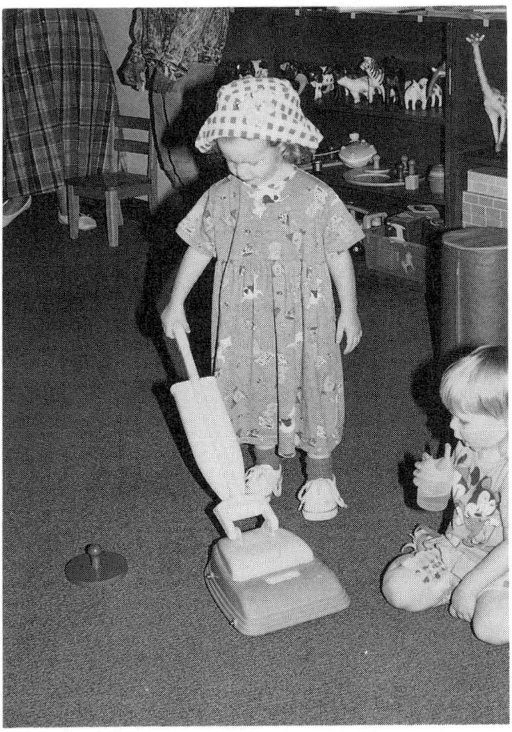

In the last chapter we saw environment/behavior relationships change in two ways. Repeated presentation of a stimulus led to the cessation of a response which is known as habituation. In the second type of change, the response came to be elicited by a new stimulus. This is respondent learning. Both relationships were concerned with a small class of behaviors called reflexes that are elicited by a *preceding* stimulus. No new responses developed, only changes in the relationship of existing reflexes to stimuli. While these are significant adaptations, they do not account for the major changes in development brought about by the environment. To understand how most nonuniversal behaviors are learned we must understand the principles of operant learning.

What is Operant Behavior?

Skinner (1938) chose the term ***operant*** because it connotes a key feature of this type of behavior: It is behavior that **operates** on the environment and thereby effects it. These effects on the environment determine the operant's frequency and define it. On the other hand, it is the preceding stimuli which determine the frequency of respondent behavior, and coupled with the relatively fixed form of the response, define it. For example, the operant, cleaning, is defined in terms of its effects on the environment. If you are cleaning your eyeglasses, the cleaning behavior has the effect of making the world clearer. Furthermore, if the cleaning behavior removes smudges from the lenses you are more likely to engage in cleaning behavior in the future. However, if the cleaning behavior has the effect of scratching the lenses, you are less likely to engage in that behavior in the future.

Consider now the respondent behavior of pupillary constriction. The number of times your pupil constricts is determined by the number of times a preceding light stimulus (e.g., a flashlight) stimulates your pupil; its frequency is **not** determined by any effects on the environment the response may have. That is, your pupil will constrict regardless of the consequences of the behavior. Furthermore, we define the respondent, pupillary constriction, in terms of the eliciting stimulus (i.e., the light) and the relatively fixed form of the response, **not** in terms of the effects it has. In addition, operant behavior initially is not caused by preceding stimuli. Unlike respondent behavior, operant behavior is emitted in an environment, but not elicited by any stimulus in that environment. For example, a newborn stretches out her arms, touching objects, some of which make a noise when touched.. This behavior is not elicited by any specific stimulus, it just occurs (or is "emitted") and is strengthened by the sounds the behavior produces. However, as we shall see later, operant behavior comes to be evoked by a preceding stimulus as when the child learns to reach for specific objects, like rattles, because of the sounds they produce. Although we have been considering operants and respondents as independent, there are many operant-respondent relationships. In some cases, operants may originate as reflexes. For example, crying may begin as one of three types of reflexive cries elicited by hunger, anger, or pain stimuli (Wolff, 1966). However, respondent crying may become operant crying. For example, a child initially cries in response to pain or hunger; however, when she cries and receives attention, or when she cries and gets to stay up late, she is engaging in operant crying. What follows crying (i.e., attention or staying up) is what determines the crying in these cases, not some unconditioned or conditioned stimulus.

While some operant behaviors are an elaboration of respondents, most are not. Instead, most operant behaviors originate as emitted responses[1]. They are strengthened or weakened by environmental consequences. In some cases the consequences may function universally to strengthen the behaviors they follow. For example, in newborns the presentation of milk or skin contact with mother strengthens the behaviors they follow. Other consequences are unique to individuals in terms of the strengthening or weakening effects they have on the behaviors they follow. As we develop, some consequences strengthen behaviors for some of us, while for others those same consequences may have neutral or even weakening effects. For example, a health conscious athlete may find the consumption of brewer's yeast following exercise increases the likelihood that he will exercise in the future, while the couch potato may find that its consumption weakens any behavior it follows (e.g. opening up the jar!!). For still others, it has no effect on the behaviors it follows. Consequences determine the occurrence of operant behavior. We adapt to our environments as we learn behaviors that produce strengthening consequences.

How Do Operants and Respondents Differ?

The distinction between operant and respondent behaviors is based on four characteristics:

1. Operants are Emitted, Respondents are Elicited
2. Operants, once emitted, continue to occur or not occur because of their consequences: respondents occur because of their antecedents.
3. Operants include a wider range of behaviors, respondents are limited to behavior which originated as reflexes.
4. Over time, operant learning involves the development (or ***shaping***) of new behaviors: respondent learning involves an existing behavior (UCR) being elicited by a **new** stimulus. Let us examine these differences.

1) Operants are Emitted

Operant behavior initially occurs without any antecedent stimulus causing it. It is in this sense that living organisms ***emit*** operant behaviors. "When a baby puts his hand to his mouth, the movement may be reinforced by the contact of hand and mouth, but we cannot find any stimulus which elicits the movement and which is present every time it occurs (Skinner, 1953, pg 107). On the other hand, respondent behavior is ***elicited*** by a conditioned or unconditioned stimulus. It is a direct response **to** a stimulus. The eliciting stimulus is present every time the respondent behavior occurs.

2) Operants Occur Because of Their Consequences

You are at the edge of a high cliff enjoying the seascape below. A friend sneaks up behind you and yells boo!!! The startle reflex elicited by the sudden noise causes you to jump . . . in spite of the rather severe consequences. This is respondent behavior. It occurred because a CS or UCS preceded it. It did not occur because jumping off cliffs in the past produced strengthening consequences. In this case it is the UCS (shouting boo!!) which causes the behavior.

Consequences are crucial to operant behavior. We perform responses because they are followed by certain consequences (called reinforcers) and do not perform other responses that have no consequences or else aversive ones (called punishers.) Reflect again on our cliff jumper. If he managed to survive his plunge by clinging to a bush to the applause and cheering of his friends, he is likely to again jump off a cliff in their presence, *sans* the boo. Such cliff jumping would be an operant, influenced by its consequences. (Is this how bungie cord jumping got started?)

Consider another example of operant behavior. In the dark, we press a button and the consequence of the light going on determines the occurrence of the response in the future. If the switch is broken and no light goes on, we soon stop pressing that switch since our behavior has no consequence. If we press a switch and get a shock, rather than light, we quickly stop... again, because of the consequence our behavior produced.

As previously noted, operants occur because of their consequences. However, this seems to be contradicted by the example of flipping on a light switch. Doesn't the presence of the light switch in the dark (an antecedent event) cause us to reach out and flip the switch in the same way the "boo!!" caused the jumper to jump? No, because the presence of a light switch causes us to turn it on only because of the reinforcing consequence that follows. We flip the switch and the light comes on. Without those reinforcing consequences, the switch would not cause this behavior. This is not the case with our jumper. He will jump when startled by a loud sound, like "boo!!" despite the unfortunate consequences. Most operant behavior is signaled or guided by antecedent stimuli. With operant behavior we say that the antecedent stimulus "***evokes***" the response. The presence of an on-off switch means that pressing responses will occur more frequently than if there were only a blank wall. Yet the function of the antecedent in operant behavior is different from a CS or UCS in respondent behavior. In operant behavior, the antecedent only cues behavior, and only does so because the behavior it cues has a certain consequence. Therefore if a switch is installed backwards, we can easily learn to press the "off" side to produce light, because it is that response in the presence of the cue that has the reinforcing consequence of producing light. In short, the switch does not elicit a "pressing reflex": there is no such thing. Instead, the switch evokes a pressing response which is reinforced by the consequence of producing light.

3) Operants Include a Wider Range of Behaviors

Respondent behaviors originate as reflexes, that is as unconditioned responses to unconditioned stimuli. They are called Universal I behaviors (see Chapter 2). As a class, respondents are restricted to innate reflexes which are part of the organism's phylogenic history. Startle reflexes, orientation reflexes, and physiological fear responses are the respondents that are of the most practical significance in human development.

As previously noted, operants can originate as reflexes too, as with crying or smiling. Even changes in physiological responses such as heart rate and brain waves (EEG) can come under the control of consequences and be classified as operants. However, operants involve much more behavior than just these former reflexes. Most of what we see emitted by children are operants, determined by the consequences the behaviors have in the environment. Therefore, most of what concerns us about human development, cognitive, language, and motor responses are operants and follow the principles of operant learning. Let us now turn to what these principles are.

4) Operant Learning Produces New Behavior

Recall that development involves progressive changes in person-environment transactions. In respondent learning the response remains the same regardless of whether it is elicited by the unconditioned **or** the conditioned stimulus. The eye blink or activation syndrome remains the same and what is learned is that a new stimulus, the conditioned stimulus, now elicits that response (conditioned response).

However, operant learning over time produces a new response since the effect of consequences is to strengthen some behaviors and weaken others. ***Shaping*** of behaviors and producing complex ***chains of behaviors*** are ways that operant learning produces new behaviors. Both of these operant learning processes will be discussed in detail later.

What is a Contingency?

A contingency is a dependent relationship, expressible as an if-then statement. The movie *Field of Dreams* had a ghostly voice whisper in the wind "If you build it, he will come." This mystical theme meant that *if* the main character built a baseball field in the middle of a cornfield in Iowa, *then* the character's deceased father would come back to play in the field and resolve a family relationship. This is a simple contingency: the first term is, "If you build it," which specifies the then term: "He will come." This type of contingency is the basis for operant behavior: If this response, then this consequence. If you press the switch, then the light goes off. If you press it again, then the light goes on. Note that the consequence (light off or on) **is contingent on** the response. That is, the consequence depends on the response.

The Four – Term Contingency

We can break down the contingency between environmental events (stimuli) and behavior (responses) into four terms (Bijou & Baer, 1978). This is called the ***four–term contingency***. We will now look at these four terms. Taken in order of occurrence, the four terms are a setting event or establishing operation, a cue or discriminative stimulus, a behavior or response, and a consequence or reinforcing stimulus. This is noted in the following sequence:

S^d	$\rightarrow$	R	$\rightarrow$	S^r
Discriminative Stimulus		Response		Reinforcing Stimulus

However, to understand the development of this contingency, we must start our analysis with the most important term, the response, rather than discussing them in the order in which they occur in time.

The First Term – The Response

R

We start with the behavior of interest, the operant response. It is the central segment of our unit of analysis, the four-term contingency. Behavior is any action of living things. Operant responses can be classified in three ways.

Response Classes Based on Topography

Responses are often classified by their form or ***topography***. We talk about running responses, button pushing responses, snoring responses, and any number of other categories. These responses are placed in these categories by the "look" or form of the responses. All running responses have a similar form, as do the button pushes and snores. However, it is important to note that there is some variability within these classes. Each stride is not exactly alike, neither is each button push. Nor is each snore. They are similar, but vary slightly from each other. Yet, it is convenient to talk about running as the response, even though we are actually dealing with a rather large number of individual responses, each of which is at least slightly different in form from any other. It is the observer who conveniently lumps them together as a response class defined by topography. However, from our viewpoint, responses are more usefully classified on the basis of their function.

Functional Response Classes

A functional response class is comprised of operant behaviors that produce the same consequence. That is, they have the same function. Most functional response classes include many behaviors which vary in their topography. For example, striking a match, flipping a light switch, and opening the drapes are all members of the same functional class when they are performed because of their effect in producing light. Furthermore, each of these response topographies are also members of *other* functional response classes. For example, the response of striking a match also belongs to that class of responses which is performed because it produces heat to light a cigarette. Other topographies belonging to this class include operating a cigarette lighter and asking another smoker for a light. In short, topographically different responses can have the same meaning or function. If they have the same function, regardless of their topography, they are members of the same functional response class.

Response Classes Based on Physical Location

Lastly, operant responses may also be placed into classes based on geography, or physical location. Thus we may divide them into classes of behaviors which occur outside the skin, so called "***public events***" (Skinner, 1953) or inside the skin, termed "***private events***" (Skinner, 1953). (The latter are not to be confused with birthday parties or *bar mitzvahs*). Thus motor activities such as walking or talking are part of the class of public events. Internal operant responses, such as talking to oneself, imaging, or hallucinating, are members of the class of private events.

Response Variability and Selectionism

Recall the earlier discussion of learning as a process of selection. Recall also, that the first requirement for selection is that there be variability in the response in order that a variety of responses are available to be selected by consequences (Donahoe & Palmer, 1994). Operant behavior is certainly characterized by variability. Even simple motor responses like jumping or reaching for a glass are characterized by variability. That is, even these simple motor responses are not exactly the same each time they occur. Some jumps are higher, or faster, or more tilted than others. It is this characteristic variability of responses which allows selection by consequences (Neuringer, 1994).

The Second Term – The Consequence

$$R \rightarrow S^{r+} \qquad S \rightarrow {}^{r-}$$

Operant behaviors produce environmental effects or changes in the environment which strengthen or weaken future occurrences of the operant. A response is "strengthened" in the sense that it is *more* likely to occur in the future. Similarly, a response is "weakened" in the sense that it is *less* likely to occur in the future. There are two types of consequences: (1) one in which a stimulus is added (+) or produced following a behavior, and (2) one in which a stimulus which is present is terminated or removed (-) following the response[2]. The effect of these consequences will be to strengthen or weaken behavior.

Selection by Consequences

One way to look at the strengthening effect of consequences is that consequences select certain responses from the wide range of behaviors which occur. Recall that there is variability in behavior. Some responses produce more adaptive consequences while others do not. For example, the better jumps of a skater may be selected by the consequences of the jump – landing upright on the ice, while poorer jumps will not be selected because the consequence of the behavior is a fall. Thus, from a selectionist perspective, variation in behavior leads to different consequences, some of which strengthen and some of which weaken behavior. We now turn to how consequences strengthen behavior – reinforcement.

Reinforcement – The Strengthening of Behavior

Behavior increases in strength when it becomes more frequent, or more likely to occur. ***Reinforcement*** is any operation[3] which strengthens behavior. Behavior which has been strengthened is said to have been ***reinforced***. Note the terms "reinforcement" and "reinforced" are used consistently with their everyday meaning as in reinforcement of a building, or reinforcing a regiment of soldiers. Reinforcement is defined empirically (Gewirtz & Pelaez-Nogueras, 1992). That is there must be an observable increase in the behavior to conclude that a behavior has actually been reinforced. There are two types of reinforcement, positive and negative. This distinction is based on the consequences which lead to the strengthening (i.e., reinforcement) of the response.

Positive Reinforcement ($R \rightarrow S^{+r}$)

Positive reinforcement occurs when a response adds or produces a stimulus event and the response increases in strength. We call the stimulus which follows the strengthened response a ***positive reinforcer or positive reinforcing stimulus*** (**S^{r+}**). Below are some examples of positive reinforcement:

- Sidney shakes a rattle and hears a noise. The shaking behavior occurs more frequently as a consequence of the response producing the noise. The shaking behavior has been positively reinforced. The noise is a positive reinforcer.
- Sylvia says "thank you" and her mother responds with "you're welcome." "Thank you" is a behavior that becomes more frequent. "Thank you" has been positively reinforced. "You're welcome" is a positive reinforcer for Sylvia.
- Tommy hits Jamie and she cries. Tommy is more likely to hit Jamie in the future. Tommy's hitting behavior has been positively reinforced. Jamie's crying is a positive reinforcer for Tommy.

Note in each case the behavior has been strengthened as a consequence of the behavior producing a stimulus. Note also that it is the **behavior** of the child **not the child herself** that is reinforced. We may be tempted to say "I reinforced Johnny," but it is more accurate to say "I reinforced Johnny's behavior."

Negative Reinforcement ($R \rightarrow S^{-r}$)

Negative reinforcement occurs when a response removes, terminates, or avoids a stimulus event and the response increases in strength. Note that since reinforcement is involved, the behavior is strengthened. This correct technical usage is contrary to the everyday usage of the term negative reinforcement. In everyday language negative reinforcement is applied to situations in which the behavior is weakened. **This is incorrect**. Technically these situations are actually punishment and will be examined later. To repeat, negative reinforcement occurs when a response removes, terminates, or avoids a stimulus **and the response is strengthened.** We shall call the stimulus which is removed or terminated as a consequence of the response, a ***negative reinforcer***, ***negative reinforcing stimulus***, or ***aversive stimulus*** **S^{r-}**).

Here are some examples of negative reinforcement:

- Wally holds his hand over his eyes and shades them from the bright sunlight. The eye-shading behavior is strengthened because it terminates the bright sunlight. The eye-shading behavior is negatively reinforced. Bright sunlight is a negative reinforcer.

- Elsie unwraps an unmarked foil package from the uncharted depths of her refrigerator. An unidentifiable, overpowering fowl odor (ancient chicken parts?) wafts through the air to her nostrils. She quickly re-wraps the package. The wrapping behavior is more likely to occur under similar circumstances. Thus the re-wrapping behavior has been negatively reinforced since it terminated the negative reinforcer (i.e., the odor).
- Steve throws a tantrum when his mother asks him to clean his room. The consequence of the tantrum is that his mother drops the demand. The tantrums will be more frequent in the future. These tantrums have been negatively reinforced since they terminated the negative reinforcer (i.e., his mother's demand).

Punishment – The Weakening of Behavior

Consequences can also weaken behavior. Behavior is said to be weakened when the frequency of the behavior decreases. This weakening of behavior due to either of the two types of consequences is called ***punishment.*** We shall now examine the two types of punishment.

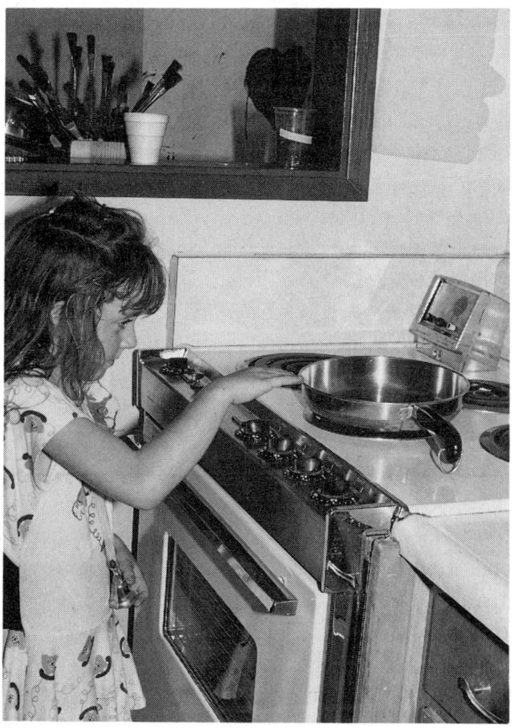

Punishment by "Hurt" (Positive Punishment)

One way behaviors are weakened is that they add or produce aversive stimuli (i.e., stimuli which "hurt") Behaviors which are followed by aversive stimuli are less likely to occur again. Some examples of punishment by hurt follow:

- Melissa grabs a pot on the stove producing a burning hot stimulus. She is unlikely to grab the pot again. The behavior was punished. The hot pot was an aversive stimulus.
- Chucky takes a swig of milk from a carton. This puts sour milk in his mouth. Chucky will not drink again from this carton. His behavior has been punished. The sour milk is an aversive stimulus.
- Amanda drives through a red light. She is stopped and given a ticket. She is less likely to drive through a stoplight in the future. She has been punished. The ticket is an aversive stimulus.

Punishment by Loss (Negative Punishment)

Behaviors may also be weakened if they have the effect of removing or terminating particular stimuli. This has been called ***punishment by "loss."*** It may also be called ***negative punishment*** to reflect the fact that the consequence is the *removal or termination* of the particular stimulus. Here are some examples of punishment by loss:

- Waldo puts his change in a pocket with a large hole in it, and the coins fall all over the ground. Waldo stops putting his change in that pocket. The weakening of the behavior is due to punishment by loss.
- Six-month-old Amy opens her hand and drops a ball which rolls to the floor below. She is less likely to let the ball go in the future. Opening of the hand is punished.
- Jake talks back to his mother and is not allowed to watch TV. Jake's talking back behavior is less likely to occur. Talking back is negatively punished.

The flowcharts (Figure 7.1 and 7.2) should help you work your way through an understanding of the technical terms. Figure 7.1 will help you decide on the name for the consequence. That is, whether a particular consequence is a case of positive reinforcement, negative reinforcement, punishment, or extinction. Because the name of the stimulus (e.g., positive or negative reinforcer) is determined in the reinforcement operation, Figure 7.2 should help you decide on the specific name for that stimulus.

We have presented these consequences as if they occur in isolation. This is not entirely accurate. Contingencies of reinforcement and punishment are complex and interrelated. Remember the first time your parents took you to the beach during the summer. Walking on the sand was punished because it produced an aversive stimulus – the burning hot sands. At the same time, hopping from wet sand to people's towels, to sand in the shadows was reinforced because it terminated the burning sensation in your feet. This shows that it is the behaviors of the person, not the person herself that are punished or reinforced. When you went to the beach for

Figure 7.1
Flow Chart for Determining the Name of an Operant Operation

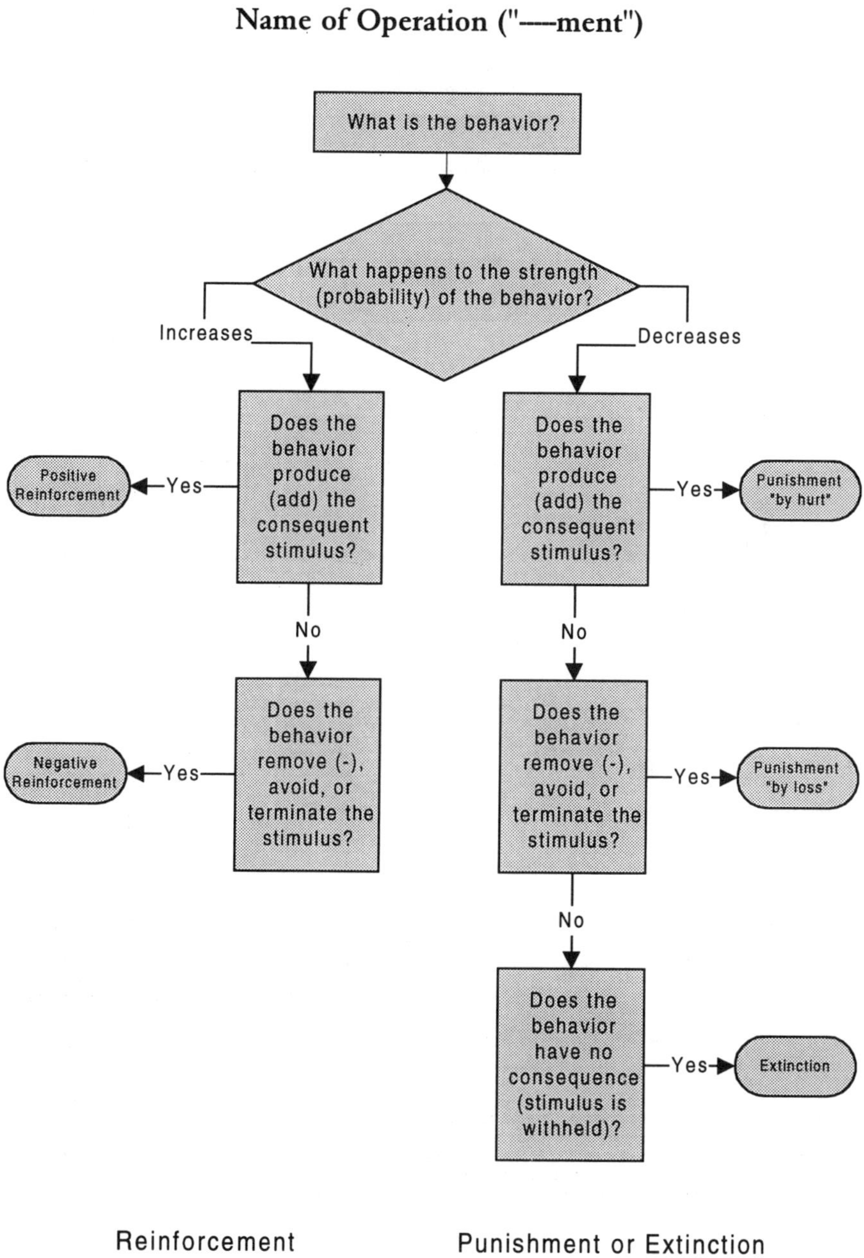

Figure 7.2
Flow Chart for Determining the Name of the Stimulus

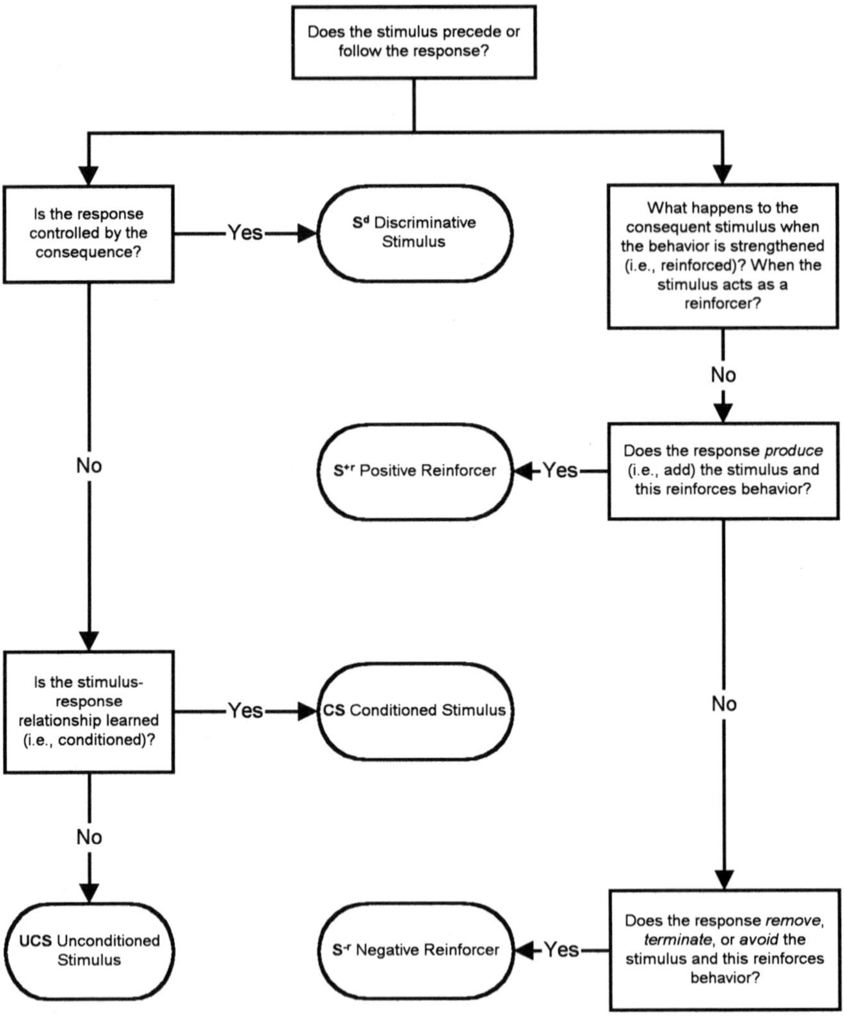

Note: The same stimulus name (i.e., positive reinforcer or negative reinforcer) can be retained when applied to punishment contingencies. Thus, *punishment by loss* occurs when a response removes, terminates or avoids a positive reinforcer. Likewise, *punishment by hurt* occurs when a response produces a negative reinforcer. Therefore, be certain whether you are naming the operation (reinforcement, punishment, or extinction) or naming the stimulus (positive or negative reinforcer).

the first time, walking on hot sand was punished by "hurt" and walking on towels or wet or shadowy sand was negatively reinforced.

Notice that in most of the examples of reinforcement and punishment discussed earlier, the change in stimulus events are naturally occurring consequences of the behavior. These consequences were not socially mediated: that is, no person attempted to change the behavior; the consequences occurred automatically. We can view the effects of consequences on behavior as a process parallel to those in natural selection (See Chapter 2). Behaviors which add positive reinforcers or remove aversive stimuli are strengthened. Behaviors which add negative reinforcers or remove positive reinforcers are weakened. Organisms have evolved these sensitivities to consequences; the ability to learn the contingencies of reinforcement and punishment in the environment make them better adapted to changes in the environments over their lifetimes. Those ancestors who had greater sensitivity to the contingencies were selected over those with less sensitivity. Although nonhuman animals are also sensitive to contingencies, it is the unparalleled ability of humans to detect subtle and complex contingencies that enables humans to learn rapidly. This colossal ability to learn is what sets the human species apart from all others (Sheppard & Willoughby, 1975).

Operant Extinction

What happens if reinforcement for a particular behavior is no longer forthcoming? If reinforcement of a behavior stops, the behavior will eventually stop occurring. If no one answers our telephone calls, we stop calling (Skinner, 1953). Likewise if we hit a key on our computer keyboard and nothing happens on the screen, we eventually stop hitting the key.

In both of these examples, the long term effects of the withholding of reinforcers is the extinction[4] of behavior. However these effects are different from the effects of punishment. With punishment the weakening of behavior is rapid (particularly if the consequent stimuli are powerful).

In operant extinction, the weakening of behavior by withholding reinforcement follows a different pattern. Generally if reinforcement of a previously reinforced behavior is withheld, the initial effect on the behavior is a rapid increase in the frequency, magnitude, and variability of the behavior. There may also be emotional behavior that is elicited by the withholding of the stimuli. This so called ***extinction burst*** may have an evolutionary significance for organisms because the increased responding may cause the reinforcement to occur again.

For example, if you press the "f" on your keyboard and it does not appear on the screen, you do not immediately stop. You press a little harder. When this does not produce the reinforcer (screen "f") you hit the key harder and more rapidly. You may even slam the keyboard. In short, there is initially a burst of activity. However, if none of this produces an "f" you stop responding. Your "f" key hitting behavior has been extinguished.

The Third Term – The Discriminative Stimulus (Sd)

$$\mathbf{S^d \rightarrow R \rightarrow S^{+r} \qquad S^d \rightarrow R \rightarrow S^{-r}}$$

We list this third because the response→consequence contingency is the crucial one for operant behavior. Yet, any stimulus which precedes the response→consequence contingency may come to evoke the response. Such an *antecedent* stimulus is called a ***discriminative stimulus*** or S^d (pronounced "ess-dee"). It "signals" or cues the response. Look at the short-hand notations above. The contingency has now become three-termed: in the presence of this stimulus (S^d) a particular response (R) will have a particular consequence (the S^{+r}or the S^{-r}). Consider the example of turning on the light switch. Because flipping the light switch produced the positive reinforcer (light), the switch itself has become a discriminative stimulus for the flipping response. The switch evokes a press that produces light. Similarly, a rattle evokes shakes that produce noise, and a seat belt evokes a buckling-up that terminates the noise. These antecedent stimuli have acquired their discriminative properties because they have been correlated with specific consequences.

Note that while there may appear to be a similarity between the operant Sd and the respondent CS or UCS, the Sd has acquired its power to "cause" behavior in a very different manner. Let us look at the case of stopping at a red light. As you approach an intersection in your car you see a red light. You automatically lift your foot from the accelerator and move it to the brake. You come to a gradual stop. Now, if the red light were a CS or UCS it would have elicited a stopping response regardless of the consequence. The stopping response would have had to originate as a reflex. Maybe in centuries to come, such a reflex will evolve *via* natural selection. But, for now, stopping at a traffic light has been acquired because of the consequences which follow. We stop because of negative reinforcement: stopping avoids having accidents and getting traffic tickets. If the consequences are changed, we may not stop at a red light. For example, at midnight, in a deserted town, a red light may not evoke stopping behavior.

At this point we have a three-term contingency, $S^d \rightarrow R \rightarrow S^{r+}$ (a positively reinforced, discriminated response) or $S^d \rightarrow R \rightarrow S^{r-}$ (a negatively reinforced, discriminated response).Yet, each contingency is affected by the context in which it occurs. Context is a central ingrediant in behavor analysis of development (Morris, 1993[5]). Thus we come to the last term, the setting event.

The Fourth Term – The Setting Event (SE)

Dad says "Come here." Dad is smiling. The Sd is a specific event, "Come here." The SE is the context in which the event occurs, the smile on dad's face. According to Bijou & Baer (1978), "a setting event influences an interactional sequence by altering the strength and characteristic of the particular stimulus response functions involved in an interaction "(pg. 26). Thus setting events are general conditions that affect the specific stimulus-response relationships.

There appear to be at least two distinct ways in which setting events affect the contingency (Michael, 1993[6]). Some setting events increase the likelihood that the

Sd will evoke a particular response by affecting the Sd→R relationship. For example, in the context of Dad's smiling, his saying "come here" (the S^d) is more likely to evoke the response than if dad were not smiling.

Some other setting events increase the likelihood that the Sd will evoke a particular response by affecting the $R \rightarrow S^{+r}$ or $R \rightarrow S^{-r}$ relationships by determining the degree to which a consequence is reinforcing or punishing. Michael (1982, 1993) used the term ***establishing operation*** (***EO***) for such a contingency altering setting event. For example, if you have eaten recently, seeing a package of dried prunes will not cause you to pick up the package. If you are food deprived, you are more likely to have the package evoke behaviors that lead to eating the prunes. Being food deprived affects the contingency by making food more reinforcing than it had previously been. Deprivation is an operation that establishes food as a reinforcer for the response. Establishing operations thus fall into the realm of motivation. They may be viewed as motivational setting events.

To recap, operant behavior can be analyzed as a four-term contingency. Within a particular context (the setting event), a particular stimulus (discriminative stimulus) evokes a behavior (response) which affects the environment (produces a consequence).

What Changes? – The Development of Reinforcing Stimuli Primary Reinforcers

One of the important developments in the progressive changes between behavior and environment is in what become reinforcing and punishing stimuli. At birth, a number of reinforcers are already functioning. We call this initial class of reinforcers ***primary reinforcers.*** This connotes that they are the first reinforcers to function. Primary reinforcers are universal, owing their reinforcing function to the genetic inheritance of the child. There are both positive and negative primary reinforcers. Among the primary positive reinforcers are: food, water, sucking produced stimulation, taste stimuli, skin temperature, rest and sleep, and air. Watson (1972) demonstrated that discovery of a contingency between the child's own behavior and its consequence may itself be a primary reinforcer. Thus noticing that an action (e.g., moving ones head) causes a consequence (e.g., change in visual stimulation) may be what reinforces a repetitive act. That is, a child may do something over and over to determine what the effects (consequences) of the action are.

Primary negative reinforcers include pain eliciting stimuli, and a range of physical, chemical stimuli. Bijou and Baer (1965) pointed out that almost any stimulus can be a negative reinforcer if it is sufficiently intense. Loud noises, bright lights, and sudden changes can negatively reinforce behaviors which terminate or avoid them.

Primary reinforcers evolved because of their adaptive significance for the newborn child (Gewirtz & Pelaez-Nogueras, 1992). Food, water, visual stimulation, and warmth are examples of primary positive reinforcers that are necessary for survival. Behaviors that produce them are strengthened. Painful stimuli, bright lights, foul odors are examples of primary negative reinforcers. Behaviors that remove, avoid, or terminate them are also strengthened. The adaptive significance of sensitivity to these consequences in terms of the survival of the species should be apparent.

Lipsitt, (1979) reported a series of studies on positive and negative reinforcers in newborns. Sucking that produced sucrose was not only stronger than that which produced water, but if the neonates were first allowed to suck to produce sucrose, switching them to water reduced their sucking below what it is when water alone has been the reinforcer. Thus this change was affected not only by the withdrawal of sucrose, but to the setting event of having the sugar first. This change in behavior produced not by the reinforcer alone, but by the context of the water following the sugar is referred to as ***behavioral contrast*** and may be a type of setting event. Lipsitt also described the behavior of neonates that is reinforced by terminating aversive stimuli.

As part of the biological inheritance of the human species, most primary reinforcers are universal. That is, all children are affected by the same primary positive and negative reinforcers. Because of individual differences in biological make-up, there will be some individual differences in responding to primary reinforcers. For example a child who is born without sensitivity to light will not respond to visual reinforcers as will the sighted newborn. More subtle differences in sensory capabilities means that individual children will be more or less affected by specific primary reinforcers. These individual differences become even greater when we consider the affects of secondary or acquired reinforcers.

Secondary (Acquired) Reinforcers

The distinction between primary and secondary reinforcers is that primary reinforcers strengthen behavior due to the phylogenic history of the organism. They are unlearned. In contrast, ***secondary reinforcers*** are learned or ***acquired reinforcers***. They are also called **conditioned reinforcers**. They are acquired because they are correlated with the other primary or secondary reinforcers. That is, they reliably signal that a response will have a certain consequence. (Note: This is the same situation that leads to the development of discriminative stimuli. Indeed, discriminative stimuli acquire the dual function of secondary reinforcers).

Unlike the essentially universal set of primary reinforcers, all individuals develop a unique catalog of acquired reinforcers. The interindividual variability in acquired reinforcers is due to the unique genetic make-up and environmental conditions each child experiences. It is due to the unique set of reinforcers that a person acquires that determines the special repertoire of behaviors of that person.

Note, however, that just as universal genetic similarities produce a common set of primary reinforcers, similar environmental experiences may produce secondary reinforcers which are shared by most members of a family, society, culture, or even species. In turn, these reinforcers produce similar behaviors in members of the family, society, culture, or species.

What Reinforcers are Acquired?

Rovee-Collier (1987) summarized what we know about what develop as reinforcers for newborn behavior. Their own mothers' voice reinforces an infant's sucking while a strange female voice or even the voice of the father does not (DeCasper & Sigafoos, 1983). Mother's smell is also reinforcing (Cernoch & Porter, 1985).

Visual stimuli require more time to become discriminated and to acquire reinforcing functions, perhaps because of relatively poor newborn acuity. Infants may be reinforced by looking at faces, Rovee-Collier (1987) concludes that the preponderance of the evidence is that faces play no special function until about four months of age (based on Dolgin & Azmitia, 1985).

Classes of Common Acquired Reinforcers

1. Tangible Reinforcers

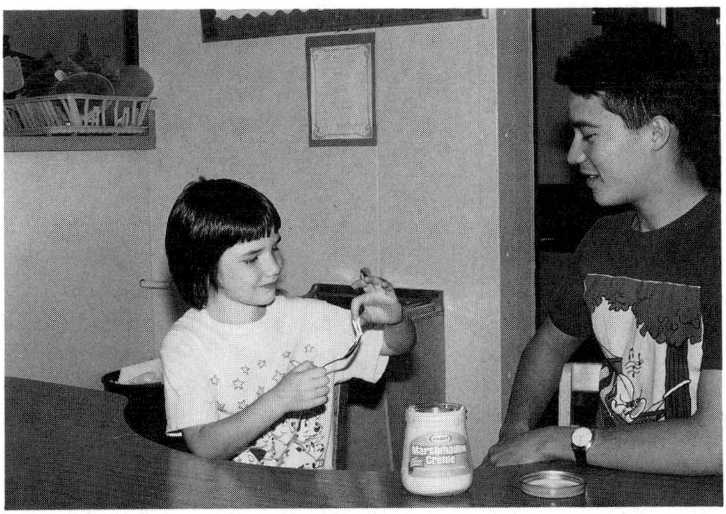

These are objects which derive their reinforcing effects because they can be touched, viewed, smelled, or manipulated in a variety of ways. This class includes items such as stickers, trinkets, scratch & sniffs, and toys.

2. Edible Reinforcers

As the name implies, these reinforcers are eaten. Most, such as cookies, crackers, and M&Ms, are primary reinforcers. The taste is reinforcing because of the evolutionary history of our species. Others, such as guacamole or liver pate are often acquired reinforcers, requiring an extensive learning history.

3. Social Reinforcers

These are acquired reinforcers which develop because they are associated with many primary reinforcers or previously established secondary reinforcers. For example, Mom's smile becomes a reinforcer because it is present when she feeds and fondles her infant.

Cooper, Heron, and Heward (1987) distinguish three types of social reinforcers. (1) physical contact (e.g., pats and hugs), (2) proximity (e.g., sitting near someone), and (3) verbal statements (e.g., "good job").

4. Activity Reinforcers

This category refers to behaviors themselves that can be reinforcing. The ***Premack principle*** (Premack, 1959) states that any high frequency behavior can be used to reinforce any low frequency behavior. So, if your child often plays Nintendo (a high frequency behavior) and rarely does his homework (a low frequency behavior), you can use the former to increase the latter.

5. Generalized Reinforcers

These are acquired reinforcers which have been associated with many other secondary and primary reinforcers, so that they are "generally" reinforcing. In other words, unlike food which is only reinforcing when you are hungry, or a coat which is only reinforcing when you are cold, generalized reinforcers strengthen behavior under many setting events. Examples of generalized reinforcers are money, Mom, attention, and the baby's security blanket.

Shaping

In working with children, very often our goal is to increase the rate of a particular behavior. For example, a teacher may want to increase the number of cursive writing assignments a student completes per week. In such a case, the teacher could use a positive reinforcement procedure and reward each completed assignment with 10 minutes of free time. However, what is a teacher to do when the student has yet to learn cursive writing? How can you reinforce a behavior that a student does not exhibit? Shaping is one answer.

Shaping is a procedure in which one reinforces successive approximations of a terminal behavior. If, for example, one is trying to teach a child to write, one can first reinforce the child's behavior of simply picking up the pencil. Once this occurs reliably, one can change the criterion for reinforcement. One now reinforces the child only when he picks up the pencil such that the lead is pointing downward. In a sense this places other, regressive, forms of pencil holding, on extinction. Since one has put the old behavior on extinction, the student will display variability in the form of the response. One form of the response is likely to be holding the pencil with the lead pointing downward. When he does so, the teacher can then reinforce him. Once the student is reliably picking up the pencil with the lead pointing downward, one then shifts the criterion of reinforcement to a behavior which is a closer approximation of the terminal behavior – putting the point to the paper. By reinforcing successive approximations of the terminal behavior (i.e., shaping), one can use positive reinforcement to teach a new behavior such as cursive writing.

Shaping does not always involve the intervention of another person, such as a teacher. Shaping often occurs as a part of normal interaction with the environment. For example, in learning to pick up a bottle, the child's first responses are likely to involve large muscle movements of both arms and hands. As the child is reinforced for these behaviors, the likelihood of a one-handed grasp occurring and being reinforced is increased. As the single hand grasp is strengthened, it is more likely that other objects, such as cups, which are smaller in size, will shape finer grasping behaviors. In this way, the environment shapes new behaviors.

The Russian psychologist Lev Vygostsky emphasized the importance of a shaping process which occurs in learning interactions. He defined the ***zone of proximal development*** (Vygotsky, 1987) as the range of behavior between what a child can achieve independently and what can be achieved with a more competent member of the culture, such as an adult or another child. The child's behavior can be enhanced through the use of ***scaffolding***. Scaffolding is the support that the parent (or other competent member, such as a teacher, or even computer) provides for the child's behavior. By successively moving the criteria for reinforcement ahead by small increments, the parent is able to shape new behavior.

Chaining

Suppose you want your child to make his own sandwiches for lunch. You cannot wait for him to make a sandwich and then reinforce him if he does not already know sandwich making. However, if he does know how to perform the individual behaviors that constitute sandwich making, we can teach him to chain those behaviors together. A ***behavior chain*** is a set of discrete behaviors sequenced in a particular order

To teach a behavior chain to someone, one must first perform a task analysis. In our example, the task of making a sandwich must be analyzed into its component behaviors. More specifically, in a task analysis one must identify: 1) the discrete behaviors comprising the chain and 2) the sequence in which these behaviors occur. Thus, sandwich making might be analyzed as follows 1) fetch the loaf of bread and mayonnaise, 2) place them on the table, 3) fetch the knife, etc. After completing the task analysis, one could then teach the student the first behavior, then teach him to perform the first and the second behavior, and so on until one finally taught him to perform all the behaviors in the appropriate sequence. This is called ***forward chaining***.

In teaching a behavior chain, one begins by providing an S^d which evokes the first behavior in the chain. In our example, one could say "Fetch the bread and mayonnaise." Having these items in his hands serves as a reinforcer for the fetching behavior. However, the bread and mayonnaise also serve as S^ds for the next behavior, placing them on the table. Similarly, seeing the loaf and mayonnaise on the table is a reinforcer for placing them there, and they are also a S^ds for performing the next behavior in the chain. In this way, each response produces a reinforcer and, simultaneously, an S^d for the next behavior until all of the behaviors in the chain have been performed.

Chains of behavior also develop without specialized teaching or training. Consider the following example. Kate has learned to push a button to turn on the TV. She has also learned to climb up on to a chair. She has learned to push a chair around. One day you observe Kate push a chair over to the TV, climb up on it, and turn on the TV. Without being trained to do so, Kate has chained three discrete behaviors together in a sequence. What causes this chain to emerge?

In order to answer this question, we must first consider another process. In the sandwich making example, we used forward chaining. We taught our student the first behavior first, then chained it to the performance of the second behavior until all the behaviors in the chain had been learned in the sequence in which they are to occur. Notice, in forward chaining, the reinforcer and Sd for the initial response (getting the bread and mayonnaise) is rather weak. In contrast, the final reinforcer (eating the sandwich) is much stronger. The new procedure, backward chaining takes advantage of this fact.

In backward chaining, the trainer may perform all the behaviors except the final behavior in the chain. All that is left for the student to do is the final behavior which is immediately and powerfully reinforced by the taste of the sandwich. Once the student can reliably perform the final behavior, the trainer would then require the student to perform the last two behaviors in the chain. Then the student performs the last three, in sequence. Eventually, the student learns the first behavior in the chain and can now perform the entire chain. The major advantage of this approach is that during the first lesson the student immediately contacts the highly reinforcing consequences of eating the sandwich. This does three things. First, the response is quickly strengthened by establishing the relationship between the response and the consequence. Second, the antecedents of the last response quickly become Sds for its occurrence. Lastly, because of their role as S^ds, the antecedents of the last response become conditioned reinforcers for the next-to-last response.

Let us return to our earlier question about how Kate developed her chain of behaviors. The reinforcer that holds the chain together is a TV show (All My Children?) Pushing the button is reinforced by this. Touching the button is an S^d for pushing it. It also becomes a reinforcer for a response (climbing on the chair) which is reinforced by touching the button. At this point you should be able to follow the chain back to its initial S^d. Can You? What would happen to Kate's chain ofbehavior if the TV broke?

Operant Learning and Dynamical Principles of Development

With this we conclude our look at the basic processes of development. Recall that learning is *a* process involved in all development. That is, even in basic sensory abilities, exposure to a species typical environment is necessary for change. Recall also, that learning plays *the* role in nonuniversal behaviors and universal II behaviors.

However, to understand how such seemingly simple processes of learning can produce the complexity of human behavioral development, we must revisit the principles of dynamical systems.

In chapter two, we discussed how and why development involves the reciprocal interaction of the organismic and environmental factors. Specifically, we concluded that the process of development involves the coalescence of genetics, interactional history, current physiological conditions, and current environmental conditions coming together to organize behavior.

Coalescent Organization Revisited

Behavior is assembled by the task and the context (Thelen, 1992). Another way of saying this is that the coalescence of factors occurs through the contingencies of reinforcement in effect for the child. Under certain setting events, a bright shiny object will evoke reaching. The form of the chain of behaviors of reaching, will determined by the coalescence of many factors including the (in-part) genetically influenced shape of the arm and hand, the presence of gravity, the history of reaching for visual stimuli and the consequences of reaching both past and present. All this is assembled by the environmental contingencies presented by the environment. We go from one phase of reaching (e.g., two-handed) to another (e.g., one-handed) as the coalescence of factors enables the child to reach and grasp the object with one hand. Hundreds of tiny influences come together through the contingency of reaching-feeling the object to produce phase shifts in the organized pattern of behavior we call reaching. *Shifts-happen!*

Another Look at the Emergence of Dynamic Attractors

As you remember, the patterns which emerge are called attractors. They have a characteristic topography or form based upon the limits imposed by the coalescence of factors involved. That is, at a particular time in development reaching may be limited by physical strength and lack of skill to picking up objects with two hands. The development of increased strength due to physical changes in bones and muscles, coupled with skills learned through environmental contingencies, lead to one-hand reach-grasps. Yet, even a basic behavior like reaching for and picking up an object is organized by the consequences. Think about your own reaching. If the task is to pick up a pin, what will the form of your response be? What if the task is to pick up a thirty-pound boulder? What if you need to pick up a thirty-pound dumbbell? What determines the form of the response?

Remembering the Importance of Leading Parts or Control Parameters

While many factors coalesce to produce behavioral development, some play a larger, more important role than others. Some factors disproportionately affect development. You have learned the term, "leading parts" (Horowitz, 1992) or "control parameters" for this principle. In backward chaining, the final reinforcer is a control parameter.

The Issue of Nonlinearity

We often assume that reinforcement has linear effects. That is, every reinforcement adds the same amount to the strength of a response. However, you have recognized that this assumption is often not true. Reinforcements and punishments may have little effect on behavior at first and then a single reinforcement (or punishment) may have a suddenly large effect on the behavior. Thus the effect of contingencies may be nonlinear.

Nonlinearity also appears in shaping. Very seldom do the successive approximations to the final goal involve evenly spaced steps. More frequently, the approximations are nonlinear. Early steps may be very small whereas, later steps may be larger leaps. Consider children playing a hiding game. One child has to find a hidden toy. Approximations to finding it are reinforced by "You're getting warmer!" and punished by "You're getting colder!" At first we are likely to see small movements around a local area. Then, the child's searching behavior may involve larger movements and progress towards the goal may be much faster. At the end of the search, approximations may again involve smaller steps.

Learning and Dynamical Systems in Summary

While learning, especially operant learning, is a process in development, it plays a key role. The contingencies of reinforcement and punishment "assemble" behavior into loosely organized patterns, or attractors. It is the function of behavior which determines its form. Forms are continually developing as the effects of biological, historical, and current environmental factors combine to make behavior function more efficiently at producing reinforcement and avoiding, terminating, or escaping punishment. Psychological development is a process of adapting to our environment and it is learning which provides the flexibility to do so.

Footnotes

[1]We choose here to use the term "response" which is the conventional behavioral terminology. Ferster & Culbertson (1982) caution that using the term "response" for operant behavior may have misleading connotations. Operant behavior is affected by its consequences, not responses to stimuli as respondent behavior is. We have considered using B to stand for behavior with C for consequence and A for antecedent. Thus our contingency would include the ABCs. However, the **Sd®R®Sr** notation is more widely used and will be the convention used here.

[2]Notice the shorthand notation for the consequent stimulus is either S^{r+} or S^{r-}. These are the technical names for the consequent stimulus. S^{r+} may be read as "positive reinforcing stimulus" or "positive reinforcer. S^{r-} is read as "negative reinforcing stimulus," or "negative reinforcer."

[3]Reinforce***ment*** is an *operation* involving contingencies that strengthen behavior. A reinforcer***er***is a stimulus which follows the behavior and strengthens it. Depending on whether the consequence of the behavior is to add or remove the stimulus, the stimulus is called a positive or negative reinforcer, respectively.

[4]The operation in which reinforcers are withheld is called operant "extinction." However, behaviors become "extinguished," not "extincted."

[5]Morris (1993) argues that behavior analysts have adopted two types of contexts in their system. The first type is, as used here, concerned with general setting conditions which alter the other three-terms of the contingency. Morris feels this "context-as-place" is what most people mean when they use the word "context." However, Morris also points out that behavior analysis is also contextualistic because it adopts the second sense of the word context--"context-as-time." This sense of "context" places current behavior squarely in the context of a history of interaction, a basic behavioral systems view which is entirely consistent with developmental psychology.

[6]Michael (1982, 1993) uses the term "Establishing Operation" and identifies both the evocative and contingency altering effects of certain events or operation. The term setting event is used here based on the terminology used by Bijou & Baer (1961).

Chapter 8

Cognitive Development

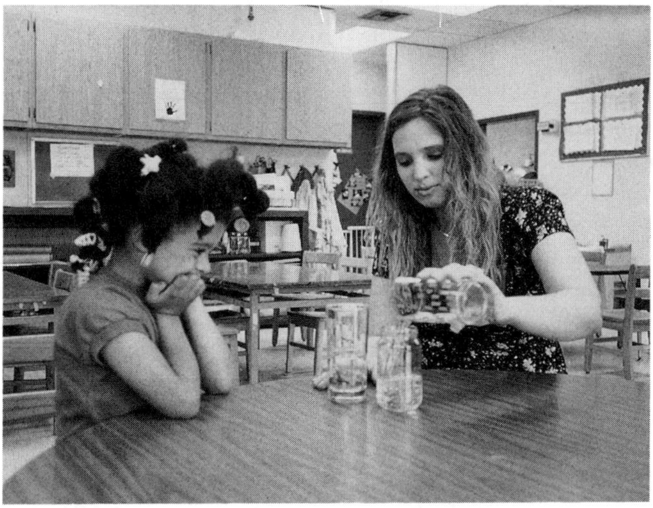

"Cogito, ergo sum"

"I think, therefore, I am." This famous quote from the French philosopher René Descartes (1596-1650) underlies the prominence of thinking as the most important human characteristic. What are thinking and thought? How shall we treat them from a natural science viewpoint? How do they develop? Do you exist because you think, or do you think, because you exist? These are questions undertaken in this chapter.

Cognition means "the act or process of knowing" (Random House). For most of us, knowing means thinking. For Skinner and other behavior analysts, thinking is an action: It is behavior. In this view, the only difference between cognitive acts and other operants is their location. Cognitive behaviors are private events occurring inside the skin. **"Cognitive processes are behavioral processes; they are things people do"** (Skinner, 1989, pg. 17).

Skinner (1953) identified two aspects of cognition: ***knowledge*** and ***ability***. He treated these as operant behaviors. Bijou and Baer (1961) added a third category of cognition, ***problem solving***. Cognitive development involves the changes in our knowledge and abilities over our life spans. We will examine the development of these behaviors from the viewpoints of behavior analysis and dynamical systems. However, to put the study of cognitive development into historical perspective, let us look at the first systematic theory of cognitive development, Jean Piaget's.

Piaget's Theory of Cognitive Development

Piaget's Worldview

Piaget transformed developmental theory. It is interesting to see how this theory emerged from Piaget's early training and the existing worldview of his day. Jean Piaget was born in Neuchâtel, Switzerland in 1896. His godfather was a professor of philosophy with a specialty in logic. Although he also studied logic , the young Jean's real interest was biology and he published his first scientific paper at the age of 10! (It was his observations on an albino sparrow.) By age 22 he had received a Ph.D. in biology and had published over two dozen papers in his specialization.

This combined background in biology and logic would emerge in his study of child psychology. The dominant theory in the field of biology during his time was the still new and controversial theory of Charles Darwin. Darwin's theory of natural selection inspired Piaget's thesis on mollusks. Piaget studied the patterns of whorls on populations of freshwater snails. Using Darwin's theory he explained how the structure of the snail's shells evolved due to natural selection. Snails in a particular ecosystem had different patterns of shells which allowed for better adaption to the existing environmental conditions.

The basic idea of adaptation would mark his viewpoint when he turned his interest to psychology. In Paris from 1919-1921, Piaget studied at the Sorbonne and worked on the development of intelligence tests with Theodore Simon. Simon, with his colleague, Alfred Binet, are credited with developing the first standardized intelligence tests. Yet, Piaget wasn't happy following the restricted format of the test. He became interested in pursuing wrong test answers given by children to try to identify the logic used in producing the errors. This use of the ***clinical method***, led him to intensive questioning of just a few young children. Among the subjects studied were his own children. From this method, developed a theory of what children know about the world and how they come by this knowledge.

What Changes? – Structure

Piaget was interested in changes in biological structure over evolutionary time. The structure of his snail shells changed in form as they adapted to changes in the ecology. Therefore he looked for and found a parallelism in the development of knowledge. He inferred change in the structure of thought. He believed that the structure of knowledge, or mental structures, developed over an individual's life span (note that this is another parallel of natural selection). Piaget called these mental structures ***schemes***.[1]

For Piaget, schemes are mental representations of the world. Schemes may be actions, images, or symbols that are used to interpret interactions with the environment. These mental representations are the child's knowledge of the world. Changes in these schemes produce changes in the child's knowledge of the world. The schemes that are the representation of the world in infancy are not only fewer than in adulthood, but their type and organization are different as well. For Piaget, development included qualitative, not just quantitative changes. Piaget based his stages of cognitive development on cognitive behavior that resulted from the emergence of increasingly more complex, and more highly organized schemes.

Types of Schemes

What does the newborn know of the world? What form does its mental structures take? Piaget believed that the child's first representations of the world were its reactions to stimuli in the form of its reflexes. Thus the child's first schemes were ***behavioral schemes.*** Remember, a reflex involves the relationship between a stimulus and a response. Behavioral schemes are mental representations in the form of actions. So Piaget called his first stage, between birth and about two years, the sensorimotor (*i.e.*, stimulus-response) stage.

As development continues, behavioral schemes are expanded to include behaviors other than just reflexes. This process, termed by Piaget as circular reations, extends other (*e.g.*, operant) stimulus-response relations into more complex and more highly organized behavior schemes. Bruner (1968) called the mental representation of the world by actions, ***enactive representation.*** For an example of a behavioral scheme, think of what you would **do** if someone asked "what's a slinky?" You would probably hold your hands palm up and alternate moving them up and down. That is a behavioral scheme for a slinky.

During the second year the child begins to represent the world first with images and then through language. Bruner called the use of images, ***iconic representation,*** with language being labeled ***symbolic representation.*** Unlike behavioral schemes, images and words do not involve the actual physical activity they represent. Symbolic schemes are representations of the things they stand for, not the things themselves. These are Piaget's ***symbolic schemes.*** In Piaget's view they enable increased ability to represent the world resulting in increased knowledge. Asking you to close your eyes and think of what a slinky looks like would evoke an iconic representation of it (an image). Asking you what the object is called would evoke a symbolic representation – "slinky." Both the image and the word are examples of symbolic schemes.

Piaget's last category of schemes are the ***operational schemes.*** In Piaget's view, an operation is a set of mental tasks that follows certain logical rules. Addition, subtraction, and negation are operations. So is reversibility, transforming something into another thing and then changing it back.

According to Piaget what develops is not only the type of schemes (starting with simple behavioral to symbolic and then operational ones) but also the amount and complexity of schemes. Our mental representations of the world become not only more numerous, but more organized as well. As we develop, our representations increase from "mommy" to "girl" and "women." Our representation also takes on a ***hierarchical*** organization: "mommy" fits under the class "women." With time the differentiation of the world produces highly organized structures of schemes. Your knowledge of the world is determined by your schemes. Thus, as your schemes become more organized and differentiated, so does your knowledge of the world. Now we turn to the question of "how" development occurs.

How do the Structures Change? – Functions

In the biology of Piaget's day, ***adaptation*** was the basic process for change in biological structures. Piaget saw a parallelism to his study of the development of knowledge. For Piaget, mental structures also changed through a process of adaptation. Biologists saw physical structures changing by adapting to the physical environment. Piaget saw mental structures changing through adaptation to the intellectual environment.

Adaptation = Assimilation and Accommodation

Biologists saw adaptation occurring through the action of two reciprocal and complementary processes: assimilation and accommodation. Both are necessary to produce changes in physical structures. Let me use an example to illustrate.

Imagine that you are really starved after a busy morning at school. You go to the cafeteria and to your delight you find that there is a special sale on chocolate decadence cake. It seems that the baker thought it said six cases of flour, not six cups, and they have about a dozen cakes too many. In order to sell them, whole cakes are on sale for $1.00 a cake. Not being one who could turn down a bargain (or chocolate decadence, for that matter) you purchase one of the cakes.

Now, what do you do? Not being of reptilian ancestry, unhinging your lower jaw is impossible. You are going to have to do something to be able to take the cake (environmental input) into your existing structures (mouth, esophagus, stomach, intestines). You begin to modify the input to put it into a form that will fit the existing structure: you must **assimilate** the cake.

What is the consequence of this? (I am all too familiar with this). Your existing structures assimilate the portion of input that readily fits into current structures. (Biologically this process would parallel digestion). Yet, often (and unfortunately for those watching their weight) some portion, usually the fat, of the input does not fit into existing structures. So the structures change or **accommodate** this new input. In the case of the cake, thighs, hips, and stomach are often the accommodating structures. Thus development is the result of the complementary action of both assimilation and accommodation.

Piaget applied these processes to cognitive development. Both assimilation and accommodation are necessary for changes in schemes to occur. Assimilation involves taking environmental information into existing structures (*i.e.*, schemes). For this to occur, aspects of the information inconsistent with existing schemes are ignored, modified, or changed. For example a child who already has the symbolic scheme "car," sees a motorcycle go by. She says "car" and sees it as a car. She has assimilated the motorcycle into her existing scheme.

Yet, what the child saw was discrepant from the existing scheme – car. This thing had only two wheels, the rider was open, and it made a different sound. These discrepancies make the existing schemes change to accommodate the experience. Thus, the scheme for car becomes enlarged or perhaps organized into different but hierarchically organized schemes involving cars, motorcycles, and vehicles.

The result of this reciprocal action of assimilation and accommodation is adaptation. The child's knowledge and ability fits better with his/her environment. Yet, the more we know, the more we need to know. The environment of the neonate is a good deal less demanding than that of the adult. A few simple behavioral schemes (the reflexes) are all the newborn knows or needs to know. However, by assimilating new information it allows accommodation to make for increasingly more numerous and complex schemes. Thus, this active interaction between what the child knows and what it needs to know produces, in Piaget's view, changes in cognitive development.

Equilibrium – Disequilibrium

What motivates adaptation? Piaget's view is that it is the mismatch between what the child knows and what it needs to know that causes assimilation and accommodation. This ***disequilibrium*** is the normal state, whereas ***equilibrium*** is only achieved temporarily when the cognitive structure matches what there is to know in the environment. If the discrepancy is too large (*e.g.*, teaching an infant about nuclear physics) no assimilation can occur. If there is no discrepancy, (*e.g.*, play) everything is assimilated, but accommodation does not occur. Cognitive development occurs when schemes change because there is ***optimal discrepancy*** between what the child knows and what it needs to know in the environment. This optimal discrepancy occurs naturally as the child actively interacts with its environment. The reciprocal changes in the child's existing knowledge and what it needs to know fits our dynamical model of development. Not only is the child affected by the environment, but the changes in the child now affect the environment as well.

For Piaget, the structures known as schemes are what change to produce development. In contrast, the processes that produce the changes; adaptation through assimilation and accommodation, remain the same over our life spans. They are ***invariant***. They work in the same manner **across the life span** to produce more numerous, complex, and organized schemes. It is the alteration in the schemes that produce the changes in cognitive behavior that Piaget categorized into his stages of cognitive development.

Piaget's Stages of Cognitive Development

Piaget saw cognitive development occurring in four stages. It is necessary to complete each stage before the child could progress to the next. These stages are determined by the type of schemes that the child possesses. The stages occur in the following order.

Sensorimotor Stage (Birth – 24 months)

Behavioral (or sensorimotor) schemes dominate this stage. It has six substages:

1. Reflexes (First month) - Reflexive Behavior.
2. Primary Circular Reactions (1 - 4 mos.) - Repetitive behaviors that are centered on the child's own body.

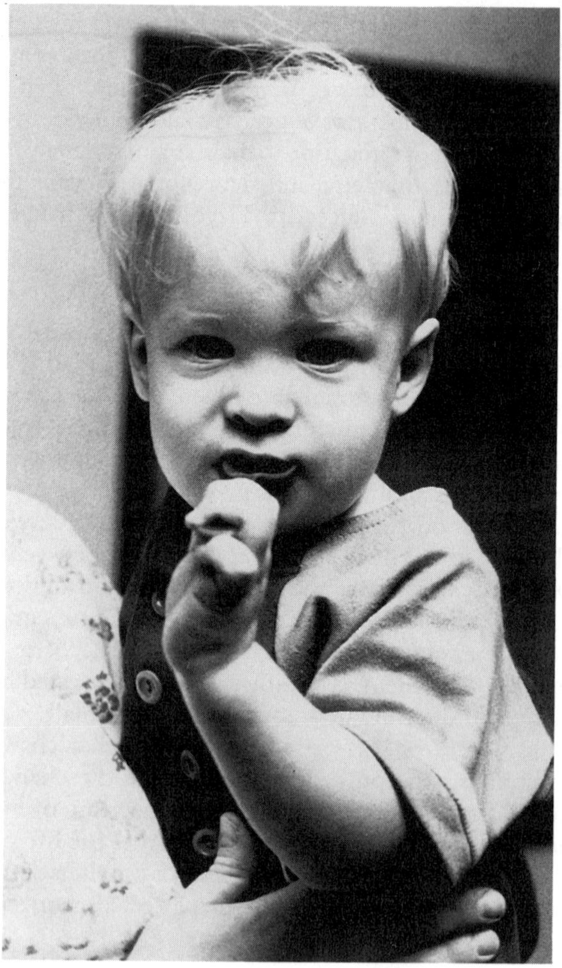

3. Secondary Circular Reactions (4 - 7 mos.) - Repetitive behaviors that produce consequences from the external environment.

4. Intentionality (8 - 12 mos.) - Consequences of the behavior are more organized. Behavior seems to occur to produce a specific consequence.

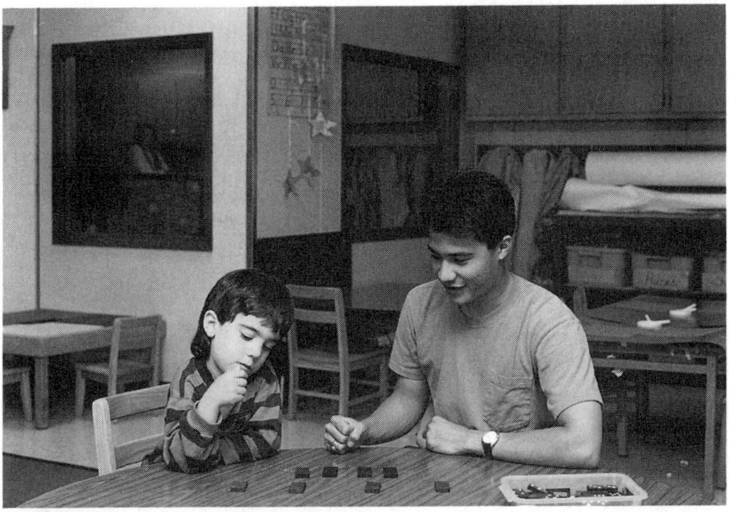

5. Tertiary Circular Reactions (12 - 18 mos.) - Child accidentally produces a consequence and then varies response to determine what behaviors produce the consequence. Curiosity begins and is influenced by the ability to use symbols.
6. Symbolic Problem Solving (18 - 24 mos.) - Emergence of mental representation. Child can anticipate the whereabouts of objects placed out of his hands.

Preoperational Stage (2 - 7 years)

The child enters this stage poised on the use of symbolic schemes, particularly language. Now with symbolic schemes, the child's representation of the environment becomes more sophisticated and increasingly more flexible. The stage has two substages:

Preconceptual Period (2 - 4 years)

In this period the child's thinking is naive and primitive compared to adult thinking. The child thinks by using *transductive reasoning*, thinking from specific to specific, unable to generalize. With transductive reasoning the child does not make cause and effect connections. Thus, the sun rises because it is daytime. Other characteristics of preconceptual thought are animism (giving human characteristics to inanimate objects), and egocentrism (seeing things from one's own point of view).

Intuitive Period (4 - 7 years)

The child's thought shows a simple form of reasoning. Still egocentric, the child guesses rather than uses true logical operations to explain events. Without being able to use the operations of conservation, the child may not know that the liquid from a tall glass maintains its amount when poured into a flat dish. Instead the child guesses that the tall glass had more, because the child guessed and centered on the height. Also, without the ability to use operations of addition or subtraction the child has difficulty with problems involving class inclusion. When asked if there are more flowers or more roses in a field, the child might guess that there are more roses because he fails to see that roses are part of the class of flowers.

Concrete Operations Stage (7 - 11 years)

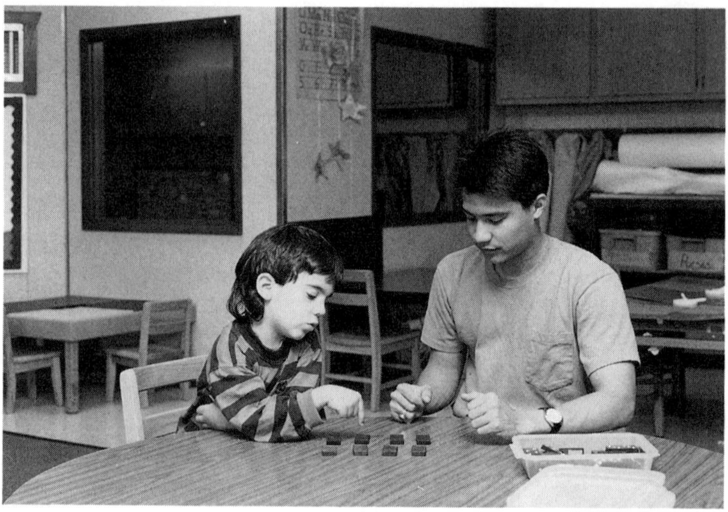

As schemes become more numerous and organizationally complex, a new class develops. These classes are called operational schemes. These represent the abstract rules that apply to the relationships among objects and events. Schemes for operations such as conservation, class inclusion, and seriation mean that now the child can use more adult like logic. Now when presented with the problem of the glass and the dish, the child can apply the operational schemes and conclude that the amount is the same in either. While the preoperational child's reasoning was from specific to specific, the concrete operational child can use ***inductive reasoning*** allowing her to go from the specific to the general. The child's world is no longer a sequence of still pictures showing the beginning and end states. Operational schemes turn it into a motion picture in which children can view the transformation of the beginning into the end.

Formal Operations Stage (12 years and up)

During this last stage the schemes are most highly organized and developed. ***Abstract reasoning*** characterizes this last stage. The difference between concrete and formal operations is that in the earlier stage the child can only apply logical operations to real (*i.e.*, concrete) objects or events. In the latter stage the child can apply them to abstract or theoretical ideas. Thus at this stage, thinking is most flexible. The term "formal" refers to the ability to follow the *form* of the argument without being tied to its content.

Piaget and Function

Schemes have been presented as if they are real things – as if they have a physical existence. They do not. Piaget inferred schemes from the behaviors children gave in responses to their environments. When presented with problems or with questions, children behaved or gave verbal explanations that had an underlying consistency. Piaget attempted to explain this underlying consistency of their behavior (motor or verbal) by attributing the behavior to schemes. Yet no one has ever seen a scheme, and though attempts have been made to find a neurological equivalent in the form of a cell assembly or neurotransmitter, none has yet been found. Thus, Piaget's schemes are really descriptions of behavior, not explanations.

Piaget's emphasis on the development and organization of schemes makes it a largely structural theory. Yet, in his last years Piaget put more emphasis on the **processes** of development (Belin, 1989). In this brief treatment of Piaget's theory I have also tried to emphasize the functions of cognition. Establishing Piaget's process of cognitive adaptation as parallel to the process of adaptation in phylogenic development is consistent with the viewpoints introduced in this book. In the following sections, cognitive development will be explained through observable events. This type of explanation follows a behavioral approach to cognitive development.

Behavioral Approaches to Cognitive Development

Behavioral psychologists are often accused of being unable, or unwilling, or merely uninterested in analyzing cognition. Yet for years behavioral psychologists have addressed the development of knowledge and thinking. Still, their approach is different, focusing on the functions of cognition, rather than its structure. The focus is on the behavior of learning, not structure.

Behavioral psychologists apply the same principles of learning to cognitive development as they do to other behaviors. They are interested in cognitive **behavior**, not some hypothetical structures such as schemes. **What develops is behavior, not hypothetical constructs.** For behaviorist's, cognition is behavior that is related and influenced by the environment. The unique thing about **cognitive behavior** is its location. It takes place within the skin. It is a private event.

Knowledge and Ability

For Skinner (1953), cognition is behavior in relationship to the environment. Skinner (1968) identified two types of behavior we call cognition. First there is **knowing about things**. This is what we call ***knowledge***. We "know" how much is two and two. We "know" who the first president was. We "know" what a reinforcer is.

The second meaning of knowing is **knowing how to do things.** This is what we call ***ability***. We are able to add 2 + 2. We are able to find the name of the first president. We are able to change a flat tire.

Bijou (1975) defined knowledge as a class of behavior specified by a particular stimulus. For example, a stimulus ("how much is 2 + 2?") is a cue for the response ("four") that is reinforced. Bijou identified four subcategories of knowledge:
(a) simple discriminative behavior (e.g., taking orange juice when offered a choice between orange juice and tomato juice); (b) conceptual or abstract behavior (*e.g.*, collecting only round stones along the seashore and ignoring their size and color); (c) describing past events (*e.g.*, one's birthday party); and (d) describing how things work (*e.g.*, how to wind up a toy so that it will propel itself). (Bijou, 1975, p. 833).

Bijou (1975) defined ability as two operant classes. The first class defined is an operant sequence of a certain order, as in solving a problem. Second, Bijou defined an operant with a characteristic response topography (*i.e.*, form), as in riding a tricycle. These abilities are cued by certain classes of discriminative stimuli. Bijou (1975) lists three sources of antecedent stimuli for preschool children: (a) the anatomy and physiology of the child's own body (*e.g.*, hopping, skipping, and jumping); (b) physical objects (*e.g.*, cutting with scissors); (c) people (*e.g.*, participating in a game) (Bijou, 1975).

In sum, behavior analysts see cognition as behavior in relation to environmental events. Cognition or thinking is not a thing. It is not a scheme. It is something that a person does in relation to the environment. In knowledge, emitting the right response under specific stimulus conditions is reinforced. Cognition, as all other behavior, is effected by the contingencies in which it occurs. In abilities, certain forms of the response are differentially reinforced. Bijou described some cognitive response classes and their antecedents. Yet, what reinforces cognitive behavior?

Natural & Contrived Consequences

Strengthening stimuli that are an inherent consequence of a response are called ***natural reinforcers*** (Skinner, 1982). The odor that is a consequence of opening a bottle of perfume, or the sound made from beating a drum are examples of natural reinforcers. Much cognitive behavior is strengthened by natural reinforcers. Thinking is strengthened by the answers it produces, reading by understanding what is read. Hopping, jumping, and skipping are reinforced by the bodily sensations they produce.

Some cognitive behaviors are strengthened by stimuli that are not naturally occurring consequences, but external to the response. These are called ***contrived***

reinforcers (Skinner, 1982). We often set up environments to extrinsically reinforce cognitive behaviors in others (e.g.,when we teach) through the use of praise or feedback. Sometimes we extrinsically reinforce ourselves (i.e., when we employ self-control) by saying to ourselves "good job" or treat ourselves to a cup of coffee for a job well done.

What Reinforces Cognitive Behavior?

There are many reinforcers for **knowledge** responses. Many of these are natural reinforcers, but some are contrived. Below, each of Bijou's (1975) examples of knowledge classes is addressed through a $S^d \rightarrow R \rightarrow S^r$ contingency sequence. In each case, the child is said to "know" when he makes a response that produces reinforcement for each stimulus situation. For example, the child "knows" the difference between orange and tomato juice when he reliably chooses one over the other.

Discriminative Stimulus	Response	Reinforcer
a) Glasses of orange & tomato juice	Drink orange juice	Taste of orange juice
b) Stones of size, shape, & color	Pick up round stones	See round ones
c) "How was your party?"	"It was great!"	Friend smiles & nods
d) Girl looks at toy car	"Twist the key, like this"	Car goes

Notice that some of these sequences involve natural reinforcers (a, b, and d) and one (c) involves **a contrived** reinforcer (although it could be argued that a smile is a natureal consequence os such an exclamation). Whenever looking at any contingency, we also must note the importance of the fourth term, the ***setting events*** that form the context for these knowledge interactions. For example, if it were not morning and the person were not thirsty, the discrimination producing orange juice would not have occurred because the stimulus (taste of the juice) would not reinforce the response (drinking the juice).

Abilities involve producing certain sequences or forms of behaviors in relationship to the environment. Again, there may be either natural or contrived reinforcers

Discriminative Stimulus	Response	Reinforcer
a) Anticipation of vacation	Hopping	Sensory stimulation
b) Scissors & paper	Manipulating scissors on paper	Paper doll
c) Boys & girls playing game	Spin the bottle	A kiss

for these behaviors. Referring to Bijou's (1975) examples of abilities the following contingency sequences might occur.

Problem Solving

In summarizing Skinner's analysis of problem solving, Reese (1994) described a *problem* as lacking the behavior needed to produce reinforcement. ***Problem solving*** is defined as emitting behaviors that change the situation in such a way that the behaviors which produce reinforcement will occur. For example, a child cannot open a box because she lacks a key. This is a problem because unlocking behavior will not be reinforced. The child may solve the problem by prying the lock open with a nearby screwdriver. Thus, by changing the situation so that the screwdriver was not used in the customary way, but rather in a novel way, led to reinforcement.

To solve a problem, two steps are involved. The first is to change the situation so that a solution is obtained. The second is to emit the problem solving behavior so that reinforcement of the solving behavior may occur. Behaviors which change the situation are called ***precurrent behaviors*** (Skinner, 1974). Precurrent behaviors may include simple responses such as feeling, looking at, listening to, smelling, or tasting an object. Precurrent behaviors may also be more complex, such as putting objects (or words) in a group, rearranging the order of things, or using plans or *algorithms* to serve as discriminative stimuli for behaviors producing the correct solution. The use of algorithms, or sequences of operations, may occur often in mathematics, as when there is an arithmetic problem such as, "how much is 395 divided by 17?" This is a problem because the answer that will produce reinforcement from the teacher is not immediately available. However, by engaging in the precurrent behavior of going through the steps of the long division algorithm, the correct response can be obtained and reported.

Exploratory Behavior

Bijou and Baer (1965, pg. 5) explained ***exploratory behavior*** as "a sequence of operant interactions that is strengthened and maintained by contingent ecological stimuli under specifiable setting factors." An ***ecological stimulus*** is one involving the physical properties of the various objects, social stimuli, or biological stimuli in the child's environment. An environment rich in ecological stimuli has many shapes, textures, colors, smells, and other stimuli. Ecological stimuli are the properties of natural reinforcers. They strengthen behaviors that produce either positive ecological stimuli or the avoidance of aversive ecological stimuli. Turning the handle on a jack-in-the-box produces the jack. Shaking a rattle makes a sound. Ecological stimuli are natural reinforcers for exploratory behaviors.

James Gibson (1979) introduced a concept called ***affordance*** which is very similar to the ecological reinforcer idea. Affordances are the various properties of objects "at the ecological level that specify how the object relates to the observer and what responses are possible or appropriate" (Schwartz, 1984, pg. 34). In other words, the various visual, tactile, auditory, and other sensory characteristics of the environment intrinsically and automatically reinforce unique responses to them.

The different characteristics of stimuli reinforce different responses, including different perceptual responses. Consider the following as an interaction between the characteristics of ecological stimuli and the reinforcement of exploratory behaviors they provide: When an infant up to 7- or 8-months-old detects a potentially graspable object within reach he grasps it, bangs it, shakes it, passes it from hand to hand, and above all, he carries it to his mouth and sucks it. He is only rarely observed to explore it, visually or tactually. It is suggested that the object is perceived as *affording* grasping, manipulation, noise making, and sucking. Similarly, objects in the intermediate but nonreachable distance afford looking and listening but not reaching and grasping. These appear to be pleasurable activities in themselves (Schwartz, 1984, pg. 51).

If you reread the above quote (pg. 230), but this time substitute the word "reinforce" (or "reinforcing") for the word "afford" (or "affording"), you will see how similar Gibson's idea is to the ecological reinforcer notion of Bijou and Baer. In both cases, inherent variability in characteristics of the environment provide automatic reinforcement for exploratory behavior (Guerin, 1990).

This is not to suggest that exploratory behavior cannot be encouraged by contrived reinforcers and setting events. Besides providing environments rich in a variety of ecological stimuli, adults and peers may prompt and directly reinforce children's explorations. For these children, exploratory behavior may emerge as a functional response class and the child may be described as "curious about things." Conversely, adults may limit exploratory behavior by prescribing to the child what to do, rather than have the child learn about the environment from the natural reinforcers in it.

Exploratory behavior leads to increased contact with the environment. This may lead to the development of knowledge and ability behaviors, including **perceptual** behaviors. In addition, exploratory behaviors may be the precurrent behavior to problem solving. Behaviors which may originate as exploratory behaviors may become strong knowledge or ability responses through reinforcement traps. That is, in the process of emitting an exploratory behavior, the natural reinforcement it produces may increase the likelihood that the same response will occur again. For example, in exploring a rattle, the child may move it and it makes a sound. The child is likely to repeat the movement over and over again.

Creative Behavior

It is difficult to define creative behavior. Definitions have included: (a) novelty of the response, or (b) novelty of the product, (c) diversity of responses (e.g., "How many ways can you think of to make a house of cards?"), or (d) the quality of response or product (e.g., "That was really creative!" versus "That was really garbage!").

Creativity has been studied as behavior in relation to its environment. Holman, Goetz and Baer (1977) identified three characteristics of most studies of creativity, novelty, originality, and uniqueness. Taken together they involve "newness." Yet, the phrase "there is nothing new under the sun" applies to creativity. Creative behavior is not entirely new, but involves unique combinations of stimulus and response elements.

If creative behavior involves the unique combination of behaviors, under what conditions does creative behavior develop? Two have been identified. First there is the development of a large repertoire of knowledge and ability responses. With many behaviors available, many more combinations can be made. Creative people know about many things and/or can do many things. Still a large repertoire of knowledge and ability is not sufficient for creative behavior. Many well-read and well trained people are not very creative. The second condition is necessary as well. This involves a history of reinforcement for making new combinations of knowledge and abilities. Both a history of knowledge and ability along with a history of being reinforced for unique combinations leads to creative behavior.

In a series of studies, Goetz and her colleagues were able to increase the diversity of children's block building (Goetz & Baer, 1973), easel painting (Goetz & Salmonson, 1972), felt pen drawing, and lego building (Holman, Goetz, & Baer, 1977). The procedures involved selection of a behavior in the children's repertoire (e.g., block building) and then reinforcement of new forms. This produced an increase in new forms that were different from the ones that were previously reinforced. Thus, creativity becomes a generalized class of responses.

The behavioral approach to cognitive development has been to consistently treat it as behavior in relation to the environment rather than as a structure. As discussed, behavior analysts have applied the four term contingency to explain the development of cognitive behaviors.

Skill Learning: A Dynamical Systems Approach to Cognitive Development

Theorists have introduced theories of cognitive development which are compatible with a dynamical systems approach (e.g., Fischer, 1980; Fischer & Pipp, 1984; Commons & Rodriguez, 1993). Among the main features of these theories is the view that cognitive development involves a hierarchical system of skills in which later skills emerge from earlier and more simple skills. These theories retain some of the observations of cognitive development first made by Piaget, but are more consistent with behavior analysis and a natural science position. Commons and Rodriguez call their theory ***General Systems Theory***. The twelve stages of General Systems Theory are logically deduced from analyzing the tasks involved in complex cognitive behavior. A second approach, called ***Skill Theory*** developed by Fischer in 1980 shall be examined in some detail.

What Develops? – Operant Response Classes

Fischer believes that Piaget's concept of schemes is more accurately viewed as operant response classes (or "sets") in relation to the environment. Rather than mental representations of the world, skills are behavior-environment relations. The relation between Piaget's schemes and Fischer's skills may be easy to see at the sensori motor level, where action in relation to the environment is involved. However, Fischer (1980) points out that thought and language, are also behaviors.

If I ask you to imagine a dog riding a bike, this may evoke an image in you. What is this image, or iconic scheme? Fischer and behavior analysts share the view that producing an image is an operant just like other behaviors. The image is the product of the response in the same way that when you sit, your lap is the product of that response. Sometimes it is difficult for us to analyze our thinking as behavior. Instead, we accord thoughts special status by using words like image, consciousness, or thought. Because of our special treatment of private events, it is difficult for us to view private behavior as fitting the four-term contingency. The image seems real to us.

Psychologists have attempted to analyze cognitive behavior through the use of a computer analogy. This approach, known as the ***Information Processing Approach***, is a broad theory which assigns computer metaphors to humans. It is suggested that humans have structures which perform tasks that are similar to the components of computers which also process information. Thus, we may have short term memory storage that is similar to computer RAM, long term memory similar to a hard disk drive, and a brain that is like the CPU of the computer.

We are often misled into viewing memory storage as a thing, but in humans, memory is a function or process. Memory is something you do. It is responding to a discriminative stimulus that was presented externally some time before. Perhaps a computer analogy can help clarify things here. You can call up to the screen a picture of your dog, Sally, that you have on your hard disk. Thus, we are able to take the image from long term memory, process it, and view it. How is the image stored in the graphics file on your disk drive? Is it a small image of the dog? Of course not. It is a series of electronic charges at specific locations on the disk. The computer acts on the electronic code to produce a very real image of the dog, but the actual image of the dog is not stored on the disk.

However, we must not lose sight that the computer is only a metaphor for humans, although, from the way we talk to (and about) our computers ("It's *thinking,*" "What's it *saying*?", etc.) one might think that they are living creatures. Humans are living things and living things behave. Some of this behavior takes place within the skin and we call it cognition. Memory is one type of internal cognitive behavior. Other cognitive behaviors can be directly observed. Those external behaviors often take place publicly. For instance, public verbal behavior is called language.

Behavior-environment relationships develop into classes of behavior from these internal and external interactions. These classes develop into organized patterns of behavior. At our most fundamental level of analysis (Level I) contingencies produce individual behavior-environment relationships. At Level II, contingencies act to organize systems of behavior-environment relationships. Emergent behaviors coalesce into a more organized systems of behavior. These organized behaviors are called response classes or ***skills*** and are the structural aspect of skill theory. Skills build upon each other with later structures emerging from earlier ones.

Structures change as a result of interaction with the environment. There are various ways in which skills emerge. Some ways will result in linear combinations of skills, as in chaining. Other ways will produce nonlinear, qualitative changes that may appear similar to the qualitative changes suggested by Piaget. The ways in which skills change will be discussed below.

Knowledge, and problem solving, not just abilities, are skills. A hierarchical organization of behavior develops into skills in many areas, or ***domains.*** Examples of domains are social skills, expressive language skills, and knowledge of mathematics. More advanced skills emerge from the strengthening of more simple behaviors by environmental contingencies. As Fischer (1980) summarizes: "The child masters specific skills, builds other specific skills upon them, and transfers skills from one domain to another. This mastery process involves qualitative changes in skills, but the specific changes occur gradually, not abruptly (pg. 483)."

How Skills Develop – Functions

Skills, as organized classes of behaviors, are strengthened by reinforcing contingencies. As indicated earlier, much cognitive behavior is automatically reinforced by the natural contingencies of the act. That is, perceiving is reinforced by what is seen, jumping is reinforced by the feeling the behavior produces, and reading is reinforced by the content of what is read (e.g., reading a "Wet Paint" sign produces negative reinforcement). For Fischer (1980), "because an action always involves a particular object or thing, a skill must be specific to particular objects or things" (pg. 483).

However, recall that skills are not just individual behaviors, but are functional response classes in which the behaviors produce the same consequences. For example, reaching for a peach involves a series of eye-hand movements which must be coordinated. Early attempts are less successful but shape the coordination of these behavior-environment relationships.

Behaviors are organized into skill classes through consequences in a number of ways. Fischer (1980) has identified five ways which he called ***transformational rules.*** These rules are ways in which a more simple skill can be shifted or "transformed" into a more complex one. It should be emphasized, that no one factor determines these rules. It is the coalescence of factors, especially of the strengthening of behaviors through interaction with the environment that produces these phase shifts. Remember, *shifts happen!*

Transformational Rules

According to Fischer (1980), two environmental conditions must be met for changes to occur. One is that the environment must be able to reinforce the more complex skill if it is to emerge. This would mean that the new skill would be reinforced and not be extinguished. The second property is that the environment must provide a context for the more simple skills to come together. For example, an environment which encourages a child to consider both the height of a container and the width of a container (e.g., through the presence of objects with clear differences in these dimensions, or by a teacher pointing out the differences) would enable the attainment of volume conservation, in which both dimensions must be considered simultaneously. The five transformational rules identified by Fischer (1980) are: intercoordination, compounding, focusing, substitution, and differentiation.

- *Compounding.*

We have already examined examples of compounding when we looked at the process of chaining. Compounding is the addition of one skill to another. It can be noted as a+b. An example would be the compounding of touching a glass and closing the hand around the glass. These are two separate behaviors that are assembled in a chain. For compounding to occur, all individual skills must already be in the person's repertoire. Compounding is considered a linear (i.e., additive) change.

- *Focusing.*

Consider the following situation. You place two rows of little balls rolled from clay in front of a four-year-old. One row has five pellets in it, and the other has six. To make the task more difficult, you space the pellets in the row of five further apart so that it makes a longer row. You now ask the child "Which row has more?" The child points to the longer row. You assume that the child, because he is at the preoperational stage, cannot focus on more than one dimension of the problem (i.e., he centers on length, but ignores quantity). Now you take away the clay. You now make the same configuration, but this time you substitute M&Ms. Now the child chooses the shorter row. This result, similar to that obtained in a study by Mehler and Bever (1967), illustrates how the environment contributes to the development of a more complex skill through focusing attention between two or more properties. In this case, focusing on only one dimension (i.e., length) was sufficient for reinforcement when the discriminative stimulus was a set of clay pellets. Changing the Sd to an edible reinforcer changed the focus which enabled the development of a new skill involving the consideration of two dimensions (i.e., length and quantity).

- *Intercoordination.*

One of the fascinating aspects of Piaget's theory to most adults is the inability of the older preoperational child to show conservation of amount. In spite of being able to correctly tell an experimenter which of two glasses is taller, or separately, which is wider, when confronted with the task of saying which glass has more liquid in it, the child fails miserably. Even pouring the liquid from one glass into the other, a demonstration that erases any doubt for an adult, does not help the child. What is missing is the ability to intercoordinate the two separate skills of height and width estimation that are necessary in determining conservation of amount.

Intercoordination is the combining of two or more skills, but the way in which they combine is not just an addition of the two skills. The combination that results is qualitatively different behaviors. That is, the skill of being able to see the amount of water in each glass is a different quality of skills than either of the two prerequisite skills of comparing height and width. Thus, in intercoordination of skills, the changes are nonlinear. Fischer (1980) represents this in the formula $a \times b = d$.

Fischer suggests that, as with compounding, intercoordination is a product of the coalescence of organismic and environmental conditions. Organismic conditions include the history of the organism which produced the more simple skills. As with compounding, current environmental conditions which evoke and reinforce intercoordination of skills are necessary. However, simple compounding is insufficient to produce reinforcement that the more advanced skill requires. The process of intercoordination is necessary for providing reinforcement of the advanced skill.

- *Differentiation.*

This is the counterpart of both compounding and intercoordination. When classes have been assembled by contingencies, the individual components may also be disassembled by contingencies. That is, once a class of behaviors have been combined it enables their individual components to function separately. The result is that the individual components may be reassembled, through intercoordination or compounding, into new skills which were not possible before differentiation. Differentiation occurs through differential reinforcement.

- *Substitution.*

In substitution, all but one member of a skill occurs. In the place of that one member, a new element is put in its place. For example, a child who can grasp a peach will learn to substitute an egg for the peach in the same skill of reaching. The substitution may encompass either stimulus or response classes. Substitution may be the basis for generalization (Fischer, 1980). By plugging in a new response to an existing stimulus, a new discriminative stimulus to an existing response, or both, we are able to form new generalized stimulus or response classes. The process of substitution is at work in the development of generalized imitation, selective imitation of language (Chapter 9), and in the development of stimulus equivalence classes. Later in this chapter, we shall see the relevance of substitution to emergent complex classes, or stimulus equivalence classes when we examine relational frame theory (Hayes, 1991; 1994).

Levels of Cognitive Skills

At the basic level, the constant interaction of organismic (including leaning history) and environmental factors produce continual changes in development. Underlying these changes are the environmental contingencies which bring about changes in the four-term contingency. Many changes are small additive steps, as when a child reaches farther for an object, or grabs a larger peach. Other changes are qualitative and nonlinear. There is a sudden change in the topography of behaviors such as when grasping changes from two-handed, to one-handed. The dynamical principles of behavior (outlined in Chapter 2) bring about the transformations described above and result in the qualitative changes.

Fischer (1980, 1984) developed a progression in the development of cognitive behavior which shows a great deal of agreement with Piaget's observation of cognitive developmental stages. However, significant differences between the two approaches are noted below.

Fischer's skill theory specifies four **tiers** based on the types of behaviors (i.e., reflex, sensory-motor, representation, abstraction) that are involved. Reflexes are placed at Level 0.[1] The remaining three tiers are further divided into four levels. These levels overlap specific skills which creates the opportunity to begin a new tier. For example, the skill at Level D-Tier 1 is the same as the skill at Level A-Tier 2. This overlapping process produces a total of ten skill levels within the three tiers. Because each level is built directly upon the previous one, there is a hierarchy of cognitive skills, with later skills emerging from earlier ones. Therefore, to reach a higher level of cognitive skill, one must first accomplish the simpler ones. Finally, because these skills are assembled by the events in the environment, there will be independence between the levels of skills for different domains and for different individuals.

Tiers of Cognitive Development

Sensorimotor Tier

Fischer (1980, 1984) used the term ***tier*** to indicate qualitatively different classes of behaviors. The first tier is called the ***sensorimotor tier***. These are stimulus-response relationships which involve the learning of four-term contingencies for overt behaviors. Within this tier are four levels. Once the fourth level of the sensorimotor tier is developed, the relationships result in a qualitatively different kind of behavior, representation.

Representational Tier

At this tier, the child is able to act upon objects or events as if they are independent agents (Fischer, 1980). That is, representation is the production of a symbol that stands for an object. Overtly, we may draw a picture or write a word which represents a doll. Within the skin, we can produce a stimulus which represents the same object. The picture, word, or thought is not the object itself; it stands for the object it represents. At this tier, there are also four levels. At the highest level of the representational tier, the person can represent complex relationships between systems of stimuli. This final representational level also becomes the first level of the next tier of skills, abstraction.

Abstract Tier

An abstract class involves the ability to relate variations in one representation to variations in a second representation (Fischer, 1980). This is labeled abstract thinking. For example, if Ben and Jerry contemplated making "Moon Pie Madness" ice cream on the surface of the moon, they would have to intercoordinate many aspects of ice cream making and space travel. As we shall soon see, abstract cognitive skills involve complex relationships between representational systems.

Levels Within a Tier

Each of the three tiers (sensorimotor, representational, and abstract) contain four levels of behaviors (labeled Levels A-D in Figure 8.1) These levels are the same for each tier, making the theory rather parsimonious. Skills at each level form the basis for progression to the next level. The fourth level at each tier produces skills which are the same as the first level of the next tier. Thus, the tiers overlap and are continuous. Yet, at the fourth level, the changes in skills are not simply additive. Rather, changes in behavior are nonlinear and qualitatively different from the other three levels in the tier. Thus, the development of a new tier occurs.

Fischer (1980, 1984) uses a metaphor from geometry to illustrate the relationships within each tier (See Figure 8.1). The lowest level is represented by a single dot and the highest by a three-dimensional cube with dots at its connection points. At the highest level of one tier, the complex systems represented by the cube becomes the dot itself at the lowest level of the next tier.

A further note on levels: Even though a high level skill may occur, the lower level skills do not disappear. For example, even though we may be capable of engaging in abstract behavior, we may still use sensorimotor reflexes. Let us now look at the four general levels of skills within a tier.

Level A – Single Classes

Within a tier, the most basic skill involves responding to a single class of stimuli, or a single response class. This level of a single class is represented by a single dot. Examples are touching a mobile or calling a single person "mommy."

Level B – Mapping Between Two Classes

As the child develops more and more single response classes, the possibilities of combining the classes increases. Combinations of two classes through compounding produces a more complex skill. This occurs when the characteristics of one response class are related to, or "mapped" onto another. Fischer (1980) called this relationship between two simple sets ***mapping***, and used a line connecting the dots to represent this. Examples of mapping are the relating of reaching for an object with grasping the object. After repeated trials, a coordinated reach-grasp response emerges. Another example is the combination of the responses to "mommy" with the combinations of the responses to other women, so that the child responds to other women in a different way than he did to either class alone.

Level C – Systems

The systems level is reached when the child can relate two or more subclasses of classes to each other. That is, individual components of one class may be

Figure 8.1

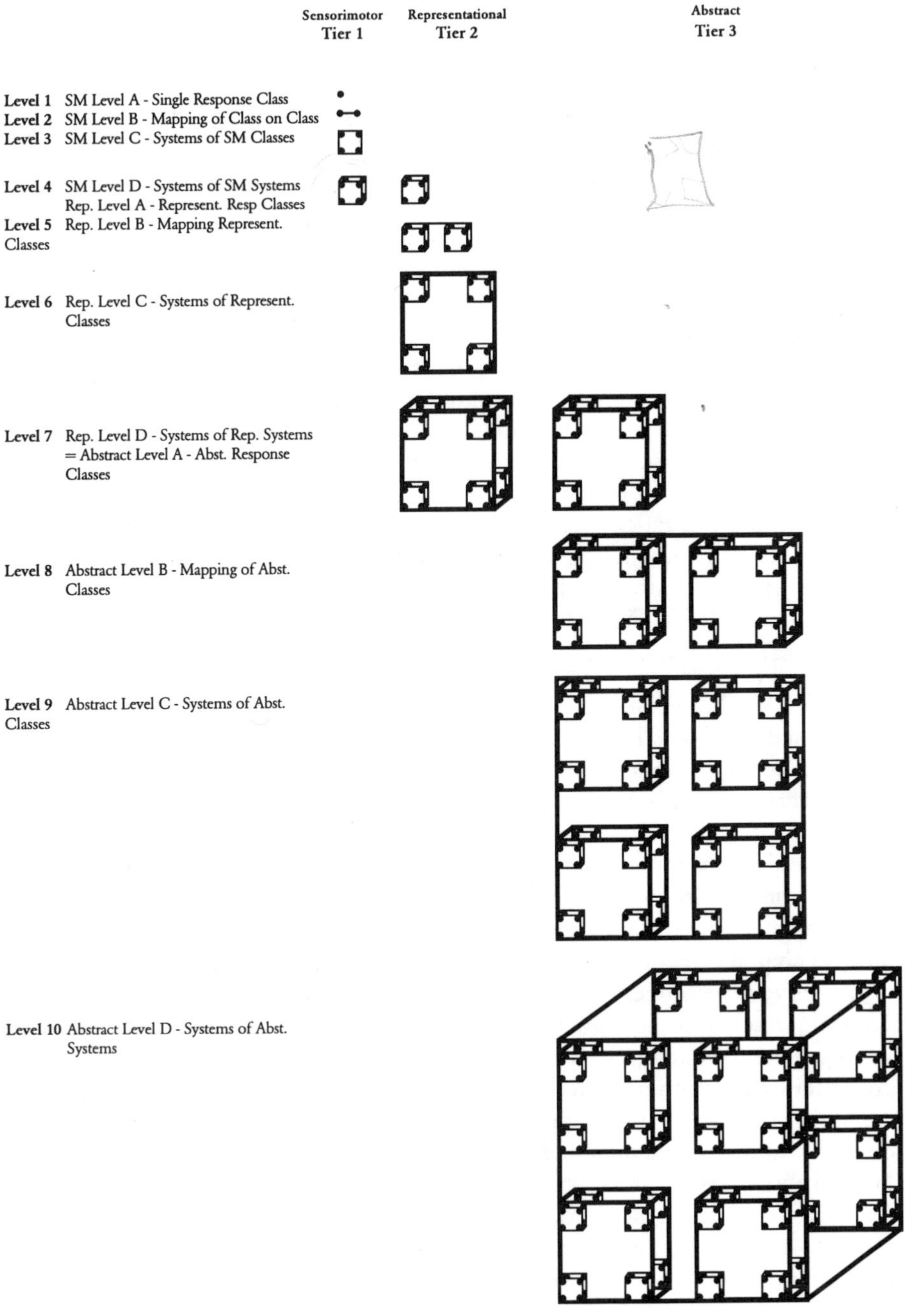
Sensorimotor
Tier 1
Representational
Tier 2
Abstract
Tier 3
Level 1 SM Level A - Single Response Class
Level 2 SM Level B - Mapping of Class on Class
Level 3 SM Level C - Systems of SM Classes
Level 4 SM Level D - Systems of SM Systems
Rep. Level A - Represent. Resp Classes
Level 5 Rep. Level B - Mapping Represent. Classes
Level 6 Rep. Level C - Systems of Represent. Classes
Level 7 Rep. Level D - Systems of Rep. Systems
= Abstract Level A - Abst. Response Classes
Level 8 Abstract Level B - Mapping of Abst. Classes
Level 9 Abstract Level C - Systems of Abst. Classes
Level 10 Abstract Level D - Systems of Abst. Systems

combined with the individual components of another. For example, being able to adjust reaching when there are subtle changes in the visual input (e.g. darkness) requires the acquisition of an entire system of reaching-grasping behavior. This level is represented by a four-sided, two-dimensional square.

Level D – Systems of Systems

At this level, the child can relate two or more systems to each other in complex ways. Intercoordination between simple systems has changed the individual complex systems into interrelated systems. Fischer calls this type of organization "systems of systems." At this level, whole systems themselves are related to other systems so that the whole is a system which is composed of lower level systems. This is represented by joining the simple squares (i.e., systems) into a three dimensional cube.

The levels are hierarchical. That is, higher level systems are built from the lower level ones. Therefore, the systems of systems that are at Level D of each tier is the single class that is at Level A of the next tier. In this metaphor, the cube of one tier is the single dot of the next tier. This is represented in Figure 8.1. The result is a progression of levels of cognitive development in which more complex skills emerge from earlier ones. In Fischer's view, the result is eleven levels of cognitive skills (Levels 0-10). Starting from reflexes as individual environment-behavior relationships in Fischer's Level 0, though systems of abstract systems at level 10, each class of behaviors organizes into skills through the levels specific to each tier.

These are listed in Figure 8.1.

Comparing Fischer's Levels with Piaget's Stages

At first blush, the astute reader may no doubt find some resemblance between Fischer's skill levels and Piaget's cognitive stages. Indeed, there are some similarities, but there are important differences as well. Let us look at the differences.

What changes? Skills versus schemes. In Fischer's theory, skills are operant behavior classes. Changes occur as relationships between response classes become more complex and more organized. The structures are the relationships between response classes. In Piaget's theory, schemes are mental structures. They are hypothetical structures; they are mental representations.

How do changes occur? Environment versus organism. Both Fischer and Piaget see cognitive development as the result of an environment/organism interaction. However, Fischer places much more emphasis on the role of environmental contingencies in shaping behavior (Bjorkland, 1989).

Consistency between domains of development: Declage versus synchrony. By emphasizing the role of the environment, Fischer finds that different skills are likely to develop at very different rates. Fischer's theory suggests, for example, that reading skill is likely to develop at a very different rate than mathematics skills or social skills. This lack of consistency across domains was called ***declage*** by Piaget and was thought by him to be the exception rather than the norm. Piaget believed, instead, that there was great consistency or ***synchrony*** across different cognitive domains like math, language, and social skills. Thus, in Piaget's view, the child was at a specific level of cognitive development, and the schemes at this level brought a consistency to behavior in all domains. This belief is in contrast with Fisher's view that differences among domains is common.

Individual differences versus universal stages. Based on the unique combination of organismic and environmental factors, Fischer's theory predicts that there will be large individual differences in the development of cognitive skills. In addition, Fischer's theory also supports equifinality, in that different individuals who reach the same cognitive skill level may have reached that level through different combinations of organismic and environmental factors. On the other hand, Piaget's theory emphasizes that all persons pass through the same sequence of stages at about the same time.

Skill Theory and Dynamical Systems

There are several points of agreement which make Fischer's skill theory especially attractive from a dynamical systems view of development. Some of these features are listed below.

Ever-changing, dynamical systems. The relationships between response classes constitute systems and systems within systems at the highest levels within each tier. Thus, Fischer's skill theory is itself a systems theory. What changes is the relationships between the systems.

Nonlinearity. Cognitive skills are built upon earlier skills. In many cases, the changes are small and proportionate to the amount of environmental experience. Fischer refers to such changes as ***microdevelopmental*** changes. In a dynamical systems approach, this principle is explained as the line of trajectory a behavior is apt to remain in. Examples would be the learning of a new name for a dog or adding the four-times table to multiplication skills. However, sometimes, small changes can produce qualitatively different changes. New levels of cognitive skills suddenly emerge as factors coalesce. Fischer would call these nonlinear changes, ***macrodevelopmental*** changes. Changes from one skill tier to another are macrodevelopmental changes. These nonlinear changes of behavior parallels the definition of phase shifts in a dynamical systems approach.

Skills as dynamic attractors. Skills are classes of behaviors which fit our view of dynamical attractors as consistent patterns of behavior organized by the coalescence of organismic and environmental factors. As such, skills should be "loose assemblies," which in their initial formation are easily perturbed. This can be seen in the characteristic of cognitive skills to be easily disrupted by environmental conditions such as stressors or ambiguous stimuli, especially as a child is first acquiring the skill. For example, the child who is just "getting" conservation of amount, may be thrown off by the adult asking a leading question such as "are you *sure* there is more in the tall glass." As skills become more strongly organized, it may be more difficult, but not impossible to disrupt them.

Equifinality. In emphasizing the reciprocal transactions of organismic and environmental factors in producing cognitive development, the skill approach stresses that there may be many paths to development. A corollary of this is that there will be individual differences in the levels of cognitive skills obtained.
Transactions. This approach emphasizes the reciprocal interaction of organismic and environmental conditions, including genetic-constitutional make-up, learning history, and current environmental conditions. Change occurs from the coalescence of these factors under an individual's unique developmental history.
Levels of Systems. It is important to keep Fischer's own cognitive skill levels separate from the levels of analysis used to understand development introduced in Chapter 1. As a whole, the emergent behaviors that constitute the organized skills of Fischer's theory are analyzed at our Systems Level II. Underlying the emergent behaviors of this level of analysis are the basic process of System Level I. These basic processes include both organismic and environmental ones, but especially the contingencies of learning which are the province of behavior analysis. Therefore, we next look at the affinity of cognitive skills theory and behavior analysis.

Skill Theory and Behavior Analysis

Cognitive skills as operants

The skills approach is consistent with behavioral principles. Fischer sees cognitive skills as operant response classes. His Level A skills are simple classes of sensorimotor, representational and abstract behaviors. As we move up his hierarchy, classes become combined in additive (compounding) and non-additive (intercoordinating) ways. Fischer's five methods for change are consistent with behavioral principles of change as well. These five principles themselves may be seen as a higher level of analysis (i.e., System Level 2), which are built upon the basic principles of the four-term contingency.
The four-term contingency. As operant classes, cognitive skills are analyzed by using the four-term contingency detailed in Chapter 7. Skills may be simple classes of individual responses or they may be organized into compound classes or complex systems of response classes. These response classes are controlled by their consequences. Complex classes and systems emerge because they have more access to reinforcing consequences. Simple response classes have a specified and limited amount of reinforcement. Many cognitive skills produce automatic reinforcement. That is, the consequence of knowledge or ability response produce some natural consequence. Because increased knowledge and ability responses enable better manipulation of the environment, the attainment of these skills allow complex problem solving responses.

The cognitive operant classes and systems come under the control of discriminative stimuli. Consider the word "stop." What is the response that it cues? A particular stimulus, such as the word "stop" may control whole classes or systems of responses. Stopping is not a simple response with a single form. "Stop" is a stimulus which specifies a relationship between any number of possible responses and the consequences of stopping. Furthermore, "stop" may mean one thing under one setting event (e.g., "stop that, you're hurting me") and another if the setting event differs (e.g., "stop me if you've heard this one").

Stimulus Equivalence Classes. Recently, much attention has been drawn to the study of ***stimulus equivalence classes*** (Hayes & Hayes, 1992; Fields, 1993). A stimulus equivalence class (or ***equivalence class***) is a group of stimuli which have the same function as discriminative stimuli. Because each stimulus in the class may be substituted for any other stimulus, they are functionally equivalent.

Stimulus Equivalence Classes

An important characteristic of equivalence classes is that functional equivalence emerges without direct training. For example, if a child learns that his pet named "Raffles" is a dog, and he learns that "canine" is the same as the word "dog," he may say that Raffles is a canine without anyone directly teaching him the Raffles-canine relationship. This four-term contingency relationship, called ***transitivity***, is the most difficult of the three relationships that must appear to say an equivalence class has been formed (Sidman, 1986). The other two relationships are ***identity or reflexivity*** (i.e., Raffles is Raffles, regardless of the context) and ***symmetry*** (i.e., taught that Raffles is a dog, the child can say that the dog is Raffles). When all three relationships, identity, symmetry, and transitivity are displayed, an equivalence class can be said to have emerged. Sidman (1986) has used simple formulas from mathematical set theory to describe these relationships:

Identity: $A = A$

(e.g., Raffles is Raffles, is Raffles)

Symmetry: $A = B$ then $B = A$

(e.g. Raffles is this dog; then this dog is Raffles),

Transitivity $A = B$ & $B = C$ then $A = C$

(e.g., Raffles is a dog. A dog is a canine. Then Raffles is a canine).

Some Speculation on Stimulus Equivalence and Cognitive Skills Theory

The contingency relationships of identity, reflexivity, and transitivity are complex, emergent behaviors assembled by functional consequences. Commons and Rodriguez (1993) have suggested that levels of cognitive skills (classified by General Systems Theory) are related to equivalence relationships. The same is likely true for the cognitive skills suggested by Fischer's theory. It is possible that identity, reflexivity, and transitivity are different levels of cognitive skills. If we apply Fischer's four levels of cognitive skills to equivalence relationships, we may see the following possibilities.

Level A: Single Classes = Identity
Level B: Mapping Between Classes = Symmetry
Level C: Systems of Classes = Transitivity
Level D: Systems of Systems = Complex Transitivity (analogy and metaphor)

This is very preliminary. Equivalence classes have only been found in verbal humans, suggesting that language is necessary. However, it is possible that the kinds of equivalence relations studied require Tier 2 representational skills, and that sensorimotor equivalence may be possible, but not yet fully understood (c.f., Commons & Rodriguez, 1993). Likewise, there may be higher order equivalence classes which develop at the Abstract Tier levels. Commons and Rodriguez, (1993) found complex equivalence relationships in adults which were equivalent to cognitive functioning at the tenth highest of twelve possible stages. This stage was called ***metasystematic***, meaning systems of systems, and was a level of cognitive skills beyond Piaget's formal operations stage.

Thus, several different lines of theorizing suggests the likelihood that cognitive development may be understood as a process involving a hierarchy of skills.

Speculation on Skill Transformation Rules and Behavior Analysis

Steven Hayes (1991, 1994) has proposed a theory to explain the emergence of equivalence classes in human behavior. This theory is called ***relational frame theory*** because in Hayes' view, what is learned in equivalence classes are relationships between stimuli not individual cases. It is as if the rest of the contingency is like a picture frame, and a new, but related stimulus can be inserted in the place of the original one. For example, once the Raffles/dog and dog/canine relationships have been established, "Raffles" can be put in place of "dog." Of interest here is the similarity of the process in relational frame theory with the process of substitution in cognitive skill theory. As research in these theories continues, there may be other similarities that can be identified between Fischer's cognitive skill theory and the study of equivalence classes by behavior analysts.

In the next chapter we will look at the development of communication, and in the particular function of language. We will again rely heavily upon a skill learning approach in this area.

Do Parents Teach Equivalencing?

It has already been suggested that equivalence relationships are automatically reinforced by naturally occurring consequences in the environment. As part of the child's natural environment, what influence, then, do parents play in the development of equivalence skills? In the next chapter, data are presented in detail on how parents teach language skills to their infants and toddlers. Are equivalence skills such as identity, reflexivity, and transitivity intuitively taught in caretakers infants interactions?

Fields (1994, personal communication) has observed such equivalence training in the interactions between his sister and her children. Hayes (1991) describes some possible training of reflexivity in how the concept of "Daddy" and other objects is taught. First, the child is taught identity in the following manner:

The child is oriented toward Daddy and asked 'who's that?' If the child says "Daddy" celebration ensues. If not, the child may again be prompted "Is that your Daddy?" If the child shows any sign of acknowledgment (e.g., a smile when the name is given), the child is fussed over. Even before the child can speak, parents to some degree assess whether Daddy has control over the word "Daddy." The child may be oriented toward Daddy and asked "Who is that? Is that your Daddy?" If the child makes a face that indicates agreement, the child may be tickled or playfully shaken and be told, "Yes, that's right, that's your Daddy!" The child in other words is taught to pick the sound "Daddy" (and later to produce it) in the presence of Daddy (Hayes, 1991, page 25-26).

In this case the child is able to pick A (word "Daddy") given B (object Daddy). A similar type of interaction may be responsible for teaching symetry:

> The child will be asked "where's Daddy" while Daddy is not immediately in the child's view. Young children will be carried around the room to face various persons and objects. Given the question, signs of recognition when the child is oriented toward Daddy are followed by parental signs of excitement. Signs of recognition elsewhere are followed by retraining: "No, that's not Daddy, that's the doggie!" Later the child will have to search the room visually without assistance, or for a more mobile child, may have to look behind objects, to find Daddy given the question "where's Daddy?" (Hayes, 1991, page 26).

To summarize, Hayes suggests a model for parent-child interactions that should result in the development of equivalence relationships. To put this model to a test, the Hayes' recruited their son, Charlie, to serve as a subject in a series of experiments (Lipkens, Hayes, & Hayes, 1993). Charlie participated in this research for an 11 month period. Training began when Charlie was 16 months old and ended when he was 27 months old. Charlie was shown line drawings of familiar (e.g., baby, ball) and novel stimuli (e.g., strange and prehistoric animals). Familiar (e.g., "cat", "dog"), and novel (e.g., "ui", "neus") spoken words were also used as stimuli. Charlie's task was

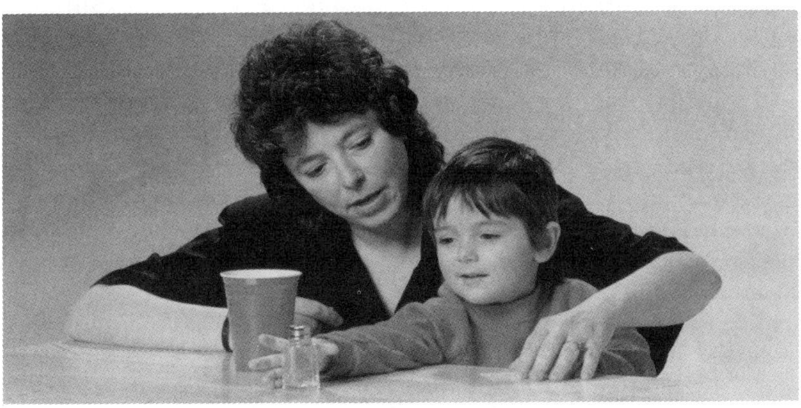

Linda Hayes Tests Charlie's Equivalancing Skills

to learn relationships between visual stimuli and spoken words. The studies were conducted to see if Charlie would form symmetry and transitivity relationships.

The emergence of symmetry was shown when Charlie, who had been trained on spoken word-pick picture relationships (e.g., "Where is the pig. That's good.") was able to produce the name of the object to a question (i.e., "What is this?"). The symmetrical relationship is said to have emerged because the picture-spoken word relationship for the pictures had not been trained. A similar procedure led to the development of transitivity. In this case, training involved the relationships between a picture and the name of the object (e.g., "This is a dog"), and a second relationship between the same picture and the sound the animal makes (e.g., "This animal goes 'woof')." Charlie demonstrated transitivity when, given the name of the animal he was able to make its sound (e.g., "What does a dog say?"). Notice, that again, the relationship, this time of transitivity, emerged without direct training.

The Charlie studies demonstrate that equivalence may be taught given appropriate environmental conditions. Further research is necessary to determine, as suggested by Fields, Hayes, and others, that parents intuitively teach equivalencing to their children. So far, much of the interest in the development of equivalence classes has focused on language, or skills at Fischer's representational skills level. It is likely that the learning of equivalencing begins earlier, even at the sensorimotor level. The form of possible sensorimotor relationships is more difficult to conceive than the representational ones that have been so extensively studied. Nevertheless, Commons and Rodriguez (1993) have suggested that there is evidence for equivalence relationships from studies of non-language using animals (e.g., Zentall, Edwards, & Hogan, 1993; Zentall & Urcuioli, 1993) and human infants (e.g., Watson & Ramey, 1972).

Sidman (1994) has taken the position that equivalence relations are a fundamental part of all natural phenomena. Therefore, when a child learns a concept, identity, symmetry, and transitivity are automatically present. What needs to develop through experience is the discrimination of equivalence into the three distinct relationships. That is, through experience, the child who sees stimuli as equivalent must learn to treat identity, symmetry, and transitivity as special cases. This is in contrast to the view of taken by Hayes (1986, 1991) who views responding to stimuli in relational ways as the result of experiences. Thus, "equivalencing" is a term for behavior involving responding to stimuli using identity, symmetry, and transitivity relations. That is, equivalencing equals relational responding.

Novak and his associates (Novak, 1995) have presented some preliminary data that mothers actually do provide conditions for the training of equivalencing. They looked at mothers' interactions with their children during toy play when children were 11, 15, 19, 24, and 30 months of age. Already at eleven months (the earliest age at which they recorded), mothers were providing their children with relational training. For example, mothers would not only label an object, but they would also ask the child "What's that?", requesting the child to label the same object. This "provide a label - request a label" sequence suggests that mothers actually *do* engage in the same kind of identity relational training suggested by Lipkens, Hayes, and Hayes (1992).

Since child language skills are not well developed at eleven months, these same mothers also provided non-language relational trials too. That is, they would constantly pick up a toy, manipulate it, and either hand it to the child to manipulate it or ask the child to do so. This "manipulation - request for manipulation" sequence provides the same type of identity relational training, but at a sensory-motor level. At eleven months, in most mother-child pairs, manipulation relations were more common than labeling relation trials. By the time their children are nineteen-months-of-age, labeling relations are the most frequent strategy used by all mothers who were observed, but other strategies, continue to be employed.

Finally, the data also suggest that symmetry and transitivity relations may also be taught by mothers who point out, play with, describe, and ask their children to do the same. Thus, the multiple experiences with objects provided by the experimenters to Charlie are observable in mothers actually playing with their infants. Thus, there seems to be support for the contention that the ability to develop functional and stimulus equivalence classes in children is a skill which emerges out of massive numbers of trials provided by parents with their children.

Why are equivalence relationships important to the study of development?

As emergent phenomena, the development of equivalence classes is consistent with a dynamical systems view. They help us understand that complexly organized, hierarchical behavior-environment relationships can emerge from the basic processes of development, particularly, from a history of environmental contingencies. Furthermore, equivalencing may be seen as a skill which is consistent with the principles underlying the development of all cognitive skills. Finally, researchers and theorists find equivalence relationships as being important to our understanding of language development and communication. After all, language enables us to represent complex relationships between a multitude of environmental features of our environment. Many of these relationships in language emerge, rather than result from direct training.

The next chapter continues to look at the development of skills in the area of communication, including the verbal behavior we call language. Skill theory will be again presented as a way of understanding the development of language as emergent behavior.

Footnotes

[1]Fischer has subdivided his reflex tier into the same four levels as he had done with the other tiers, at this point it is difficult to relate these reflexive levels to the operant levels presented in detail here. This task will be left for some future analysis.

[2]Piaget used the French noun "schéme" which frequently is translated into the term "schema" (plural is "schemata." In later years, Piaget (Piaget & Inhelder, 1971) reserved the term "schéma" for mental images. Thus, most psychologists now use the term "scheme" as the equivalent of Piaget's term for mental representations in general. (See Fischer, 1980).

Chapter 9

The Development of Communication

Most introductory textbooks in developmental psychology devote a chapter to ***language*** development. Such chapters often describe the development of verbal behavior in terms of the structure of verbal behavior's products. For example, a child's developing speech may be described as a progression from single-word utterances (i.e., simple structure) to multi-word utterances (complex structure). In addition, the ability to speak and understand utterances with varying structure is attributed to mental structures possessed by the language user.

In this chapter, however, instead of focusing on the **structure** of linguistic and mental entities, we shall focus on the **function** of language (see structural and functional knowledge, in Chapter 2): communication. In this context, "to communicate" means to change via verbal behavior the relationship between a person's behavior and some part of the environment. For example, if I tell you "it's raining," I have temporarily changed your behavioral relationship with umbrellas and raincoats; you are now more likely to reach for them. We will first look at the two significant theoretical viewpoints that have attempted to explain communication development. Then we will look at a transactional view of how communicative behavior develops.

Structure versus Function – Clashing Theories

The traditional debate in this area has focused on language. Throughout the nineteen-sixties and eighties, a war (Hebb, 1973) raged in the field of language development. On one side were structuralists (cognitive theorists, who called themselves psycholinguists). In the other corner were functionalists (behavioral psychologists). The war began when Noam Chomsky, an MIT linguist, wrote a searing review (Chomsky, 1958) of B.F. Skinner's book, *Verbal Behavior* (1957). In the subsequent counter-reviews, (e.g., MacCorquodale, 1965) both sides claimed to have won. Only in recent years does there appear to be some rapprochement, much of it due to the emerging worldview of a transactional perspective. The battle has been said to have been between the "miracle theory" (i.e., psycholinguisitics) and the "impossible theory" (i.e., behavioral theory, see Chapter 2). Psycholinguistics was deemed the miracle theory in that language "just happened" in human children without formal training – seemingly a miracle. Behavioral theories were deemed impossible because operant principles did not seem adequate to account for language development. Let us turn our attention first to psycholinguistics.

A Structural Approach – Psycholinguistics

A major reason for the gulf dividing these theories was that each was looking at language in a fundamentally different way. Psycholinguists emphasized structure. They saw language as an idealized system of ***symbols***. Led first by Chomsky's linguistic theory, they began to focus on word order, or ***syntax***, as the basic structure of language. They were much more interested in the structure or form of language, rather than its actual usage (i.e., function). Instead of focusing on what children actually said, psycholinguists focused on determining ***linguistic competence***. This was the hypothetical, rather than real ability of the child to form language constructions. Mispronunciations, grammatical errors, and dysfluencies that real children made were often seen as errors and were less important than the consistent structure that language had. Structure was what was important and the structure of the language was thought to reflect the structure of the mind. Competence was what children were **capable** of doing with language, not what they actually **did**. Although children often spoke ungrammatically, they were seen to know all there is to know about the structure of language, and to develop this competence by the age of four or five. No wonder this is called the Miracle theory.

Nativism

The reason for this emphasis on syntactic structure was Chomsky's argument that language structure was constrained by the structure of the mind. That is, humans have certain ***linguistic universals*** in language that are emitted by the structure of thought. For example, all languages have subjects and actions (nouns and verbs) because the structure of thought causes our language to talk about these things. The structure of syntax follows a grammatical set of rules because of the constraints of the human mind to impose a certain order when we speak, and to understand a certain order when we hear. Therefore, language is a part of the biological nature of humans. This view is called ***nativism*** (Chapter 5).

As nativists, psycholinguists invoke biology as the primary mechanism for language acquisition. They argue that children in all cultures know all the basics there are to know about their language structure by the time they are 4 or 5 years old. To do this with little formal teaching, children must have a type of ***language acquisition device (LAD)*** in their heads. The human mind has the structure to hear a limited number of utterances in early childhood and despite the variability in what they hear, deduce the rules of language. These rules enable the child to generate an unlimited number of novel yet grammatical utterances from then on. How can that happen?

The Child as Linguist

Psycholinguists suggest that children learning their native language are like little linguists discovering a new language. Children are said to follow the same process linguists use. This involves (1) listening to the sounds that are made and the situations in which they are made; (2) forming a hypothesis about what the sound means; (3) testing this hypothesis by using the sound in a situation; and (4) confirming or weakening the hypothesis. For the child, as for the linguist, language learning involves testing hypotheses about the relationship of sounds to events. For example, the child hears "mama" frequently. Mama is nearly always present when she hears this sound. Thus the child forms the hypothesis: "mama" is Mama. Now the child tests the hypothesis by waiting to see that when she hears "mama" her mother will come. When the test is confirmed, the child has acquired the word.

The LAD

Psycholinguists argue that to acquire words with such apparent ease, the child must have a specialized mechanism that takes linguistic input (sounds and sights), processes this information, and produces rules that lead to language. The rules are seen as important since language is viewed as a ***generative*** process. Language is not merely imitative or rote, but characterized by an infinite number of grammatical utterances. A finite (i.e., limited) set of rules can produce an infinite number of novel, yet grammatical utterances With a LAD, all children in a normal species typical environment (one with normal linguistic information) can not only understand an infinite variety of utterances, but can say an infinite number of grammatically correct utterances as well. Again, a miracle.

Changes in Emphasis

The focus of psycholinguists has shifted over the years. The initial emphasis was on how syntax determined meaning. Grammars which specified the rules developed by children to produce meaningful utterances were developed. Chomsky argued that ***surface structure*** (the actual ordering of words as spoken) was determined by ***deep structure*** (the underlying meaning). He first proposed a phrase structure grammar that parceled language into tree diagrams revealing the structure of the sentence as consisting of nouns, verbs and other components hierarchically organized. Later he proposed a transformational grammar in which specialized rules, called transformations developed. Transformational rules expanded the generativity of language by providing the simple rules for changing a basic sentence into another form (e.g., active to passive or question).

Researchers questioned the importance of syntax in determining meaning. Snow (1972) argued that when a child says "mommy sweater," we know the meaning of the utterance not by the deep structure of the utterance, but by its context. If the child is cold we derive one meaning, if the child points to mommy's sweater, we infer another. This study of the relationship of the situation or context to meaning is called ***semantics*** and has been the focus of cognitive psychologists in recent years.

An even more recent trend is the emphasis on ***pragmatics***. Pragmatics deals with the way language is used. Taking turns or using language to ask for things in different ways (e.g., a request with "please" versus a demand) are examples of pragmatics. At this point the emphasis is no longer on structure, but on function. That brings us to a look at an approach to language that emphasizes function, verbal behavior.

A Functional Approach – The Analysis of Verbal Behavior

It was Skinner's 1957 book that set off the language "war." In it he presented verbal behavior as "behavior reinforced through the mediation of other persons" (Skinner, 1957, p. 2). What this means is that verbal behavior is the same as any other operant behavior – it is determined by the four-term contingency. The thing that makes verbal behavior unique is that it must be reinforced by someone who understands it. "Thank you," "danke," and "merci" are reinforced by people who understand the words.

Verbal behavior is not limited to vocal speech in Skinner's analysis. Sign language, written language, even body language can be verbal behavior if they are mediated by people who understand the function of the behavior. Your pet dog or cat may use verbal behavior toward you when it pokes its food dish across the floor and you reinforce that **verbal** behavior by filling it with food.

Skinner listed several categories of verbal behavior. These categories were based on the functional relationship between the behavior and the environment, not structural categories like nouns and verbs. The primary verbal behaviors are described below:

Mand. The mand is operant behavior under the control of a setting event such as deprivation or aversive stimulation and reinforced by the stimulus that reduces this deprivation or aversive situation. Saying "water," "agua," "wawa," "I want water please," writing the word "water," using gestures, a certain kind of cry, or even a puppy pushing its empty water dish with its nose are all examples of mands. (1) They are controlled by deprivation of water; (2) getting water reinforces each response; and (3) the response will be reinforced only if there is another in the environment who will mediate reinforcement (i.e., give the water). Notice that what is paramount here is not the form the response takes, but rather its function. A mand is a functional response class. Anything can be a mand if it is reinforced by the thing that it names.

Tact. Tacts are a class of verbal operants in which a response of a given form is evoked by a particular object or event or property of an event (Skinner, 1957). In other words, tacts are specific responses that are controlled by a discriminative stimulus and reinforced by the verbal environment. In a simple sense, tacts are labels, words, or other symbols that stand for something. Thus "cat," "That's a cat," or "gato" are tacts that the verbal community reinforces (perhaps by saying "yes, that's right") for labeling certain furry little animals. Note, unlike the mand, the object itself is not the reinforcer, the response of a listener who understands and provides a consequence is.

Echoic. In echoics the controlling stimulus is verbal (remember, not necessarily vocal) and the response matches the form of this stimulus. Imitation is an echoic if the child's response matches the model's. For example, if the mother says "chair" and her daughter repeats this, the daughter's utterance is an echoic.

Textual. A textual is a verbal response whose discriminative stimulus is written or printed. Reading the word "stop" is a textual.

Intraverbal. An intraverbal is a verbal behavior whose controlling stimulus is the speaker's prior verbal behavior. Chains of verbal behavior (the sentences we speak) are intraverbals. For example, if I say " Ask not what your country can do for you...," your response ("ask what you can do for your country") is an intraverbal.

Autoclitic. This final category is comprised of a heterogeneous class of verbal responses. This is Skinner's most complex category. Autoclitics are verbal behaviors that are based upon or depend upon other verbal behavior (Skinner, 1957). Skinner identified several types of autoclitics. Autoclitics are what gives language its style and complexity. Syntactical word order, grammatical tagging (e.g., walk*s*, walk*ed*, walk*ing*), assertion ("I'm *sure* its going to rain today"), and negation ("He is *not* stupid") are some of the subcategories of autoclitics (Winokur, 1976). Another sub-category, called qualifying autoclitics, are seen in the difference between a speaker saying "It's going to rain today" and "I ***think*** it's going to rain today." "Think" is an autoclitic that qualifies the strength of the speaker's conviction that it is going to rain.

This is a necessarily brief overview of Skinner's work. It is important to emphasize again the major distinction between verbal behavior and language seen by cognitive psycholinguists. For Skinner, verbal behavior is something people do, not a thing that they have. Grammar is a description of behavior, not an explanation. Skinner's theory focuses on function, psycholinguists focused on structure. With the change of focus by psycholinguists to more emphasis on syntax and pragmatics has come an interest in function, or process. Perhaps it is time to call a truce in this language war. The rest of the chapter will look at a dynamical systems view of communication.

A Dynamical Systems Perspective

Our dynamical systems viewpoint leads us to look at the ever-changing reciprocal relationships between our genetic make-up, history of interactions and environment to explain communication.

What is the role of genetics?

While other organisms communicate among themselves and with other species, animal communication is limited compared with human communication. The complex communications behaviors we have that we call language are unique to humans. It is obvious that we have a common genetic basis for a physiology that enables us to develop such flexible communication skills. The evolution of our vocal apparatus enables us to produce a range of sounds which can be produced with the great precision necessary for vocal language. The localization of certain speech functions in specialized areas of the cortex has been known for centuries. Yet, we still know very little about the physiology of language. One may speculate that we may just inherit to a much higher degree than other organisms a genetic make-up that enables us to learn the environment/behavior relationships necessary for acquiring and manipulating symbols.

At any rate, at this time we cannot identify the specifics of neurology that lead to language development. We may never be able to do this. For the purpose of psychological analysis, we do not need to engage in reductionism. Using the unique biological capabilities of the human organism as a universal base, we can look at language in terms of its functional relationships to the environment.

The Functions of Language

The main function of language is communication. Language develops because of its increasing effectiveness in obtaining reinforcement from the environment. We can adapt better to our environment with language behaviors than we can without them. For example, with language we can get things that are not present; we can talk about things that no longer exist. We can produce positive reinforcers and avoid or escape negative reinforcers by asking for them.

The neonate comes into this world with perceptual systems that enable it to interact with a world rich in verbal behavior. Among the Universal I behaviors the newborn possesses are the ability to detect human language sounds. This is not such an easy task. Speech is an ephemeral thing. The sounds the child hears quickly change and then are gone. In addition, unlike written language, speech sounds are streams of sound and these streams are constantly varying. The child must be able to detect the boundaries between one basic unit of sound (a ***phoneme***) and the next. It is likely that the ability to chop up the stream of speech into language units is an important Universal I behavior. The research of Eimas and his colleagues (Eimas, Siqueland, Jusczyk, & Vigorito, 1971) on "pa" and "ba" (described earlier) suggests that infants can do this during their first month.

Besides the ability to detect differences in speech sounds, children may show differential reactions to speech sounds at a very early age. Watson (1973) found that auditory stimuli were more reinforcing for girls than visual stimuli. For boys the reverse was true. DeCasper and Fifer (1980) showed that neonates will suck at a specified rate to turn on a recording of their mother's voice. Taken together the evidence is strong that very young infants perceive variations in human speech and that some speech sounds may be reinforcing.

Neonates also come into the world with a built in repertoire of communication behaviors. Most notable is the cry. Wolff (1969) identified three types of newborn cries: hunger, pain, and "mad." For neonates these cries are reflexes, each elicited by particular stimulus classes. They also differ in form, with the pain cry being particularly high pitched, loud, and irritating – a sound which no parent could ignore, thus obtaining its evolutionary survival function.

Cries may begin as reflexes, but quickly the functions of crying expand. By the third week of life, infants are developing a ***fake cry***. Wolff described this as having a different form and function than the reflexive types. Fake cries are combinations of low moans and intermittent cries and do not seem related to the aversives that elicit the others. Fake cries are reinforced by attention or, Wolff suggests, the intrinsic reinforcement of the sound of the fake cries themselves.

Of course operant crying can become the bane of the new parent. Infants may quickly learn that a cry is an effective way to produce a positive reinforcer – her parents presence. Do parents who respond to their crying children reinforce such operant crying? As with most transactions, the answer is not simple.

A correlational study by Ainsworth, Bell, and Stanyon (1972) found that mothers who were the quickest to respond to their infant's crying had the children who cried the least at the end of the first year. Why should this be the case? A study by Gewirtz & Boyd (1977) showed that mothers who responded quickly to their infants cries were able to respond to other more desirable cues that the infant makes. Mothers who delay responding to their babies cries inadvertently wind up teaching their children that longer and more intense crying is necessary to receive parental attention. In both cases, the children have learned to use vocal behavior to produce changes in their environments. They have learned the function of communication.

Around 3-5 weeks of age infants begin ***cooing***. Coos are vowel-like sounds that appear to occur under pleasant setting events. Somewhat later, true babbling occurs (3-4 months). Babbling sounds include most of the basic sounds of language. The same sounds appear in the babbling of all children. Those exposed to **any** language and those, as in deaf children, who are exposed to none. This early part of babbling appears to be a Universal II behavior. At this point the babbling of infants all over the world consists of the same set of sounds. Somewhere around six months of age the babbling of children exposed to different languages and of deaf children begin to develop on different paths. Due to environmental experiences, the sounds that hearing children produce becomes more and more restricted to the sounds in the language to which the child is exposed. The babbling sounds of non-hearing children begin to disappear. At this point babbling more clearly comes to resemble operant behavior. It is also at about this point that the child begins to gain control over volume, pitch, and phrasing.

Near the end of the babbling period, ***echolalic babbling*** appears. This is where the baby babbles, but has developed the intonation of adult language. The effect is that someone in the next room might think the child is talking even thought the sounds are nonsense syllables. Near the end of this time (10-12 months) infants coin their own words, and begin to use their own sounds for certain functions (mands?, tacts?). These are called ***vocables***. At about this same time (10-12 months) children begin to use gestures to stand for things, such as waving to signify "bye-bye" (Acredelo & Goodwyn, 1988). Finally around 10-12 months infants begin to use their first true words.

Do Prelanguage Sounds Lead to Language?

Most parents assume that crying, cooing, and babbling are the building blocks of language development. Psycholinguists do not necessarily think they are. Instead, their view is that these ***prelinguistic sounds*** are necessary for the child to perform, but do not get shaped into words themselves. Instead, their view is that the ***prelinguistic stage*** is a time for effectively exercising the tools for real language. However, behavioral psychologists see the prelinguistic sounds as shaped into later language in a continuous manner.

Who Shapes Babbling?

If babbling does become language, who does the shaping? Certainly the drift in babbling across languages and in the hearing impaired suggests an environmental role, but the question remains: "who dunnit?"

The most obvious agent for shaping babbling is the parent. At first blush this appears to be the case. Mom and dad hover over their baby, smile and laugh and tickle whenever their little one emits a babble. Rheingold, Gewirtz, and Ross (1965) and Weisberg (1963) showed that infant vocalizations could be increased with contingent social reinforcement. The studies involved a researcher who would smile, tickle, and say "tsk, tsk, tsk," whenever the infant vocalized. With this contingent social reinforcement vocalizations increased.

So there is evidence that adults can reinforce infant vocalizations. But how important is their role in real life? Consider the difficulty of trying to shape a babble into a word. It would require much skill and an enormous amount of reinforcement to accurately shape this behavior. While parents do some of this, they do not do it at the level required to shape all the sounds of the child's language. Parents simply do not stand over their infants, accurately differentially reinforcing every correct sound and ignoring incorrect ones. This is one reason why psycholinguists called the behavioral approach "impossible theory." There must be another mechanism.

Automatic Reinforcement

Automatic reinforcement has been proposed as that mechanism by behavioral psychologists (Bijou & Baer, 1965; Vaughn & Michael, 1982). In automatic reinforcement, the native speech sounds become acquired reinforcers and, the child herself, in uttering one of the sounds, hears the sound, thus "automatically" reinforcing the motor behaviors that produced the sound. The process is as follows:

(a) During parenting, the parents use the sounds of the child's native language;
(b) Because of their association with other reinforcers provided by the parents, these sounds of the native language become secondary reinforcers themselves;
(c) When the child babbles, by luck it emits one of these sounds (a response);
(d) The consequence of the response is hearing the sound (the secondary reinforcer);
(e) The response (producing the sound) is automatically reinforced (by the sound produced by the babbling behavior).

In this view the child's babbling is shaped by a combination of automatic reinforcement and some parent shaping. The parent provides models of native language utterances which become secondary reinforcers that reinforce the baby who emits the sound itself.

Early Stages of Language Development

Symbolic Gesturing

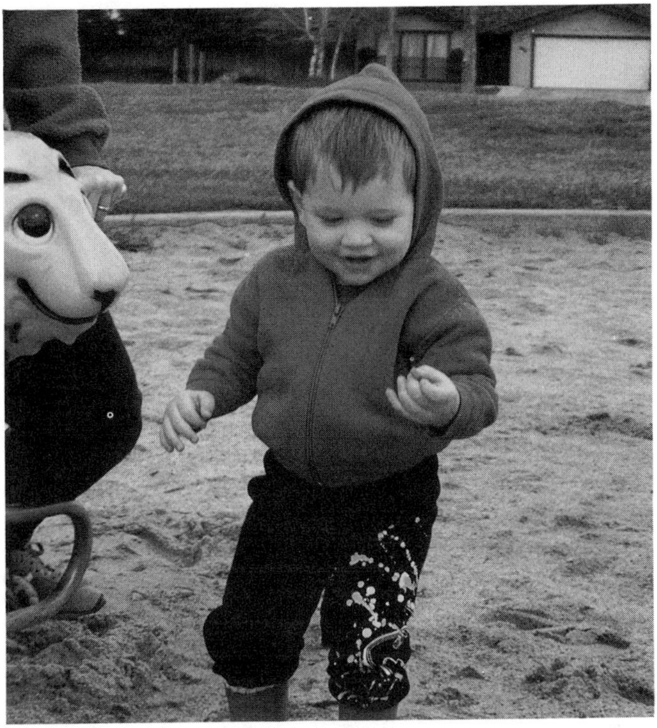

Brandon makes the symbolic gesture "bug."

True words are symbols arbitrarily selected by a community to stand for concepts. At about the beginning of the second year, the time that true vocal words first appear, children begin using gestures to represent their environment in the same manner as words. For example, a child may flap his arms to represent a bird or blow through his mouth to mean hot. This has been called ***symbolic gesturing*** (Acredolo & Goodwyn, 1990). Table 9-1 shows the symbolic gestures used by Kate Acredolo and compares these with her age at appearance of the symbolic gesture and the age at appearance of the equivalent true word. Notice how, in all cases, the use of a symbolic gesture precedes the acquisition of the equivalent word by many months.

The development of both symbolic gesturing and real words seem to coalesce around the functions of communication. Indeed, the first functional class of symbolic gestures to emerge are those symbols requesting things, followed by symbols describing attributes of objects, and then by symbols functioning as labels (Acredelo and Goodwyn, 1988). The same order and relative timing for the functions

Table 9.1
Kate Acredolo's Symbolic Gestures from 12 -14 months of age

Signs	Descriptions	Age Sign Acquired	Age Word Acquired	How Acquired
Flower	sniff, sniff	12.50	20.00	Imitation
Big	arms raised	13.00	17.25	Trained
Elephant	arm extended from nose	13.50	19.75	Trained
Anteater	tongue in and out	14.00	24.00	Trained
Bunny	torso up and down	14.00	19.75	Trained
Cookie monster	palm to mouth plus smack	14.00	20.75	Trained
Monkey	hands in armpits, up-down	14.25	19.75	Trained
Skunk	wrinkled nose plus sniff	14.50	24.00	Trained
Fish	blow though the mouth	14.50	17.50	Imitation
Slide	hand waved downward	14.50	17.50	Spontaneous
Swing	torso back and forth	14.50	18.25	Spontaneous
Ball	both hands waved	14.50	15.75	Spontaneous
Alligator	palms together, open-shut	14.75	24.00	Trained
Bee	finger plus thumb waved	14.75	20.00	Trained
Butterfly hands	crossed, fingers waved	14.75	24.00	Trained

Adapted from Acredolo & Goodwyn, 1985

of requests and timings occurs with vocal words (Griffiths, 1985, cited in Acredolo & Goodwyn, 1990). It is also the same sequence suggested for the acquisition of Skinner's mands (which function as requests) and tacts (which functions as descriptions and labels).

Organized by the functions of communication we see the coalescence of symbolic language usage appear. It requires physiological changes, but also a long history of interaction with the environment. Symbolic gestures may coalesce first because of advantages they have in developing (See Acredolo & Goodwyn, 1990). Some of these advantages may be physiological (dexterity of the arms and hands versus dexterity of the vocal apparatus), but some advantages are due to the consequences they produce. For example, gestures are present for a longer time than sounds and are present when the reinforcement is applied. Sounds are reinforced after they are no longer present. Furthermore, gestures may look like the things they represent and therefore be directly prompted by the object they specify. Such symbolic gestures may have a higher probability of leading to reinforcement by the environment because their meaning is obvious.

The advantages to symbolic gestures are, however, limited and true words begin to dominate the communicative repertoire of the child. Vocabulary is not limited to what can be visually represented. True words are arbitrary symbols so an infinite number of words are possible.

First Words

The child's first true word emerges around the time of the child's first birthday. Nelson (1973) looked at the first fifteen words of children. Names for items, including "mommy", "daddy", and pet names were most common. These, when used as names would be considered tacts. What Nelson called "action words" such as *give, bye-bye,* and *up* were almost as frequent. Many of these "action words" would fit the category of ***mands*** when used to obtain the thing.

The Holophrastic Stage

During this stage children use single words to stand for entire concepts. A child may say "wawa" when it means "I want water," "That's a glass of water," or "There's water on the floor." Snow (1972) suggests that it is the parent who decides what the child means and responds appropriately. Here the function of language (here tact or mand) is ambiguous with the parent using the context to interpret what the child means.

The Telegraphic Stage

Between 18 and 24 months the child begins to put words together to form sentences. At first these are two word utterances such as "Mommy sweater," "Cookie allgone," or "More wawa". Because these utterances are missing some unimportant words, they are deemed ***telegraphic speech*** in that they resemble the messages sent when people have to pay per word.

Why do children increase the mean length of utterance from one to two and then from two to three words? Why do they leave out words, rather than add words in grammatical sequences? The answer is in the communicative function of language. Two word utterances are more effective in obtaining reinforcers from the social environment than one word utterances. "More wawa" is more likely to obtain the reinforcer than is "wawa;" which an adult may interpret wrongly. Then why do we not use fully adult grammatical speech right away?

The answer is that language learning is very difficult. The ***law of least effort*** suggests that we do the least effortful behavior that is reinforced. In a way the telegraphic speech child is paying for every word, in effort, not in money. Early in development the child's environment is very supportive of language learning. Patient parents reinforce ambiguous utterances and try to clarify them. Later when the child's language is stronger the environment will be less tolerant.

Language Development as Skill Learning

Some (*e.g.*, Brown & Hanlon, 1978) have suggested that parents play little direct role in language development. They suggest that parents are more likely to reinforce the truthfulness of an utterance, but not its grammaticality. Others suggest that imitation has no important role either. They argue that imitation can only lead to mimicry and not produce the generative quality that distinguishes language. Those who take this position tend to be nativists and look for the innate Language

Acquisition Device (LAD) to explain the miracle of language. Others have looked elsewhere.

Ernst Moerk (1988) has found the LAD – and discovered that it is really a LADY – the child's mother. Moerk's point is that there is ample evidence that the environment, mediated particularly by the mother, shapes language development.

Moerk (1986) identifies four behavior characteristics of mothers in teaching any skill to children which aid in informally teaching language to their children. These four characteristics of skill teaching evident in the language interactions of the mother are:

1) *High Intensity of repetitions of each of the sentence types by the caretaker.* Since young children usually do not employ rehearsal strategies themselves, repetition by the mother is very important for learning. The intensity of repetitions has three aspects (Moerk, 1986).

- Repetitiveness. Mothers are likely to repeat their modeled utterances over and over again, sometimes with minor variations.
- Priming (or Prompting). Mothers initiate retrieval of utterances in the child by asking the child to name an item or to talk about a subject.
- Combining massed practice with spaced rehearsals. Mothers enhance language skills by massing three-to five repetitions of an utterance closely together. Then, they back off, allowing the child to rest. As Moerk (1986, page 210) describes this intuitive approach to skill learning by mothers: "The principles guiding maternal techniques seem to be: (1) Initially, the item has to be repeated, densely spaced to be retained in the child's short-term memory long enough in order to be analyzable and transferable to long-term memory. (2) It should not be repeated so often as to lead to fatigue or loss of interest. (3) After several repetitions with short intervals, the speed of forgetting declines and the rehearsals can be reinstated after longer and longer intervals. After a certain degree of learning, testing might replace modeled reinstatements."

2) *The effects of frequency of repetitions by parents on their children.* Findings (e.g., Brown, Cazden, and Bellugi, 1969) show that there is a relationship between the frequency of use of a sentence type by parents and the order of appearance of the sentence type by the child. Although Brown has subsequently argued that no such frequency effects exist (Brown, 1973; Cazden and Brown, 1975), Moerk (1986) has re-analyzed the same data and found clear evidence for the effects of parental frequency on the emergence of child language.

The high level of teaching techniques evident in mother-child dyads makes the role of environmental shaping not only seem "possible" but likely. For example, analyzing tapes of one of Brown's mother-child dyads Moerk (1983) estimated that the child (Eve) would have encountered each major sentence type about 100,000 times per month. The same child responded to all the sentence types between 500,000 and one million times per month! In looking at the language of his own children, Bell (1903) found that his two daughters (age 3 year/6 months and 4 years/

4 months) spoke 15,230 and 14,996 words per day , respectively. Brandenburg and Brandenburg (1919) counted 14,930 words per day for their 4 year/4 month old daughter. Moerk (1986) points out that this is about 1,000 words per working hour and nearly half a million words per month! Given the enormous number of language trials experienced by the child, this theory no longer sounds so "impossible."

3) *Knowledge of Results (Feedback to the child).* According to Moerk (1986) caretakers provide frequent feedback to the child. Both positive feedback (or positive reinforcement) and negative feedback (or punishment) is provided and the findings, are that mothers give either positive or negative feedback on utterances in from 33% (Rogers-Warren and Warren, 1980) to as many as 40-50% (Rondal, 1978) of their utterances. While positive feedback may take the form of praise, it need not be limited to this. Indeed, behaviors of the caretaker which demonstrate understanding of the child's utterance (such as giving the child the requested toy, or using a more complicated utterance repeating in part what the child said) can serve as positive reinforcement for the child's utterance.

Likewise, negative feedback need not be a verbal rebuff, such as "No!" Instead, parents provide negative feedback to the child in many ways, including corrections and expansions. Moerk (1983), again analyzing Brown's data, found that mothers may correct their infants' grammar around 50 times per hour or nearly once every minute.

Maternal corrections do not just punish the child's incorrect utterance. This feedback also serves as a prompt (i.e., an S^d) to try again with the mother modeling the correct expansion of the child's utterance. In the data, Moerk found that not only do mothers correct their infant's grammatical errors most of the time, but if the mothers correct the child or give them eye contact, the children recommunicate their messages nearly 100 percent of the time. In contrast, only about three percent of messages **accepted** by the mother are restated by the child.

4) *Information acquired by the teacher, of the learner's failure or success, which allows the mother to modify her talk.* Language learning is a dynamical process involving two way transactions. In the process of influencing the child's behavior by her own, changes she has produced in the child's behavior affect her behavior as well. Mothers are sensitive to the child's level of language skills as shown in their ability to predict with high precision the level of their children's language abilities (Berko-Gleason, 1976; Rondal, 1979).

This maternal sensitivity to the level of their child's language skills allows them to adjust their modeling and feedback to levels which keep them just steps ahead of the child. Early on this appears in the baby-talk or ***motherese*** used by the mother in interactions with her child. Motherese can be seen as a universal characteristic of mother-to-child interactions which is shaped by the pace of the child's ability to respond to the mother.

The Role of Imitation

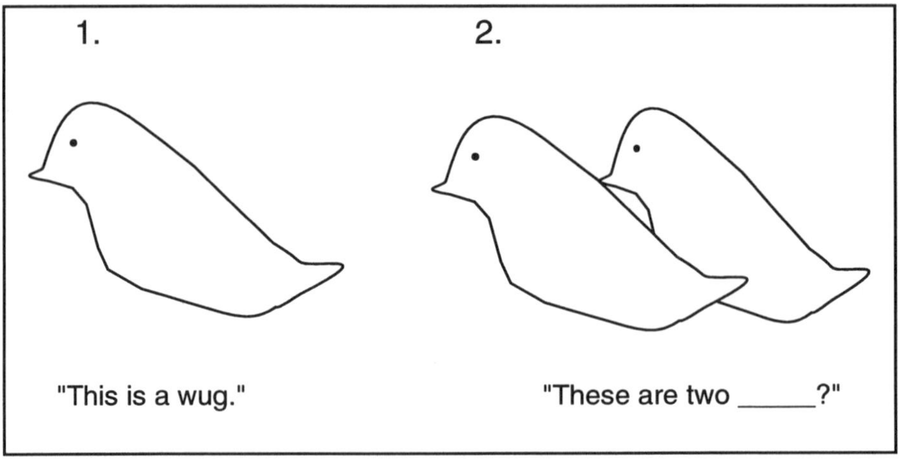

Some have argued that imitation plays a very small role in language development. They base this on logical grounds: if language is generative, characterized by an unlimited number of novel, yet mostly grammatical utterances, then mimicry cannot play a role. They argue that if imitation were a process in language development, then children would first have to hear all the utterances they would later produce.

This argument was attacked on logical and empirical grounds. Whitehurst and Novak (1973) conducted a study in which children heard sentence phrases (e.g., prepositional) with a consistent syntax (e.g., "The boy is on the bike," "The squirrel is in the mailbox") to describe a set of pictures. The children were prompted to repeat the modeled sentence and were reinforced when they did. No phrases were provided for a second set. Instead children gave their own descriptions to this novel set of pictures. The results showed that the children produced their own utterances to the novel pictures. These utterances contained the same **type** of phrases as learned on the training pictures but were novel in terms of their content. Whitehurst and Novak (1973) called this behavior that matches some part of the model's utterance (i.e., syntax) but is novel on another (i.e., what is being talked about) ***selective imitation.***

Selective imitation may explain the learning of regularities in language that include the use of plurals, tenses, and adjectives as well as sentence structure. For example, look at the single figure below. It is a picture of a wug. Now look at the next figure. It shows two ...... You probably said two "wugs." How did you know that? Did anyone ever teach you that two of them are "wugs" and not "wuggen" or "wuggi." Berko (1958) used this "Wug Test" and showed that children say "wugs" too (or, make that, "two wugs.") Caretakers model the "s" sound for nearly all plural nouns and correct for misuse. Children have a history of learning to add "s" for plural.

Selective imitation and not a biological LAD may be responsible for the universal errors that appear in children's misuse of verb tenses and plurals called ***over-regularization.*** In English, verbs, such as walk, touch, and smell are called "regular" verbs because they follow a standard rule: the "Ed" sound is added to them. Verbs such as go, run, and see are called "irregular" because the past tense (i.e., went, ran, saw) do not follow a rule. Some irregular verbs, such as: "to be" ("am," "are") "go" are very frequently modeled by caretakers and their individual frequencies are high. Thus, children often use the appropriate past tense of frequently used irregular verbs (i.e., "was," "were," "went"). However, increasing vocabulary means that many regular verbs are acquired through the teaching techniques of the caretaker. Thus, next, children begin to apply the regular past tense form "-ed" more and more. At some point selective imitation of the regularized form "-ed" is applied to the irregular verbs so that the child now says "goed" instead of "went" and "runned" instead of "ran". This is over-regularization. The effects of caretaker teaching, including corrective feedback results in a mixture of irregular and regular forms, so the child may now say "wented." Finally, appropriate use of both irregular and regular verbs appears. Similar sequences occur for plurals and adjectives (Reich, 1986).

The Role of Reinforcement in Imitation

Several studies have been conducted to show how this expanded view of imitation makes it more likely to view imitation as an important part of language development. Poulson, Kymissis, Reeve, Andreatos, and Richards (1991) looked at generalized vocal imitations in infants 9 to 13 months of age.

Generalized Imitation was first studied by Baer & Sherman (1964) and demonstrates that imitative behavior can be a functional response class that is established by reinforcement of some, but not all imitated behaviors. For example, in the Baer and Sherman study children were reinforced for imitating some of "Jimmy the Puppet's" behaviors, such as head touching, and opening their mouth. They were never reinforced for pressing a lever, but when after the other imitative behaviors were reinforced, the children also imitated Jimmy's lever pressing even though this behavior continued to be nonreinforced. Poulson, et al. (1991) extended this to language by demonstrating that reproduction of adult verbal sounds (e.g., "EE", "DAH," "EH") which had never been reinforced would occur if imitation of other sounds (e.g., "OO," "MAH") were reinforced. Reinforcement was contingent descriptive praise (e.g., "Good baby! You said "OO.") Thus the study shows that reinforcement need not be given for every verbal imitation for generalized verbal imitation to play a role in language acquisition.

Poulson's study suggests that not all imitations must be reinforced, but that generalized imitation of language will occur if imitation is intermittently reinforced. Still, some have suggested that reinforcement is not important in language development (e.g., Brown & Hanlon, 1970). They argued that parents are more likely to reinforce the truthfulness of children's utterances (e.g., "It rain") than their grammatical correctness (e.g., "It is not raining now".)

In contrast, Whitehurst and Valdez-Menchaca (1988) argued that differential reinforcement of language is important and necessary. As evidence, they conducted a study in which 2- and 3-year-olds were exposed to a foreign language (either Spanish or English). If children used the foreign language word to name the toy, their response was reinforced by receiving the toy. One group was differentially reinforced in this manner throughout the study, while a second group received reinforcement for naming in both languages and was later switched to differential reinforcement for use of the foreign vocabulary.

The results showed that differential reinforcement with the named toys increased spontaneous use of the foreign words. In addition, formal assessment using tests showed that comprehension and production of language was significantly increased by differential reinforcement. Whitehurst and Valdez-Menchaca concluded that the role of contingent reinforcement was significant. Virtually no spontaneous use of the new language occurred without differential reinforcement, but with it, a great deal of usage occurred.

Note that the type of reinforcement used here was not praise or feedback. Instead, the response was reinforced by the object requested. This fits Skinner's definition of the "mand" (although it is also a tact since they named an object actually in front of them). Hart and Risley (1968, 1974, 1975) made effective use of this type of contingency in enhancing several categories of language, including descriptive adjectives and compound sentences, of educationally challenged children.

While mand type contingencies have been shown to be effective forms of reinforcement for verbal behavior, other parentally mediated reinforcement contingencies may be effective, as well. Petersen and Sherrod (1982) found mother frequently provided approval to children's utterances during free play. Moreover, there was a significant correlation between the amount of feedback provided by the mothers and their child's mean length of utterance. Caufield (1988) found mothers with children just beginning to learn language were much more likely to provide praise for words and to criticize non-words. Thus in the early stages of language, mothers are most likely to use contingent reinforcement and punishment.

This is apparently the case even in the development of symbolic gesturing. Once Kate Acredolo began to spontaneously use symbolic gestures, her mother, Linda began a "game" from which Kate learned at 13 months, the gestures of sniffing as a reference for a flower and arms-over-the-head for "big" (Acredolo and Goodwyn, 1990). Soon, other adults joined in modeling gestures, pairing them with objects, and providing feedback. By age 17.5 months, Kate had acquired 29 signs, more than half of which had been intentionally taught by her parents (See figure 5-1).

Reinforcement for verbal behavior takes many forms, including praise, automatic reinforcement, correction, and obtaining the consequences specified by the verbal behavior itself. When mothers use expansions, they are simultaneously reinforcing what the child has uttered, but providing a model for a successive approximation to adult speech, a clear form of shaping. Taken together, these types of reinforcers seem to play an important role in the acquisition of language.

Finally, Moerk (1990) found strong evidence for the existence of three-term contingency patterns in mother-child language interactions. Early in language development, child behaviors which were followed by maternal agreement were likely to be repeated Thus these maternal consequences functioned as reinforcers. The most common three-term contingency, occurring in 30 percent of the interactions was a sequence in which the mother used a vocabulary word (S^d) which evoked the use of the word by the child (R) which was consequated by mother's agreement (S^{+r}).
Thus, the following contingency is likely in language interactions:

S^d	→	R	→	S^{+r}
M: "Ball."		C: "Ball."		M: "Yes, that's right."

Later on, expansions by the mother are increasingly likely to follow the child's utterance. Expansions may reinforce the correct part of the child's utterance (as occurs in selective imitation) but may punish an immediate child repetition. The data show that maternal expansions often terminate an interaction as in the following sequence (Moerk, 1990):

S^d	→	R	→	S^{+r}
M: "What is the child doing?"		C: "Running."		M: "She is running."

Thus, maternal expansions which occur frequently in the later stages of language development, may serve to strengthen the child's response, but may punish responses that are too difficult for the child at the time. However, expansions are observed by Moerk (1990) to function also as discriminative stimuli in the form of prompts. Thus expansions are often followed by child verbal behavior which, is followed by maternal agreement. This is just one set of three-term contingencies (i.e., $S^d \rightarrow R \rightarrow S^{+r}$) observed to occur in mother child language interactions.

In sum, there is ample evidence that the mother-child dyad plays a crucial role in language skill, learning (Moerk, 1983, 1992). From a dynamical systems perspective, language development is the result of an interaction between a specialized organism and a specialized environment. The organism has a physiological structure which facilitates linguistic interactions with the environment. The caretaker is a leading part who disproportionately influences the development of communication by providing environmental contingencies which are constantly adjusted to the improving skills level of the developing child.

lie w/ WORDS more than gestures. Ch. 16 Gen 4, DePaulo '92

Box 9

Interactive Storybook Reading and Language

One of the most enjoyable, yet most important things parents can do with their child is to read to them. Reading to a child promotes language development, and establishes reading as a significant reinforcer for the child. While any type of reading may be beneficial, storybook reading provides an especially rich opportunity for language learning interactions. Russ Whitehurst and his associates noted this while working with language delayed children and developed a procedure they called "dialogic reading". The term "dialogic" comes from the word "dialog" and suggests that reading can involve an interactive dialog between child and parent, rather than just a parental monolog. They reasoned that this "hear-say" method, in which the child first hears some of the story and then is prompted to say part of it, fits the skills notion of learning in which the child learns language by active participation.

Dialogic reading involves seven steps designed to maximize language interaction (Whitehurst, Falco, Lonigan, Fischel, DeBaryshe, Valdez-Menchaca, & Caufield, 1988) These steps are:

1. Ask open-ended "What" questions, such as "What's this?" or "What's it doing now?"
2. Follow the child's answers with more questions. This confirms or reinforces the child's utterances and at the same time prompts more language.
3. Repeat what the child says, such as "Yes, that's a turkey." This again confirms and reinforces the child's response.
4. Help the child as needed such as by providing the answer. This prevents the frustration of extinction and models the correct response.
5. Praise and encourage the child.
6. Shadow the child's interest. For example, if the child seems to really like a particular animal in a story, spend more time on that character.
7 Have fun. This final step reinforces the child's language, and particpation in the interaction. Furthermore, it helps make reading a reinforcer.

Whitehurst, et al. (1988) showed that with two training sessions, mothers using dialogic reading over a six week period could significantly increase their two-year-olds' language skills. In fact, with just one month of dialogic reading, children's vocabulary measures increased an equivalent of 6 and 8 months, and the length of the child's utterances also significantly increasesd.. Subsequent studies have shown similar results (e.g., Branscum & Novak, 1995). The method has been adapted to slightly different formats. For example, Valdez-Menchaca and Whitehurst (1992) taught the dialogic reading method to teachers in a Mexican day care center. In turn, the teachers used the method in reading with individual 2-year-olds in their centers for 30 sessions that lasted 10-12 minutes each. The results were similar to previous studies: children participating in the dialogic reading sessions showed significant increases on standardized tests of receptive and expressive vocabulary. In addition, dialogic reading produced significant increases in measures of actual language production skills, such as the mean length and complexity of utterances.

In my own research I reasoned that if dialogic reading works in one-on-one situations between parent and child and between teacher and child, perhaps it would work in small groups with one teacher working with a few children at a time. My research group embarked on a series of studies using the "multilogic reading technique" with preschool and school-aged children with English language deficits (Novak, Staggs, & Jones, 1993, Novak, 1993). Two of the studies involved children classified as "Limited English Proficiency" because their parents spoke little or no English and their school language tests identified them as such.

The steps in the dialogic method were maintained, but the procedure modified to fit the small group setting. This involved arranging the children in a semi-circle in front of the teacher (who was an undergraduate or graduate student). The teacher would read a sentence or two while showing the book and then call on one of the children to answer "what" questions. The teacher followed this with the dialogic steps, randomly calling each child so that all children were part of the interaction. Our results showed that after six weeks of reading, the child's verbal expression increased in complexity and length. However, receptive vocabulary did not increase. The size of the group did matter, for there was a significant difference in the four-children groups versus groups with eight children. Never-the-less, it seems possible to use interactive storybook reading with small groups of children. Furthermore, the method was used successfully with school-age children with language deficits.

So far, most of the research has shown dialogic and multilogic reading to be effective in increasing some language skills in children. It seems particularly to enhance productive language skills. Moreover, teachers who learn to use an interactive reading style often report difficulty in abandoning it for a more traditional, passive reading style if asked to do so. They report that the interactive style is more fun. If that is so, we wondered whether parents naturally adopt such a style and went looking for the answer in videotaped mother-child storybook reading when children were 36-months-old (Goodwyn, Acredelo, & Novak, 1995).

After coding the reading behaviors of mothers to the children during 5-

minute picture book reading sessions, we looked to see if those mothers using a style of actively evoking child behaviors by asking questions and providing feedback would have children who did better on language measures than those using a more passive, mother reading style. The results were the opposite of what was predicted: mothers using the evocative style actually had children who were poorer on language measures.

At first blush, the results suggest that in real life, an interactive reading style such as dialogic reading may adversely affect child language development as measured by both expressive and receptive vocabulary. However, this conclusion must be questioned on the basis of the direction of the correlation. That is, it is plausible that by the time the child is 36 months of age, mothers have adapted their reading styles to the level of the child's language development. That is, by the time the child is 36 months, mothers of the poorer language users may have developed a more active labeling style in order to compensate for the child's slow development. In the same manner, mothers of advanced children may use a less pedantic, more flexible style in which the content of the book is presented pretty much as it was written. Because we only have a correlation, we can not be sure which (i.e., the mother's behavior or the child's behavior) is the cause and which is the effect.

In fact, at 30 months, there is already a significant correlation (in the same direction) between the child's vocabulary development and the mother's reading style at 36 months. However, because we did not have interactive reading data at 30 months, it is not possible to clearly examine the issue of direction of cause and effect. Furthermore, the labeling style was the most effective in increasing the number and length of child utterances during the reading sessions, so it may be an effective strategy for the mothers of children struggling with language to use.

Finally, failure to find facilitative effects for dialogic reading in this study does not mean it is ineffective in promoting language. The experimental studies have demonstrated that interactive reading is effective. Although distinct styles were identified in the taping session, the presence of the styles does not mean that mothers actually employed them in frequent reading to their children. Unlike the experimental studies of Whitehurst and his colleagues, in which the amount of dialogic reading was controlled, we did not even assess the frequency of maternal reading to their children. It is possible that there was wide variation in the frequency of reading, and that this, even more than a particular style could have influenced the outcomes.

In sum, interactive storybook reading is a fun and potentially effective way for parents and teachers to promote the development of reading and language learning skills.

Chapter 10

Personality and the Self

- Who are you?
- What is your best friend like? Take out a sheet of paper and take a few minutes to answer these questions. List all the words you can to describe your best friend:
- Now, do the same thing to describe yourself as others see you.
- Finally, list all the words you can that describe yourself.

What did you find? What kind of words did you use? How many words did you use? Did the list describing yourself as seen by others differ from the one with which you described yourself?

These questions deal with personality and the self. These are areas that have been the focus of traditional areas of psychology for years. We will look at these and then consider personality and the self from a transactional perspective.

Personality

Biological Theories

Personality has been the concern of poets and philosophers for centuries. One of the earliest theories of personality can be traced to the ancient Greek physician Galen. Galen thought that personality was due to biology, specifically the fluids of the body called "humors". The four humors were thought to be in various proportions in our bodies. If one of these humors – blood, phlegm, yellow bile, or black bile – predominated, the personality would be affected. With blood predominating, the person would be sanguine (from the Latin word for blood) or cheerful. If phlegm predominated, then the person would be slow and lethargic. The word *phlegmatic*, meaning apathetic, sluggish, or cool, comes from this humor. Too much black bile would cause melancholia. The yellow bile will produce choleric behavior (i.e., anger or wrath). Notice that the explanatory role played by the humors in ancient times is similar to the role we now assign to hormones.

Since Galen's time theorists have looked at biology as the source of the unique qualities of individuals. Sheldon developed one of the most important biological theories of the twentieth century. He felt that personality was strongly determined by body type. In one of the most ambitious research projects ever done in psychology, Sheldon set out to measure the body types of males. This was published in the *Atlas of Men* (Sheldon, 1942). The *Atlas* measured hundreds of males from photographs. From these measurements Sheldon identified three body types or

somatotypes. The somatotypes were (a)***ectomorph***, (b)***mesomorph***, and (c)***endomorph***, so named because of the embryological layer from which they presumingly originated (Chapter 4). Sheldon calculated the relationship between somatotype and personality characteristics and found a strong correlation. Ectomorphs were not only thin and frail, but were also introverted, sensitive, and intelligent (remember, the central nervous system originated in the ectoderm). In fact, ectomorphy was correlated with this personality type called***cerebrotonia***. Mesomorphs were not only muscular and strong, but also athletic and energetic. This aggressive, risk-taking personality was called***somatotonia***. Finally endomorphs were round and plump, and were likely to have personality traits which included the search for pleasure and social contact, a personality type called ***viscerotonia***.

As with many correlational studies, Sheldon was unable to determine what caused this relationship; did the somatotype cause personality, did personality cause somatotype, or did something else cause both? So while the theory had some intuitive appeal and some empirical data for support, it was too broad and general. It has largely been ignored for the last fifty years.

However, in early 1995, Sheldon's name again made headlines. Eighteen years after his death, the press became aware that photographs taken of students attending a few elite colleges in the from the 1940s through the 1960s existed. These students were photographed in the nude for Sheldon's study in an attempt to relate somatotype and intelligence. For all these years, photos of thousands of nude undergraduates (among those photographed were former President George Bush and the wife of President Clinton, Hillary Rodham Clinton) were kept in the archives of Yale University. The public concern (and perhaps fantasies) surrounding the potentially embarrassing photographs led to their destruction (at least we've been told they have been destroyed!). All told, over 100 pounds of photographs were shredded.

While Sheldon's work was no longer deemed scientifically significant enough to pursue, other current personality theories retain a biological orientation. However, the biological mechanism causing personality is very general or unspecified. Instead today there is an emphasis on measuring personality characteristics for the purpose of identifying ***individual differences***. Among the most influential of current theorists is Cattell, whose 16 personality factors are thought to be due to a biological basis in the brain. Another prominent theorist is Hans Eysenck who has identified three personality dimensions: Extroversion-Introversion[1], Neuroticism, and Psychoticism. As a way of explaining this approach to personality, consider the first of these three dimensions. Extroversion-Introversion is thought to be due to the physiological arousal level of the person. A person with low arousal needs the external stimulation that the extrovert seeks to bring the arousal to a normal level. The introvert is already too aroused and avoids external stimulation.

Biological theories such as these place personality as part of the nature of the organism. Whether the source is a trait (Cattell) a type (Eysenck, Sheldon) or even a humor, it is due to a physical entity: the physiological make-up of the individual.

Furthermore, research showing that Introversion-Extroversion and Neuroticism are moderately heritable (Henderson, 1982) has encouraged the view that individual differences within the personality dimensions are the product of **genetically** determined differences in physiological make-up.

In these theories, personality is a physiological entity; it is some thing that you **have**. Measurements, in the form of personality tests (e.g., Cattell's 16 PF or the Eysenck Personality Questionnaire) are taken to determine how much of each trait or type you have. This is the most common approach to the study of personality. However, because this approach does not explain the progressive changes in individual reactions to the environment, it is not a developmental approach.

Behavioral Approaches

Many think behaviorists are disinterested in, or incapable of, offering an account of personality. If personality is meant only as a *thing,* then this is undoubtedly so. However, behavioral psychologists are interested in providing an account of personality when it is cast as a summary description of stable patterns of responding across settings. For the behaviorist, attributing a trait or type to someone is based on how that person behaves, not on what physiological structures he possesses. No one has seen a trait or type, but only inferred them from the behavior of the person. When we asked you to describe your friend, were the words you wrote down traits? Yes, in the sense that they described the characteristic behaviors of your friend. Words such as *humorous*, *smart*, and *energetic* are descriptions of behaviors that a person does across many situations, but not physiological entities. Some would have you treat these as the causes of your friend's behavior, but they are just descriptions of it. As we saw earlier, these are really descriptions masquerading as causal explanations. As such, they are circular explanations. We say a person is active, always moving, and vigorous *because* he is energetic. Yet how did we identify the trait as energetic? Because he is active, always moving, and vigorous. This is not to say that such explanations are never useful. If someone tells you that John is energetic, you can generally expect that he will work hard at most tasks he is presented. However, in labeling him "energetic," I have not identified the causes of his propensity to work hard. Our prediction is based on his previous behavior under various conditions.

Lundin (1961) defined personality as "that organization of unique behavioral equipment an individual has acquired under the special conditions of his development." Let us look at two of the important features of this definition.

First, personality is not just the sum of the person's behaviors. What leads us to call it personality is that the behaviors are **organized**. By "organized" it is meant that behaviors have a relationship to each other. This organized nature of the behaviors produces the characteristics which are unique to the individual. Rather than being the sum of individual behaviors, characteristic behaviors emerge. These characteristics called personality can be best analyzed at Horowitz's Systems Level II.

Second, personality develops under the individual's unique history of interactions between her genetic, historical, current physiological and environmental conditions. Significantly, these transactions produce a unique set of behaviors and reinforcers based on biological and learning factors. Thus, individuals labeled as introverts have different reinforcers than extroverts. It is not**just** that they engage in different behaviors.

Recall also Baer's suggestion that we behave in ways that maintain consistent environments. We do things to maintain familiar cues for our behaviors. For example, we select friends who talk about certain topics, or play familiar games. Furthermore, these friends engage in behaviors which produce reinforcing consequences for us. This makes it more likely that we will continue to seek out the same social environment. Friends also provide setting events and discriminative stimuli for the child to behave in characteristic ways. For example, a scout troop dresses in uniforms which make certain behaviors more likely to occur and be reinforced than other behaviors (e.g., helping old people across the street – even against their "will").

Is behavior totally characteristic across settings or is it situational specific? This is one of the great controversies in the field of personality theory. You probably can guess that biological theorists believe that the physiological mechanisms that cause personality produce consistent behavior across situations. They feel situations play only a minor role. In contrast, behavioral psychologists suggest that the environment plays the major role in our consistent pattern of behavior, but as situations change, so do behaviors. Behavior is specific to the situation.

A Dynamical Systems Approach to Personality

Our dynamical systems perspective assumes that both physiological and environmental factors play a role in determining the consistencies and changes in behavior. More specifically, our theory involves two types of interactions that the person has with her environment. These are ***genotype/environment interactions*** which emphasize how phylogenic characteristics of the person impact developing transactions. The second type are ***person/environment interactions.*** These show how ontogenically developed characteristics influence subsequent transactions. Both were introduced as basic processes in Chapter 3, but it is here, in the development of personality, that their roles come to the fore.

Genotype/Environment Interactions

One role for biological factors is the establishment of genotypes involved in the genotype/environment interactions described in Chapter 3. Recall there were three types of interactions, passive, evocative, and active. Recall also that it was hinted that there was a developmental sequence to the appearance of these. One way to look at the contribution of biology is initially through genotypes that react to the environment. These react first passively, then evocatively, and finally by actively selecting the environment. One area to look at for the beginning of personality may be in the initial behavioral differences called ***temperament.***

There are many theories of temperament. The first influential theory was proposed by Thomas, Chess, and Birch (1968). Studying 136 children over a 10-year

period they identified nine categories of behavioral style that they called temperamental characteristics. (Thomas, Chess, Birch, Hertzig, & Korn, 1963). These were:
Activity Level: This is whether the child generally is quiet or moving.
Rhythmicity: This is the regularity of biological patterns. It is reflected in the regularity of sleeping, eating, and elimination cycles.
Approach or Withdrawal: When touched, does the child respond positively, engaging the caretaker, or does the child withdraw and tense up?
Adaptability: Is the child able to adjust easily to changes in caretaking patterns?
Intensity of Reaction: Is the child relatively quiet and passive, or show extremes in crying and fussing?
Threshold of Responsiveness: How sensitive is the child to stimuli? Some are unfazed by relatively high levels of noise and light, others are hypersensitive, reacting at the drop of a pin.
Quality of Mood: Some children are happy, bubbly infants from the start. Others cry and are upset as in the classic "colicky" baby.
Distractibility: Some infants ignore novel stimuli, others are easily captured by them.
Attention Span and Persistence: Some infants are able to attend intently for a long time, others flit from interest to interest as new stimuli come along.

For more than two-thirds of their subjects the individual characteristics seemed to form an organized pattern in relation to the environment. Thomas and Chess (1977) identified three such patterns:
The Easy Child - These are children whose characteristics, such as moderate activity level, rhythmicity in biological functions, positive mood and others make care of the child easy. Some of these characteristics passively respond to and others evoke from the environment events that facilitate behavioral development.
The Difficult Child - This child's characteristics including negative mood, short attention span, nonadaptability react to and evoke environments that are nonfacilitative.
The Slow-to-Warm Child - This child's withdrawal, unpredictability in moods and biological patterns causes the child to respond to the environment less strongly and to evoke milder reactions from the environment than the difficult child. Development of a facilitative environment takes longer but probably will occur.

Thomas and Chess found that these characteristics tended to be long lasting. Difficult children are more likely to develop behavioral problems later (Thomas, Chess, & Korn, 1982). Yet, there is evidence that parental practices can strongly influence the development of child outcomes (Thomas & Chess, 1977). This illustrates the interaction of possible genetics, early history of interactions, current physiological conditions (e.g., mood, health) and current environmental conditions (i.e., current parental practices).

As development proceeds, temperamental characteristics become strengthened and organized into what we call personality. Now the child actively seeks environments that cue and reinforce the behaviors in their repertoires. Individual personality becomes stronger.

Individual characteristics may influence how the environment reacts to us. Some of these, such as our physical appearance, may be strongly determined by phylogenic factors. Consider the person with a babyface. Researchers, including Lorenz (1943) and Guthrie (1976), have suggested that people perceive a babyfaced person as childlike. Zebrowitz and Montpare (1992) have shown that not only can people reliably identify individuals with large eyes, a round face, thin, and a small nose bridge as babyfaced. Moreover, they perceive babyfaced adults as more childlike. That is, raters found people with babyfaces were more dependent, physically weaker, more naive, and physically weaker, more honest, and warmer than mature-faced people. Are similar effects possible due to the color of a person's skin, the gender they are, or even their physical size?

We may characterize these effects as genotype/environment effects. But since physical appearance may often be altered (as in a babyfaced person applying make-up to appear older, or a more mature person dying his hair), these are actually person/environment interactions. These types of interactions (passive, evocative, and active) may apply to the clothing we wear, as well.

What happens when environments change? Different environments evoke and reinforce different behaviors. Still we would expect to find many characteristic behaviors because if the environment is not too dissimilar it will evoke and strengthen the behaviors already strong in the repertoire. As the environment changes, so does behavior. We often hear statements such as "Johnny's a completely different child at school," or "Mary's a different person at work." Johnny is Johnny and Mary is Mary. It is their characteristic behaviors that are different in the different environments.

These are still person-specific environments for Johnny and Mary. They also influence their environments by the way they behave, even by the clothes they wear. What differences would occur if Johnny wore a school uniform versus a Bart Simpson sweatshirt and earring to school? But what if the environment is drastically different? Based on our history of interactions we will likely use characteristic behaviors. However we may not know the discriminative stimuli, and the reinforcers may not be present. For example, hostages often undergo dramatic changes in behavior. When Patty Hearst, the heiress to a huge publishing fortune was kidnapped by the radical Symbionese Liberation Army (SLA), her shy, quiet, conservative, college student behavior underwent many changes. After months in captivity she was photographed by a bank camera taking an active part in a violent hold-up. She appeared to be "a different person." After the destruction of the SLA and her return to her family Patty Hearst emerged appearing to be much the same "person" as before. What happened to her personality?

When environments are radically different, extinction of existing behaviors occurs. Changes take place in these behaviors through shaping. New behaviors coalesce, come to strength, and are organized into "a new person(ality)."

Sex Differences

Certain words are associated with one sex or the other. If you hear someone is "sensitive," "dependent," "pretty," or "indecisive," do you picture a male or a female? Which words come to mind if I ask you to describe the typical males? These are our sex role stereotypes, generalizations about each gender. As stereotypes, some may be true about one group or another, but need not be true for the individual. Some are not even true as generalizations about males or females. Let us look at these stereotypes and then how sex differences come about during development.

How Do Gender Related Behaviors Develop?

The interaction of organismic and environmental factors are clear in the area of sex role development. Gender is determined at conception by the presence of the sex gene based on whether the zygote has an XX or XY. Even before birth the differential treatment of boys or girls is already set in motion though the actions of baby showers, advertising and other environmental influences. At birth boys and girls are treated differently by parents, nurses and others. Not only are all three types of genotype/ environment interactions at work producing gender related behaviors, but societal, cultural, and parental expectations prompt and shape sex role specific behaviors as well.

Sex Role Stereotypes and Societal/Cultural Expectations

Recall Horowitz' levels of systems. We may analyze the processes that produce gender related behaviors at any of these four levels. All four systems are at work simultaneously to produce the behaviors typical of boys and girls. To understand how the four levels produce these behaviors we start at the highest level. The society and culture determine which behaviors will be shaped in their children.

In most cultures it is expected that males will develop an instrumental style and females an expressive one. However, this is not universal, and exceptions exist. societies promote their sex roles in many ways. Families, religious and social institutions, and media reinforce and model expectations about how boys and girls are supposed to behave which are consistent with existing sex role stereotypes. These create expectations in parents and others about appropriate gender related behaviors. How do these expectations translate into the development of gender related behaviors?

Parental Expectations & Reinforcement

Societal and cultural expectations are transmitted through the transactions between the child and parents. These transactions constitute Horowitz's System Level III. Because of the gender of the child, the parents have societally based expectations about what behaviors the child should do. Rubin, Provenzano, & Luria (1974) conducted a study in a hospital nursery with the parents of newborns. With only brief exposure to their neonates (not enough to detect real differences) both mothers and fathers described their daughters in language that was different from those who had sons. Although independent observers could record no such differences, daughters were described as smaller, weaker, and crying more. Sons, on the other hand were described as more active and more vocal. Again these were perceived differences, or expectations, not observed differences.

The existence of such differences in expectations in the first days of life suggest the importance of societal and cultural expectations. These differences are translated into transactional differences suggested in a study by Lyberger-Ficek and Sternglanz (1975). They observed that nurses in an infant nursery interacted differently with girls than with boys. Nurses were more likely to give more attention to boys not only when they were crying, but when they were quiet as well.

The power of expectations is also illustrated in a classic study by Rothbart and Maccoby (1966). These authors recorded a child's voice making statements. Parents were asked to write down their reactions to what the child said. Half of the parents were told that the voice belonged to a boy, the other half was told it belonged to a girl. Fathers who were told it was a girl were more permissive than those told it was a boy. The reverse was true for mothers. Thus parents have different expectations for the same behavior in boys than in girls.

Reinforcement of Gender Appropriate Behaviors

The emergence of gender appropriate behaviors requires differential reinforcement. Boys are reinforced when their behaviors are consistent with the expectations of parents, teachers, peers, and others.

Reinforcement is generally not given for behavior which is inconsistent with the sex role stereotype. Cross-gender behaviors may be punished by the environment. This may be particularly true with boys where "sissy" behavior is ridiculed or otherwise socially punished. Our society is more tolerant of "tomboy" girls, and such behaviors are less likely to be punished. Yet, as the tomboy enters adolescence, her cross-gender behaviors too may be punished.

The Development of Gender Specific Reinforcers

Boys and girls may be reinforced by different stimuli. Watson (1969, 1972) found that there were sex differences in the effectiveness of auditory and visual stimuli in children as young as fourteen weeks. Girls learned best with an auditory reinforcer (i.e., a tone) and boys with a visual reinforcer (i.e., a light). As development proceeds, new gender-appropriate stimuli become conditioned reinforcers. For example, in traditional families dolls are likely to be associated with positive reinforcement for girls, and trucks for boys. Thus, playing with sex role appropriate toys becomes automatically reinforcing.

Developmental Changes in Gender Related Behavior Gender Identity

By the age of two most children know their gender (Thompson, 1975) and prefer to play with toys which are traditionally associated with their particular sex (Weinraub, Clemens, Sockloff, Ethridge, Gracely, & Myers, 1984). This knowledge of one's sex is called ***gender identity***. For example, at this age girls are more likely than boys to play with dolls. By the time they are three, children act out sex-typed roles (Eisenberg-Berg, Boothby, & Matson, 1979). Thus, at this age a boy is more likely than a girl to assume the role of a fireman while playing.

Gender Stability

At around the age of five or six, children know that their sex is not going to change. This is called ***gender stability***. Furthermore, at this point, they begin to prefer and imitate those of the same sex (Bryan and Luria, 1978).

Gender Consistency

By the age of six most children have developed full-blown gender stereotypes (Huston, 1983). A final characteristic of their stereotypes is ***gender consistency*** – the knowledge that sex roles are consistent across settings.

A result of these changes is a solidification of behaviors which are consistent with their sex role stereotypes. For example, they are likely to maintain that men cannot be nurses and to ridicule any boy who plays with dolls (Marantz and Mansfield, 1977). As children continue to develop, these gender stereotypes broaden and become more divergent. As evidence of this, one study discovered that fourth and fifth graders believe that men and women differ greatly in terms of a number of stable personality traits. For example, these elementary school children viewed women in general as weak and emotional, while men were viewed as ambitious and dominating (Best, Williams, Davis, Robertson, Edwards, Giles, & Fowles, 1977).

Androgyny – Combining Roles

Some have argued that these rigid sex-roles are harmful because they limit the behavior of both males and females. Indeed, Sandra Bem (1975, 1978) asserted that individuals who possess both masculine and feminine traits are better able to adapt to different situations because of their sex role flexibility. In short, Bem endorsed ***psychological androgyny***. According to Bem, men should respond to some situations by being forceful and to others by being gentle; similarly, women should be dominant when the situation requires it, and defer to others when that is the best strategy.

In an attempt to demonstrate that androgynous individuals are more adaptable than those who are traditionally sex-typed, Bem and her colleagues first developed the Bem Sex Role Inventory to allow the differentiation of androgynous people from others. Next, in a series of studies (e.g., 1974, 1975, 1981), they tested her hypothesis. One study found that when compared to traditional sex-typed subjects, androgynous individuals were more likely to display behavioral flexibility. Specifically, they were more likely to act independently (a "masculine" trait) when the situation required it, and to act in a nurturing manner (a "feminine" trait) when that approach was most efficacious. In another study, androgynous adolescents and college students were compared to those with traditional sex-roles, and were found to have higher self-esteem and to be viewed as more likable and well-adjusted by their peers (Major, Carnevale, & Deaux, 1981; Massad, 1981; Spence, 1982). Although androgyny has had its harsh critics (e.g., those who charge that it promotes a unisex society), there remains strong evidence that individuals benefit from having both masculine and feminine characteristics (Spence, 1984).

The Self

The self is one of the oldest and most familiar concepts in psychology. How shall we look at it from a natural science perspective? What is the self? If the mind is located in the head, where is the self located? What is the relationship between the self and personality?

Skinner (1989) noted that Webster's *Third New International Dictionary* contains about 500 entries that begin with "self." As with personality, many theories look at the self as a thing, as an object. William James drew a distinction between the "***self-as-knower,***" and the "***self-as-known.***" The self-as-knower is equivalent to your listing of words to describe yourself. It is the you that *you* know. The self-as-known equates to your listing as others see you. It is the public you. It is your personality as you think others see you.

From a natural science perspective, personality is the organization of characteristic behaviors under a unique developmental history. The self is verbal behavior describing your own personality (Skinner, 1953). The self is usually private verbal behavior – your thoughts that describe your characteristics – but these self descriptions may be made public (as when I asked you to describe yourself at the beginning of this chapter). The self-statements may be made with respect to your own evaluation, with respect to how others may see you, or as evaluative statements. Evaluative statements are also called ***self-esteem.***

Self Concept and Self Recognition

The preverbal child may be said to have a self-concept. This self-concept is inferred from the child's behavior with respect to stimuli pertaining to self. Lewis (1987) concluded that there is little evidence for self-recognition before eight months of age. Thus the child does not differentially respond to his picture or to himself in a mirror at this age. It is not until 12 months of age that children show self-awareness, which Lewis takes as the emotional reaction to seeing themselves in a mirror.

But under what conditions do self-recognition and self-awareness develop? Let us look at a history which will produce self-recognition.

First, parents constantly speak the child's name across a wide range of situations. The child also learns "you" and "your." These verbal stimuli accompany situations involving the child's image in pictures and in the mirror. For example parents ask "Who's that?" and then say "That's Mary." The child's image of itself in a mirror or a picture becomes discriminative behaviors with respect to itself. Behaving in front of the mirror produces different consequences than behaving in front of a picture or another person. The movement of a part of the body is accompanied by a change in the stimulus. In the presence of a mirror, the child makes a response and is reinforced by a corresponding visual cue. With the parents' labeling of the stimulus in the mirror with the infant's name or "you," the self-recognition develops into self-awareness.

Parents encourage their children to provide self statements. They ask, "How do you feel?"; "What do you think?"; "Why did you do that?" Hayes (1988) has suggested that this produces ***literality***. That is, the parents prompt and then strengthen the equivalence between the child's self-statements, behaviors, and physiological responses. Thus, children behave as if their thoughts were the same thing as their physiological conditions. The words "I am afraid" become attached to the physiological condition of fear.

Parents also encourage the development of ***reason giving*** (Hayes, 1988). They ask "Why did you do that?" and reinforce the child's verbal response "I did it because . . ." If a child breaks a dish, the parent is likely to ask "Why did you break that?" and expects the child to state a reason by making an "I- statement". Since parents reinforce the child for providing the I-statements, either by agreeing (*i.e.*, positive reinforcement) or by terminating further demands for an answer (negative reinforcement), reason giving becomes a strong response for the child and the reasons become secondary reinforcers. Thus the child will engage in reason giving I-statements even without reinforcement from the parents because they are automatically reinforced (see Chapter 9). It is reinforcing to give reasons. Reason giving continues throughout life. As adults we continue to give reasons for our behavior and treat the reasons as the actual causes of our behaviors.

Reason giving I-statements may start out as public verbal behavior that is reinforced by others. However, it becomes private behavior because it is self reinforcing and because revealing self-talk is often punished as we get older. Some of the reasons given attribute the cause to external events ("It was too heavy," "I didn't see the ball on the stairs," "The other driver cut me off."). Besides being external, these causes are specific to the event. Other causes refer to our own, more permanent, characteristics ("I'm not very strong," "I'm hyperactive," "I'm not a good driver.") Rotter (1966) distinguished between these two stated sources of cause as external or internal ***locus of control***. Furthermore, Rotter (1966) thinks that some children are characteristically "externalizers" and others "internalizers" because they have learned to attribute causes to either an external or internal source.

Stable vs. Unstable Traits

Those viewing the source of control as being an internal condition also view these causes as being stable. That is, a cause due to a trait of the self is rather stable. For example, if the child attributes his failure to his lack of intelligence, he is unlikely to behave in a way to change his performance. In short, he is more likely to give up trying. On the other hand, causes that are external are viewed as more likely to change. So if the child attributes his failure to bad luck, or a hard test, then he is more likely to try again. These unstable causes are not seen to be part of the characteristics of the self.

Self-Efficacy Beliefs

Bandura (1977) used the term ***self-efficacy beliefs*** for self statements about the ability to succeed in accomplishing specific behaviors. Bandura found self-efficacy statements to be central in coping with stressful situations and to underlie all successful therapeutic interventions. He proposed that the development of self-efficacy beliefs originated from four sources. First was the actual successful accomplishment of tasks. A child who is successful has a history of success. Second, observing a model be successful sets the occasion for a child to imitate the behavior and become successful, as in the child who sees an adult fold a paper airplane, and the child follows. Third, others can use verbal persuasion, encouraging the child by providing efficacy statements, such as "See, now you can do it too!" Finally self-efficacy beliefs are enhanced (or weakened) by the emotional arousal of the child. The child who is excited may be more (or if too excited, less) likely to make self-statements about being able to accomplish a task, such as jumping a stream or speaking in front of an audience.

Self-Esteem

Self-esteem includes the evaluative statements about what we can do and how we appear to others. A person with a high self-esteem emits self statements with high positive value, such as "I'm good at math," "I'm pretty good looking," "People really like me." A child with a low self-esteem makes self-statements of high negative value "I'm dumb at math," "I'm ugly," or "People don't like me." Like most self-statements, these are likely to originate from others in the child's social environment: parents, siblings, or teachers. They attribute good or bad outcomes to enduring internal characteristics of the child (e.g., personality, intelligence, aptitude). Positive statements are associated with other positive reinforcers (good math grades, praise) and the statements become positive self-reinforcers when the child emits them privately.

The low self-esteem statements become self-reinforcers as well. Saying the child is dumb "explains" why the child got bad grades and terminates the aversive situation. Likewise "ugly" explains unpopularity and is negatively reinforcing. Pejorative statements by others become negative self-reinforcers because they terminate aversive events.

Self-Control

A final topic dealing with the self is called self control. This area deals with **resistance to temptation**. In this situation the child is faced between obeying a societal rule (e.g., "Don't eat the candy.") and yielding to the sweet siren call of sugar coated chocolates. Some explanations of children who can resist temptations such as these rely on internalized states or conditions, such as "high ego strength" or a "strong superego." However, from a dynamical systems perspective, we may see the child's dilemma as a choice between behaviors which have different consequences, and the history of the child with respect to these.

Box 10

Delay and Choice

As Andy Rooney might say: "Did you ever notice how all the candy bars are on display right at the check-out stand at the grocery store? – Did you ever notice?" Well, the store manager who puts them there understands the classic problem in self-control–that immediate reinforcement nearly always wins out over delay of gratification. One thing that managers and economists also know is that if it takes time to get a reward, the value of the reward becomes less. Kagel, Green, & Caraco (1986) call this change in the value of a reward as a function of increased time ***delay discounting***. For example, you may choose $100 now over $300 in 5 years. Why do we do this? Kagel, et al. (1968) have argued that we have learned that there is risk implicit in waiting, and that this delay discounting is an adaptive response to uncertainty in an organism's natural environment.

It turns out that an equation can be constructed which predicts the behavior of various organisms, including pigeons and humans, given various combinations of amounts and time delays. Both pigeon choice of food and human choice of hypothetical amounts of money are discounted in the same way (Rachlin, Raineri, & Cross, 1991). The formula is:

$$V = \frac{A}{(1 + kD)^2}$$

(Where V is the value of a reward, A, the amount of the reward, D the delay of the reward, and k is a constant – the larger the value of k, the greater discounting).

Len Green and his associates (Green, Fry, & Myerson, 1994) wanted to know if this same mathematical function held up in predicting the discounting behavior of young children, young adults, and the elderly. The subjects included groups of 6th graders, college students, and older adults (mean age 67.9 years). Subjects were given binders of file cards with pairs of various monetary amounts and times. One choice was always one fixed large delayed amount (either $100 and $1,000 for the 6th graders, or $1,000 and $10,000 for the adults). There were 6 different delays for these rewards, ranging from 1 week to 25 years. The immediate rewards ranged from .1% to 100% of the delayed amount with which they were compared. For example, a choice might have been between $1,000 in 10 years or $100 now.

The choices of all subjects in each age group were combined to produce ***equivalence points.*** These were the points at each combination of amount and delay in which the immediate reward matched the delayed one. These data were plotted and mathematically generated curves were fit to the data.

The results showed both similarities and differences in the age groups. All groups showed discounting (reducing the size of the immediate reward they would accept as equal to the delayed one).The same basic mathematical formula given above fit all groups. However, the constants were different. Children discounted much more quickly suggesting that they did not value the delayed rewards as much. The children were also more sensitive to short delays than adults who were more sensitive to long delays. The result is what we would call impulsivity. That is, children will accept a smaller immediate reward in place of a large delayed one, and the delays they will tolerate are very small. The older adults were the most willing to accept large delays for large rewards and discounted least.

So, the next time you pass the candy display with a child, don't try to suggest that if he waits he can have a better dessert. The child will probably discount what you're saying.

Often the need for self-control occurs when we have a choice between a behavior which has an immediate but rather small (such as the taste of the candy) reinforcer versus a behavior whose consequence is delayed but larger (praise from the adult). Much of human development involves such choices between buying a piece of candy or saving up for a new video game, or tasting the smoke of a cigarette versus not smoking and adding years to one's life. Rachlin (1976) presents such dilemmas as choices between behaviors which have small immediate consequences versus those that have large, but delayed ones. He concludes that living things follow the ***matching law.*** This law states that we closely match our behavior to the value of the consequences of each behavior.

Based on a study involving self control in pigeons (Rachlin & Green, 1972), Rachlin provided a formula that predicts the behavior of a college student faced with a choice between studying versus going to the movies. The formula states that the person will do the behavior for which the consequences has the highest value. The value of the consequences involves both the amount of reinforcement (or punishment) and the time before the consequence occurs. If both behaviors have consequences that are immediate, such as going to the movie now, or taking a final exam now, then the student should study, since passing the exam is a larger reinforcer than watching the movie. Likewise, if both the exam and the movie are the same time in the future, say one week away, the student will study. However, if the student can go to the movie now and the exam is a week away, the value of the choice switches and the student goes to the movie. The matching law explains why it is easier to give in to the temptation of eating a snack versus resisting that temptation and looking slim for swimsuit season.

How do we engage in self-control? We learn to emit behaviors which change the matching law equation. In other words, we learn to change the value of the consequences. We can do this by increasing the amount of reinforcement. We may do this by adding reinforcers for the desired behavior, such as adding self-praise ("Good, I lost three pounds this week.") or giving ourself a special reward (e.g., buying a new bathing suit). Or, we may increase the aversiveness of the undesired behavior (fining ourself for a transgression, or nagging ourself).

When we use such strategies we also are making consequences of the delayed behavior more immediate. For example, posting a particularly bad photo of an out-of-shape self on the refrigerator door makes the consequences for eating not only more aversive, but more immediately so.

The term "self" refers to many phenomena and may be used in many contexts. In this chapter we have looked at several ways in which the term has been used and noted that these often include very different aspects of the term.

The Self Revisited

In summary, taken together, the self statements we make constitute our **self-concept**. The topics of self-recognition, literality, reason giving, locus of control and self-efficacy, combine to suggest a theoretical approach to self-concept. The response class of self-statements we make regarding our publicly observable behavior may make up what James called "the self-as-known." This is the self we call "me". The class of self-statements that includes private as well as public behavior about what our behavior constitutes James' "the self-as-knower," or "I."

Footnote

[1] In Eysenck's theory, two of these dimensions are bipolar. That is, they are continua with opposite endpoints. Extraversion-Introversion mark the extremes of the first of these. The second, Neurotocism, runs from "stable" to "unstable". The Psychoticism factor has no opposite poles. It is a factor that varies in strength from person to person.

Chapter 11

Prosocial Development

Social Behavior as Operant Interactions

In our coverage of operant interactions (Chapter 7) we emphasized the four term contingency. As you recall, the contingency involved (1) a discriminative stimulus signaling (2) a response which was followed by (3) a reinforcing stimulus occurring in the context of a general (4) setting event. Recall the schematic below:

$$S^d \rightarrow R \rightarrow S^r$$
(Setting Event)

In this chapter, we focus on social transactions which also are four-term contingencies. What makes social transactions unique is that one person's behavior functions as discriminative and/or reinforcing stimuli for another. Thus we have reciprocal interactions in which one person's *behavior* functions as a *stimulus* for others. These dynamic, reciprocal interactions mutually influence the development of the behaviors of individuals in social transactions.

Consider the following meeting of two individuals, Bert and Ernie:

Bert's Contingency:			
Sees Ernie	"Hi Ernie"	E. smiles	
S^d →	**R** →	**S^{+r}**	
	(Setting Event = Walking along)		
Ernie's Contingency:			
	"Hi Ernie"	E smiles	Bert Smiles
	S^d →	**R** →	**S^{+r}**
	(Setting Event = In a good mood)		

Notice the **same event** ("Hi, Ernie") that functions as a *response* for Bert, functions as a *discriminative stimulus* for Ernie. Note also that we are analyzing one small segment of a series of interlocking chains of behavior. It is as if we are looking at a still frame of a video. If we were to resume "play" of this transaction we would note that Ernie's smile serves not only as a reinforcer for Bert's "Hi, Ernie," but that Ernie's smile also serves as an S^d for Bert's next behavior, perhaps evoking a smile from Bert. We could continue analyzing these interlocking chains until the two parted and ceased to function as the stimuli for the others' responses.

Behavior is both an event controlled by social stimuli, and itself serves as a social stimulus for the behavior of others; this is the essence of social transaction. This is our analysis of social transactions at the level of basic processes (Level 1). This chapter (and the next on antisocial interactions) is about long-term changes in social transactions (Level III). That is, here we focus on the dynamic outcomes of the basic processes: how reciprocal social interactions produce what we call prosocial transactions such as attachment, separation anxiety, and altruism.

The Functions of Social Behaviors

The child enters this world with a set of Universal I behaviors, reflexes. These enable him to transact with others. Not only are reflexes elicited by other people, but the child possesses characteristics (including "cuteness" and "cuddliness") and emits reflexes (such as the smiling reflex), which function to evoke caretaking behavior directed at the child. Ethologists suggest that such universal behaviors evolved because of natural selection. Individuals who evoked caretaking by their parents were more likely to survive the vulnerable period of infancy to grow to maturity and have offspring of their own who possessed these characteristics as well.

Thus we first examine the phylogenic basis for prosocial behaviors.

Phylogenic Contributions to Social Development

Ethologists have argued that natural selection would have favored the evolution of characteristics which would promote the development of caretaking behaviors. They argue that vulnerable human newborns would be more likely to survive if they possessed characteristics which elicited or evoked parental caretaking. Among these proposed characteristics of the child are the child's physical appearance and her initial reflexive behaviors.

Physical Characteristics

Has there ever been an ugly baby? Certainly not, if you ask parents. Neonates have unique appearances which most of us see as cute. Not only are newborns' heads disproportionately large, compared to adult proportions, but their facial characteristics are different too. Lorenz (1943) observed that the large forehead, prominent eyes, flattened nose, and small chin characteristic of newborn humans, also are characteristic of other newborn animals. It is suggested that such universal "cute" characteristics evolved through natural selection because they elicit in adult members of the species positive emotions which promote caretaking.

Social Reflexes

Included in the repertoire of reflexes that the human newborn possesses are the so-called social reflexes. These reflexes, such as smiling and crying, have the function of evoking parental caretaking. While these behaviors may originate as reflexes, they may soon develop into operant behaviors as well, since they produce reinforcing consequences.

Facial Expressions

Izard and Malatesta (1987) have reported ample evidence that most human emotional responses display a facial expression that is based on specific muscular patterns which are universal. That is the muscles involved in showing interest, disgust, and smiling are the same for all infants. Following a line of reasoning first suggested by Darwin (1872), Izard and Malatesta conclude that these universal facial expressions are the result of phylogenic contingencies that have selected genotypes for these expressions because they contribute to the survival of the infant by evoking parental caretaking.

Both the expressions of "interest" and "disgust" are present at birth, with the smile appearing three- to four-weeks later (Izard & Malatesta, 1987). An interest reflex can be elicited by novelty or a human face (Izard & Malatesta, 1987). Painful stimuli and discomfort elicit the facial expression of disgust.

Crying

Recall (Chapter 9) that at least three distinct cries can be detected in newborns: hunger, anger, and pain. Each is elicited by one of these classes of stimuli (i.e., hunger, anger, pain) and have the function of causing the caretaker to terminate the aversive stimulus affecting the infant. The adaptive significance of these behaviors is clear. Of additional significance is that crying can have an influence on parental caretaking even if the parent is at a distance. This is not true of physical characteristics or facial expressions. These require that the parent has visual contact in order to be influenced by them. Crying can evoke parental behavior from the next room (and while the parents sleep!).

Neonatal Imitation

Consider the basic problem in imitating motor behaviors. Let's play the game "Simon Says." I am the model. I raise my hand over my head, saying "Simon says, DO THIS". Go ahead, do it! If I raised my right hand, which one would you raise? How do you know that what you did matches, or looks like what I did? Did you look in a mirror to see if your gesture looked like mine? Of course you didn't. Imitation of gestures seems to require knowledge that the child's own unseen behavior matches that of the observed model. Because he felt such knowledge requires cognitive development, Piaget concluded that true imitation does not emerge until the last quarter of the first year (Anisfeld, 1991).

In the mid 1970's psychologists (e.g., Maratos, 1973; Meltzoff & Moore, 1977) first reported observations of newborns imitating adult facial and motor gestures. They videotaped the faces of newborns who watched adults model behaviors such as sticking out their tongues (tongue protrusion), smiling, or exaggerated eye movements. If a child behavior occurred in the next time interval following a model's behavior and it matched the form of the models behavior, the child's behavior was considered imitative. Children as young as two days old (Meltzoff & Moore, 1983) were said to imitate adult facial gestures. Such early appearance strongly suggests that these are Universal I behaviors that have evolved because of phylogenic contingencies.

This raises the question of whether such neonatal imitation is the basis for development of later imitation. After carefully reviewing the evidence, it does not seem that neonatal imitation is the same phenomenon as later imitation (Poulson, de Paula Nunes, & Warren, 1989; Anisfeld, 1991).

How does neonatal imitation differ from later imitation? First, it appears that neonatal imitation is more limited and less robust than originally suggested. In his review of 19 well controlled studies on neonatal imitation, Anisfeld (1991) concluded that the only behavior for which there is strong evidence for imitation is tongue protrusion. Studies attempting to demonstrate the imitation of other behaviors have either failed to be replicated or have strong methodological flaws (Anisfeld, 1991).

Second, even tongue protrusion may be elicited by a stimulus other than the behavior of a model. Jacobson (1979) showed that tongue protrusion in six-week-olds could be elicited by a ball or pen moving toward the child, just as readily as by an adult protruding his/her tongue. She concluded that rather than true imitation, it was behavior released (or elicited) by any stimulus that contained curvature and concentricity.

Third, neonatal imitation seems to disappear around two months of age. Imitation of adult behaviors disappears only to develop slowly over the first nine months (Uzgiris, 1972). Thus it appears that there is little evidence that neonatal imitation directly leads to generalized imitation (Poulson, et al., 1989; Anisfeld, 1991).

However, neonatal imitation may have been selected by phylogenic contingencies because it facilitates the development of social interaction. Bjorklund (1987) felt that one of the functions of early imitation was to focus the infant's attention on the adult's face. In our view, the neonatal behavior may facilitate the development of true imitation by reinforcing the parent's modeling behaviors. Papousek & Papousek (1981) have noted that both mothers and fathers model feeding behaviors such as mouth opening, lip movements, and licking, for their infants. Some of these modeled behaviors may act as stimuli eliciting neonatal imitation. The newborn's matching behaviors may serve as positive reinforcing stimuli strengthening the modeled behaviors of the parent. This makes it more likely that the parent will prompt further imitation. Thus, the neonatal behavior may reinforce the beginnings of the reciprocal interactions between parent and child. The development of reciprocal interactions may be a hidden skill which leads to the development of true imitation, and might form a basis for later language learning.

Ontogenic Contributions

Although phylogenically based universal social reflexes such as tongue protrusion may contribute to the survival of the human species, most social behavior is more varied than this and develops over a long period of time. Thus, we now turn our attention to how social behaviors develop over the life span of the individual. To do this, we must look at the development of social transactions.

Social Behaviors

Social behaviors are those actions of an individual which involve transactions with others. That is, social behaviors are responses of an individual which are strengthened or weakened by the reciprocal actions of other individuals or groups.

Reinforcement

Social behaviors are strengthened by the actions of others. That is, they produce social reinforcers (See Chapter 7). Recall that social reinforcers are considered secondary or acquired reinforcers – stimuli which acquire their strengthening

Box 11

The Power of Touch

Human touch can be a very powerful reinforcer. Researchers at Florida International University and the Touch Research Institute at the University of Miami have conducted a series of studies investigating the usefulness of this variable. Early on in the study of social reinforcers, researchers often used touch as part of a package of social reinforcers that also included a smile and vocalization. (Rheingold, Gewirtz, & Ross, 1959, Weisberg, 1964). However, without appropriate controls, some have argued that touch elicits, rather than reinforces behavior. That is, touching a child might elicit a sound from the child in the same manner that a tickle or pinch would. To verify that touch is reinforcing, it is necessary to keep the number of touches equal, but to vary whether the touch is contingent on the behavior of the child or independent of the child's behavior (Poulson, 1983). If the number of touches is the same, but the child only increases behavior when touch is contingent on the response, then touch is a reinforcer, not an unconditioned (or conditioned stimulus). A recent study (Pelaez-Nogueras, Field, Cigales, Gewirtz, Malphurs, Clasky, and Sanchez, 1993) showed exactly this. Ten infants from 1-1/2 to 3-1/2- months old received two types of social reinforcers. In the Touch Condition, infant eye-contact responses were followed by adult smiling, cooing and rubbing of the child's legs and feet. The stimuli continued as long as the child continued eye contact in what is called a "synchronous reinforcement" procedure. In the No Touch Condition, the rubbing was omitted. All infants showed more eye contact during the Touch Condition indicating that touch was an additional reinforcer for eye contact. In addition the touch had the effect of eliciting increased smiles and vocalizations and in the Touch Condition, children spent less time crying and protesting.

In order to investigate the type of touch that infants most preferred, the same research team (Pelaez-Nogueras, Field, Gewirtz, Cigales, Gonzalez, Clasky, and Sanchez, 1995) conducted a study comparing massage-like touch with poking/tickling touch. The massage-like touch consisted of deep but gentle circular rubs starting at the infant's legs and moving up to the abdomen and forearm. Poking/tickling touch consisted of a pattern of deep, but short nudges along the same path on the child's body. Both types of touching were delivered using the synchronous reinforcement procedure in which the stimuli were presented when the child made eye contact and were withdrawn when the child looked away.

The results from this study showed that massage-like touch strengthened eye contact more than the tickling/poking touch. In addition, massage-like touch increased smiling and vocalizations more and decreased crying compared to the poking/tickling. Since the stimulation could be terminated by the infant by looking away, the increases in looking away, crying, and protesting suggests the poking/tickling, although gentle, was, nevertheless, a negative reinforcer.

These studies demonstrated not only that touch serves as a reinforcer, but it can also elicit positive affect. Furthermore, the type of touch is important. Rhythmical, massage-like touch is more reinforcing than intrusive poking and tickling. Consequently, the same researchers wondered if they could use touch as therapy for infants of depressed mothers. Depressed mothers frequently have nonfacilitative effects on their infants. Infants of depressed mothers are likely to show less attentiveness, fewer smiles, lower activity levels, and more fussing (Cohn, Campbell, Matias, & Hopkins, 1990). And While Field, Healy, Goldstein, Perry, Bendell, Schanberg, Zimmerman & Kuhn (1990) showed that these infants would continue to act "depressed" with a "non-depressed adult stranger, that need not be the case. Pelaez-Nogueras, Field, Cigales, Gonzalez, and Clasky (1994) showed children act less depressed in the presence of an adult who is familiar with the child (i.e., a nursery school teacher), than they act than with their depressed mothers. This suggested that the interactions the child has with the caretaker elicits and reinforces the infant's negative moods.

Finally, the researchers (Pelaez-Nogueras, Field, Hossain, & Pickens, 1995) undertook a study to see if teaching the depressed mothers to use massage like touching could lead to positive affect and attention. The results showed that by using massage-like touch depressed mothers, even in a condition in which they kept a straight, non-expressive face, could get their infants to increase smiling, vocalizations, and looking at the mothers' hands. Thus it appears that depressed mothers need not produce poor emotional outcomes in their children. Certain kinds of touch can be effective in overcoming some of the nonfacilitative effects of the negative affect of depressed mothers.

characteristics because they are associated with primary and other secondary reinforcers. In this analysis, stimuli which are reliably present when behavior is reinforced become discriminative for reinforcement and therefore become reinforcing stimuli as well.

Bijou and Baer (1965) described how mothers (or other caretakers) are likely to emerge early on as social reinforcers. In their analysis, the mother is likely to provide positive reinforcers (e.g., food, water, taste stimuli, pleasant temperature, tactile stimulation, visual and auditory stimuli) and to remove negative reinforcers (e.g., roll the child off of uncomfortable hard objects, move out of harsh light, burp the child to relieve him/her of gas build-up, massage aching gums, drive away pesky older siblings or pets, etc.). Thus, by this combination of providing positive reinforcers and removing, terminating, or avoiding negative ones, the caretaker becomes discriminative for reinforcement. In addition, her/his presence and actions come to strengthen child behaviors which produce the caretaker's presence or actions. Caretakers become positive reinforcers.

Proximity

Bijou & Baer (1965) argued that at first just the proximity or nearness of the mother is reinforcing. That is, the child engages in behaviors which bring the mother near. Some of these proximity producing behaviors may originate as reflexes, especially the smiling and crying reflexes described previously. In our analysis, these behaviors soon acquire a new function, to bring the mother near.

Attention

While the mother's proximity is a reinforcer, Bijou & Baer (1965) suggest that children learn that in some situations, just having the mother nearby is less reinforcing than getting her to direct her behavior toward the child. For example, a child cries and her mother picks him/her up, or a child tugs at his father who asks "What's wrong? Thus, the caretaker's *attention,* not just *proximity*, becomes a reinforcer. From then on, behaviors which produce these directed changes in the parent's behavior (i.e., attention) become more frequent.

Attention producing behaviors have unique characteristics. They may be considered verbal behaviors in the form of mands. "Mommy!!!," a tug on the mother's arm, or even hitting a younger sibling meet the criteria for a mand in that they are emitted in a state of deprivation for the caretaker's attention and reinforced by the mother's attentional response (i.e., "What is it dear?", a look down, "Stop that hitting.") As with most mands, attention seeking behavior is more likely to occur with deprivation of the reinforcer. That is, a child is more likely to emit "Mommy", a tug, or hit another when the child is deprived of adult attention. Child-parent problems often arise when a child learns that high magnitude behaviors (e.g., cries, biting another child, attempting suicide) are necessary to produce the reinforcing attention of others. Parents often fail to see that their reaction to these attention seeking behaviors, such as yelling at the child to stop, function as reinforcers. However yelling at the child meets the criteria that define a positive reinforcer if the yelling strengthens the child's behavior which produced it. So, parents (and others too) often think they are punishing behavior when in fact they are unwittingly reinforcing it. This principle of human behavior is what underlies the saying, "It's the squeaking wheel that gets oiled."

Since attention producing behaviors are often problematic for parents, teachers, and others, finding ways to reduce these behaviors is of interest. There are three primary ways to reduce mands for attention. In the first method, extinction, we may try to ignore the behaviors and expect the behavior to slowly decrease. While this procedure may eventually work, it has several problems. First, withholding attention means that the deprivation of adult attention becomes greater and is likely to increase, rather than decrease demands for attention. Second, ignoring the behavior usually results in an extinction burst (See Chapter 7), so that the behavior in the short run is likely to escalate rather than decrease. That means a mand for attention may turn into a full-blown tantrum. Third, the increased attention seeking behavior means that it is even more difficult to ignore, thus increasing the likelihood that it will eventually be reinforced. This means that the behavior will be maintained under an intermittent reinforcement schedule (specifically, a Variable Ratio). Therefore, the behavior will become increasingly resistant to extinction and continue to occur with intermittent reinforcement. For these reasons, extinction by itself is rarely the answer to reducing attention seeking behavior.

A second method, ***Differential Reinforcement of Other behavior (DRO)*** combines the extinction of the undesirable attention seeking behavior with reinforcement of another, incompatible behavior. An ***incompatible behavior*** is one which cannot be done at the same time as the first. For example, sitting quietly with hands folded is incompatible with yelling and flailing the arms to get attention. The advantages of DRO (also called the ***incompatible response technique***) are twofold. First, a desired response is strengthened making the undesired one less likely to occur. Second, attention is provided so that deprivation of the desired reinforcer does not happen. These are the principles behind the advice, "Catch them being good!"

A third technique to reduce attention seeking behavior is punishment by hurt (Chapter 7). Parents may apply some aversive stimulus (e.g., a spanking, a threat) contingent on the attention seeking behavior in an attempt to reduce the undesired behavior. Unfortunately, as we have seen above, unless the aversive stimuli are strong and consistently applied, the long term effects may be to reinforce, rather than decrease the attention seeking behavior. The use of these aversives is likely to be unsuccessful for other reasons. First, adults may be reluctant (for moral or ethical reasons) to administer strong aversives, and to do so consistently. Second, aversives may negatively reinforce escape behaviors, so that the child avoids or escapes from the adult. This escape interferes with the positive role of parenting or teaching.

Punishment by loss (Chapter 7) is the final technique that can be used to reduce undesirable attention seeking. Recall that this involves the contingent loss of positive reinforcers. Taking away privileges, such as TV time or outside play is sometimes used by adults to reduce undesirable behavior, including attention seeking. These procedures can be effective if the reinforcer that is lost is large enough and if the punishment contingency is immediate. One problem with the procedure is that the loss of reinforcement is often delayed (e.g., "You can't watch TV tonight", "You can't go to the movies on Saturday). It has been suggested that the delays in sending criminals to prison due to complications in legal due process (refer to the O.J. Simpson trial) has rendered prison a less effective deterrent to criminal behavior than it otherwise would be.

A second type of punishment by loss is called ***time out***. In time out, an undesirable behavior is immediately consequated by removing the child from reinforcement. Usually this involves placing the child in a room or corner for a brief period of time. The purpose is to have the undesirable behavior result in the loss of the reinforcers the child was receiving. It is effective if the loss of reinforcers is immediate and brief. It's purpose is to punish the behavior, not to isolate the child. Studies have shown that time out is effective when a brief time out from positive reinforcement of three to five minutes immediately follows as a consequence of undesirable behavior. Again, the purpose of time out is to punish the behavior by a brief, contingent loss of reinforcement, not to isolate the child from his environment.

Affection

While *attention* reinforces behaviors which the provider may find desirable or undesirable, the last of Bijou and Baer's classes of social reinforcers, ***affection*** is likely to be provided for behaviors which elicit feelings of affection. Usually affection takes the form of hugs, kisses, smiles, pats, nuzzling, tickling, hair ruffling, special crooning tones of voice, and affectionate words, but the exact form will vary from one parent-child dyad to the next (Bijou & Baer, 1965). Bijou and Baer suggest that there is a great deal of variability from dyad to dyad, not only in the form of affection provided, but in the amount. They point out that parents invariably reinforce by being near and providing attention, but they need not give affection. Therefore, there may be some parents who provide little affection as positive reinforcers.

Those who do provide affection often find that because it, unlike proximity and attention, is likely to follow "desirable" behaviors, it strengthens these desirable behaviors. Contingent use of affection is an effective way to shape desired behavior:

> "The ease of giving affection for good behavior, and the natural tendency not to present it and to withdraw it when confronted with bad behavior, set up situations which strengthen selectively those behaviors which please the mother, rather than those which displease her. This line of reasoning suggests that children who are maximally responsive to affection as a positive reinforcer are more readily influenced by the mother's goals for them than are children more responsive to her attention than to her affection" (Bijou & Baer, 1965, pg. 141).

Observational Learning

If we were to ask you to say the Polish word for "good," we could wait for you to pronounce it and then reinforce you. Assuming you do not speak the Polish language, this would take a long, long time, as it is unlikely that you would emit the correct sounds in the course of a normal lifetime! Likewise, we could employ shaping, waiting until you emitted an approximation to the sounds, reinforcing you, and then reinforcing ever closer approximations to the word itself. While this would be somewhat faster, and be more likely to succeed, it would still take a very long time. No, neither of these reinforcement methods would be very effective. Instead, our success would likely be enhanced by modeling the sound "dub-zhe" and prompting you to imitate it. Imitation is the basis for what is called ***observational learning***, or changes in behavior brought about by watching the behavior (including the verbal behavior) of others.

How are we to analyze observational learning? Do we need a new set of principles to explain it? Much of the early work on observational learning was conducted by Albert Bandura and his colleague, Richard Walter, at Stanford University. Bandura and Walter published much of their work in an important early text *Social Learning & Personality Development* (Bandura & Walter, 1963). Bandura followed this description of experimental work with a systematic treatment in his book, *Social Learning Theory* (Bandura, 1977). In his early work, Bandura treated the learning of behavior through the observation of models as following basic learning principles. While he believed reinforcement of behavior was important, he felt that reinforcement affected the **performance** of the behavior, *not* the **learning** of it. This distinction between learning and performance and whether unique processes were involved became key issues in understanding observational learning.

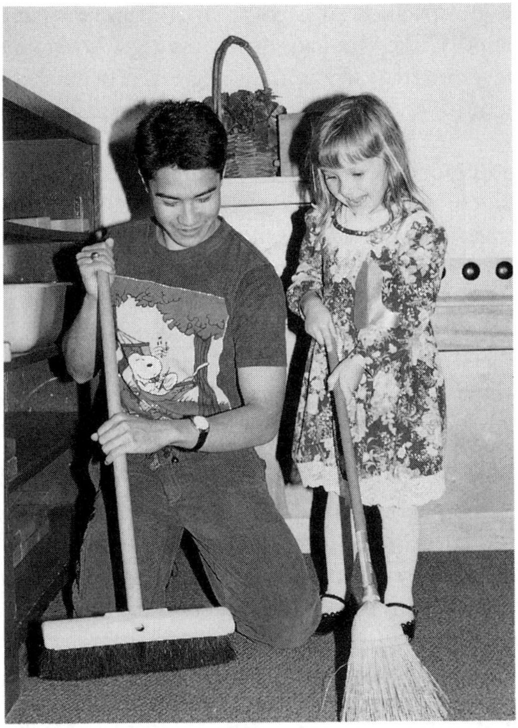

Bandura based the learning-performance distinction on his classic "Bobo" doll studies (Bandura, Ross, & Ross, 1963; Bandura, 1965). In one of these studies (Bandura, 1965), children watched filmed adults (models) emit aggressive behaviors against Bobo dolls. The adults modeled physical (e.g., kicking, hitting with a hammer) and unique verbal (e.g., "Wettosmacko") behaviors. One third of the children saw the model in the film severely punished. Another third of the children saw the model receive praise and rewards. The remaining third saw a film in which the model was neither punished nor praised.

After watching the modeling on film, the children were brought in to an observation room with a Bobo doll and aggressive implements including a hammer and knife. The children were observed in two post-modeling sessions. In the first, the *performance test*, children were not given consequences for aggressive behaviors. Under these conditions, the children in both the model rewarded and model no consequences groups *performed* significantly more aggressive responses than the children in the model punished group.

However, in the second session following the film, the *learning test*, all children were told that they would get highly attractive rewards if they could reproduce the model's behaviors. Under these conditions, the differences between the groups vanished. All three groups showed high rates of aggressive responses. Even sex differences disappeared. Girls, who had shown less aggressive behavior than boys in the performance test, emitted nearly as many aggressive behaviors as the boys under the learning test conditions. All children had *learned* the aggressive behaviors of the model.

Bandura, and other social learning theorists have used these studies to make two points. First, since all children were able to reproduce the behaviors when offered a reward, they all *learned* what the model did, regardless of whether the model was reinforced, punished, or neither. Therefore, Bandura concluded, reinforcement is **not** necessary for *learning* behavior, but only the *performance* of it. Second, Bandura theorized that reinforcement (and punishment) need not be direct, but could also be experienced by watching others. Thus, ***vicarious consequences*** (i.e., ***vicarious reinforcement*** and ***vicarious punishment***) were thought to be key aspects of observational learning which had their effects on performance of behavior.

An Operant Approach to Observational Learning

While Bandura felt new principles, such as vicarious consequences, were needed to explain observational learning, others felt that existing principles of operant learning were sufficient. Gewirtz and Stingle (1968) presented the argument that vicarious reinforcement actually does not function as reinforcement (i.e., to strengthen the behavior of the observer). Instead, they suggested that the behavior of the model is a discriminative stimulus which signals the observer that a behavior which matches the model's behavior will be reinforced. This happens because of a history of interaction in which the observer has developed generalized imitation (Chapter 9). That is, behaviors which match a models behaviors are frequently reinforced by the consequences they produce. For example, a child watches another child open a puzzle. When the observer matches the puzzle solving behavior, she too is reinforced by the solution to the puzzle. When we view the consequences to the model as discriminative stimuli rather than vicarious reinforcers, we can also understand a phenomenon known as "counter-imitation." In ***counter-imitation***, a child observers another child do something that is reinforced, but the observer does not match the model's reinforced behavior. She may even do the opposite, or counter-imitate. For example, Johnny may watch his older brother get away with cookie nabbing behavior, but Johnny doesn't try it because he has learned that his brother's behavior is punished, not reinforced. His brother serves as a discriminative stimulus that signals a matching behavior would likely be punished, not reinforced.

From this perspective, we imitate a model's behaviors when they are discriminative for direct, not vicarious consequences to the imitator. Thus if we look at Bandura's (1965) study, we can see that in the absence of offering the child contrived rewards, the child is likely to match the model's behavior if the model is reinforced by toys or by the fun of hitting the Bobo doll. This is generalized imitation. In the absence of the direct consequences to the contrary, observing a model who is punished for aggression means the child is not very likely to aggress himself. Finally, when children are offered extrinsic rewards to imitate the behavior, the verbal cue is a setting event establishing that repeating the model's behavior will be reinforced.

Observational Learning of Respondents – Emotional Behavior

In Chapter 6 we examined how we may acquire fears and other emotional responses by the process of respondent learning. As you recall, a neutral stimulus becomes a conditioned stimulus because of its pairing with an unconditional stimulus for the emotional response. However, as suggested by Bandura (1969), emotional responses may be conditioned vicariously, as well as directly. That is, emotional responses may be learned by observing them in others as well as by experiencing the conditioning procedure ourselves.

A clever study of college students by Berger (1962) illustrates vicarious respondent conditioning. The students were assigned to one of two groups. In the vicarious conditioning phase, both groups witnessed the same event: a model was seated at a table, as the light dimmed, a buzzer was sounded and then the model rapidly jerked his arm off of the table. The control group was told this was a reaction time study and the model was trying to lift his arm as soon as the buzzer sounded. The vicarious conditioning group was told that the model was receiving an electric shock when the buzzer sounded, and that the jerking of the arm was a response to pain. Thus, this group was led to believe that the model was expressing pain, and that the buzzer was associated with electric shock.

Following the observations, the subjects were tested for vicarious conditioning. Their galvanic skin response (GSR), which is a measure of sweating associated with emotional arousal, was measured to the same buzzer which they had heard when they had seen the model's performance. That is, they were tested to see if the buzzer came to be a CS for the CR. There was no changes in GSR for the Control Group. Remember, they were told they were watching a reaction time study. Apparently, the buzzer remained a neutral stimulus for them. However, subjects in the Experimental Group showed increased GSR activity. The buzzer had *vicariously* become a conditioned stimulus for those who had thought they had seen the model being shocked. This suggests that we may come to fear (or like) things by merely watching others become conditioned to them, not just by experiencing the conditioning directly ourselves.

Verbal Instruction – Rule Governed vs. Contingency Shaped

Another way that we may learn from others is through verbal instruction. Consider the following example: A child sees a new video game at the arcade. How does she learn how to play it? How does she learn what she must do to win? One approach would be to come in contact with the contingencies directly. That is, she could put her money in and play. Some of her behavior would be reinforced, some punished, and some have no consequences. Gradually, she would learn how to play the game. This could be a slow and expensive way to learn the contingencies of reinforcement. This is ***contingency shaped behavior***.

Alternatively, our game player could learn the contingencies from the rules about how the game works. By either reading the rules or by listening to skilled player tell her the rules, she could learn what behaviors are consequated and in what manner. Her behavior would be what Skinner (1969) called ***rule governed behavior.*** In Skinner's (1957) view, rules specify the contingencies of reinforcement and punishment. Furthermore, rules can usually be learned in less time than needed to derive the contingencies by direct trial-and-error experience (Skinner, 1974).

Zettle and Hayes (1982) identified two styles of responding based on the relationship between rules and contingencies. The first is called ***tracking.*** A person who tracks is sensitive to the natural environmental contingencies in effect. Rule following puts them on the right track and then they track the actual contingencies in effect. For example, a tracker may take the rule "Walk – you'll get there just as soon" and follow it until she finds that she is usually late. At that point, her sensitivity to the contingency (loosing out on some fun) will enable her to try the other behavior and to track whether it is better at producing reinforcing consequences.

In contrast to this is ***pliance*** (from the word "compliance"). Plyers learn to comply with the behavior specified by the rules, even if the rules do not accurately specify the contingencies in effect. For example, given the same rule ("Walk–you'll get there just as fast) a plyer will continue to follow the rule, insensitive to the actual contingencies. Thus tracking and pliance may be two different response styles characteristic of individuals. They are likely to develop under different conditions. One of these, the style of parental discipline used by parents is discussed in Chapter 13.

Riegler & Baer (1989) presented a developmental analysis of rule-following. In their analysis, the development of rule governed behavior relies on five steps. These steps need not occur in order, but may happen simultaneously. The steps are:

1)Early in the child's life, the parents provide stimuli for compliance. These take the forms of requests, commands, rules, etc. At first, children follow specific requests, demands, or rules given by the parent. The parent is likely to reinforce compliance of these specific rules or instructions.

2) These requests, demands, and other rules function as instructions. Because instructions specify what response will produce a reinforcing (positive or negative) consequence, they become discriminative stimuli. The result is that a child may engage in generalized compliance. That is, the child will follow nearly all instructions because of his history of reinforcement to responding to other members of this instructional stimulus class. This is maintained as long as there is a correspondence between the rules-behavior-and consequences in most cases.

3) Compliance generalizes to other aspects of the child's environment. Now the rules of grandparents, teachers, and others are followed in the same manner as the parents' rules. The child can learn to discriminate those whose rules lead to reinforcement and those whose rules do not. Thus, the child may learn to

not follow the rules of a culture (e.g., "Thou shalt not steal." — but crime pays) or for drug use where adults say "Just say no", while peers say it is fun.

4) The child generates her own rules and instructions from imitating the rule giving behavior of adults. Adults may prompt the development of this self-instruction by asking the child "What are you going to do" and by reinforcing the child's overt self-instructions. Eventually children are prompted and reinforced for making their instructional self-talk private rather than public.

5) The use of self-instructions generalizes so that they can be used in novel situations. For example, the child can say to himself "No, I shouldn't cheat on this test," without ever hearing another say that. Generalized self-instruction becomes the basis for a highly compliant child.

Prosocial Transactions – Intuitive Parenting

How do parents know when and how to interact with their children? Is there a phylogenic basis for social interaction? As noted above, there is some evidence that physical and behavioral characteristics of the infant elicit positive maternal responses. From an ethological viewpoint, it would benefit the species if respondent caretaking responses were hard-wired. However, knowing how to interact with a neonate need not require a phylogenic explanation. It is likely that, because of the social experiences the parents have had with other adults and children, parents, particularly mothers, may intuitively know how and what to do to take care of and interact with their infants.

Papousêk and Papousêk (1987) have detailed many parental behaviors directed at infants. They have identified six ways in which parents intuitively interact with their infants in order to promote learning in their infants. These six ways are:

1. Creating and maintaining an awake state.
2. Presenting a simple structure of stimuli and learning trials.
3. Providing a large number of repetitions of trials.
4. Gradually ordering of tasks so that there is increasing complexity.
5. Using adequate reinforcers.
6. Being sensitive to feedback signals indicating the child's limits of tolerance.

These characteristics that parents use intuitively in early social interactions are conditions which promote the development of learning in their infants. They are remarkably similar to the characteristics described by Moerk (1989) (Chapter 9) of parent-child interactions in the learning of language. It suggests that early on, parents already know or develop the skills necessary to teach their infants to acquire basic skills and abilities in social, cognitive, and linguistic domains.

Social Behaviors in Infancy

Attachment

Above we have described some of the characteristics of the infant which evoke caretaking behaviors from adults. We have also described how these caretaking behaviors are likely to reinforce proximity, attention, and affection producing behaviors in the infant. When the infant's proximity and security-regulating behaviors become *organized* around one or more particular caretakers, we say the child is developing an ***attachment*** (Bretherton, 1987, pg. 1063). When we say the behaviors are "organized", we mean that more than just individual behaviors occur. Instead, attachment is characterized by dynamical patterns of behaviors focused on the attachment object (i.e., the caretaker). Bowlby (1969, 1973, 1980) proposed that attachment evolved due to phylogenic contingencies in which behaviors which protected the child from predators were naturally selected. Petrovich and Gewirtz (1991) argued that both phylogenic contingencies and ontogenic contingencies, in which caretakers reinforce proximity, imitation, and identification (Commons, 1991) contribute to attachment. The combination of phylogenic and ontogenic contributions to attachment is consistent with a dynamical systems approach.

Social Cognition

In her review in the *Handbook of Child Psychology* (Mussen, 1983), Shantz referred to ***social cognition*** as "the development of social knowledge and reasoning". She went on to suggest that it focuses on "understanding the relationship between social behavior and cognitive development between thinking and behaving, between social and nonsocial knowing" (pg. 495). From a dynamical systems view, we may analyze social cognition in the same way that we analyze other cognitive behavior (Chapter 8). Therefore, we focus on three aspects of social cognition (Novak, 1987):

1. Social Knowledge: Knowing about things in social situations. For example, saying "please" when asking for something or wearing the appropriate clothes for a rock concert vs. a funeral.
2. Social Abilities: Knowing how to do things of a social nature. For example, being able to initiate conversations or being able to play house.
3. Social Problem Solving: This involves manipulating public or private events (i.e., thoughts) to produce solutions to social problems. For example, both Mary and Marisa want to swing but there is only one swing, Mary offers to let Marisa go first and to push her so that she can swing next.

Thus, in this view, social cognition it treated in the same manner as other cognitive behavior. What is special about social cognition is that in these four-term contingencies, cognitive behavior is influenced by the behavior of other individuals. This means that cognitive behavior is a function of setting events, discriminative stimuli, and reinforcing stimuli, all or some of which may be social in nature.

Separation Protests

Visit nearly any child care center or preschool at the beginning of a new year and you are certain to observe separation protests by infants and toddlers. The protests take the form of cries, whines, screams, whimpers, grabbing on to the parent's body or clothing, and pleading or imploring (Gewirtz & Pelaez-Nogueras, 1991a). Some children are particularly upset and their displays of "separation anxiety" are dramatic. Other children do not exhibit any of these protestation behaviors. As pointed out by Gewirtz and Pelaez-Nogueras, 1991a), many explanations have been offered for the causes of the behavior, including "attachment" (Bowlby, 1960), "security of attachment" (Ainsworth, Blehar, Waters & Wall, 1978), and "separation anxiety" (Kagan, Kearsley, & Zelazo, 1978). Let us look at the possibility that separation protest might develop as learned interactions between the child and parent(s).

As we have described earlier, the caretaker becomes reinforcing for many infant behaviors. Loss of a reinforcer, as occurs in separations of the parent and child at the

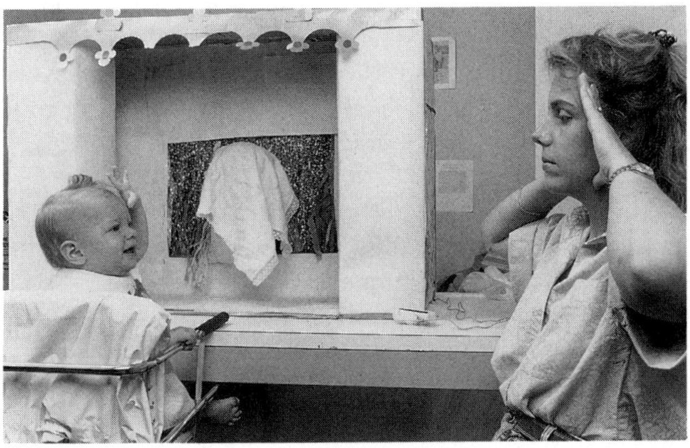

Mother gives the "palms-to-both-cheeks" cue to her infant.

start of school, is aversive to the child. The loss elicits some emotional respondents as well as evokes behavior which may function to get mother back. Jack Gewirtz and Martha Pelaez-Nogueras (1991) have conducted studies on how the mother-infant interaction influences the development of separation protests.

In one of their first studies (Gewirtz &Pelaez-Nogueras, 1991a), the researchers hypothesized that protest behaviors were shaped by contingent maternal responding to the protests. They further hypothesized that separation protests could be reduced if parents would differentially reinforce behaviors other than protest behaviors (see, DRO or incompatible response technique, above).

In the study, twenty-three infants 6 to 11months-old and their mothers were studied in a laboratory setting. Mothers were given cues by a private earphone to signal the child that she was leaving by standing up, kissing the child, waving and saying "bye-bye, I'll be right back." At this point the mother left the room for up to three minutes, at which point she returned. After a brief reunion, another separation trial was conducted.

The effects of two conditions of reinforcement, CRF and DRO were compared. In the CRF (contingent - Continuous Reinforcement) condition, every infant protest to the mother's separation cues was reinforced by the mother by stopping, retracing her steps, turning to, speaking to the child, etc. In the DRO (noncontingent

- Differential Reinforcement of Other behavior) condition, an infant's protests cued by the mother leaving, never received contingent reinforcement from the mother.

The child-mother dyads were given 6 to 8 separation trials daily for 8 to 12 days. An ABA design was used in which successive trials of a noncontingent baseline (DRO) were followed by trials of the contingent responding to protests (CRF), which in turn were followed by a return to the DRO of baseline. Analysis showed significant increases in protest behaviors during the contingent CRF trials compared to both DRO conditions.

The authors concluded that separation protests, which have been used by others as a measure of the strength of attachment, can be learned as operants. They go on to suggest that such operant learning "is very-likely trained inadvertently in the life settings in which it occurs by the maternal reactions that operate under the conception of positive, responsive, 'loving' mothering" (Gewirtz & Nogueras, 1991, pg. 4).

In viewing these typical transactions from a dynamical systems viewpoint, we must point out that while the above study demonstrates how the mother is likely to shape the child's behavior in separation protests, the interactions are reciprocal. It appears that mothers "inadvertently" reinforce protestations because in doing so, the mother is likely to reduce (at least temporarily) the whining and crying. Thus, her behavior is shaped by the child through negative reinforcement, while the child's behavior is shaped by the mother through positive reinforcement.

Fear of Strangers

The crying and screaming of children experiencing stranger anxiety is said to emerge between 6 and 7 months and to peak at 8 to 10 months (Sroufe, 1977). Explanations for its development include the development of attachments and the development of a cognitive representation or schema for the mother (Kagan, 1974).

Gewirtz and Petrovich (1991) suggest that an approaching stranger is a discriminative stimulus for the disruption of a child's ongoing, positively reinforced behavior with the mother. They cite a finding by Emde, Gaensbauer, and Harmon (1976) that infants picked up by a stranger in the mother's presence cry more than if the mother is not there. Presumably, crying in the presence of the mother is likely to cause the stranger to put the child down, allowing the previous reinforcing interaction to resume.

With experience the child learns other stimuli, such as strangers, may be associated with harm, and these strange stimuli evoke and elicit the crying we call stranger anxiety. This analysis is supported by research which shows that characteristics of the setting (e.g. a strange room) and characteristics of the stranger's behavior (e.g. threatening facial expressions, speed of approach) affect the occurrence of crying.

Social Referencing

One factor which seems to affect the child's response to strangers during this period is the behavior of familiar others, particularly the mother, but this has also been demonstrated with familiar same-age companions. As the stranger approaches, the child observes the facial expressions and physical and motor behavior of the familiar person. This looking at another's facial, vocal, or body expressions as a discriminative stimulus for one's own behavior is labeled ***social referencing***. Traditionally, it has been suggested that the child references the person's emotional characteristics and must have the cognitive ability to interpret these with respect to his/her own behavior.

Behaviorally, we view this an example of social knowledge. With experience, the child learns that if the mother is smiling when the stranger approaches reinforcement is likely. However, if the mother is cringing, crying may prevent the stranger from hurting her. Thus, the facial expression of the mother becomes a setting event which establishes the function of the stranger as being discriminative for positive or negative reinforcement. That is, if the mother is smiling, the stranger may evoke attention from the child if the mother is showing concern, the stranger may evoke crying from the child.

Gewirtz and Pelaez (1990) designed a study to see if infants could learn to respond to maternal "expressive" cues in ambiguous situations. The mother's cues were chosen arbitrarily for being neutral for the expression of emotions. These cues were either *palms-to-both-cheeks* (in which the mother held her palms against the sides of her face) or *fist-to-nose* (in which the mother held her clenched right fist to her nose). Both cues were selected because they have no preexisting status as emotional cues. This enabled them to be acquired as social referencing cues through learning.

Twenty children ranging in age from 9 to 12 months were seen daily with their mothers over a period of eight to thirteen weeks. On each trial, a covered, ambiguous object was placed before the child. This was followed by the mother giving one of two initially neutral cues when the child turned and looked at the mother. When the child turned back, the object had been uncovered and moved within reach of the child. If the child reached for the object, one of two consequences was delivered, based on the cue given by the mother. For half the children, the mothers *palms-to-both-cheeks* behavior was predictive of a pleasant consequence and reaching was consequated by a brief musical baby melody and slow movements of the object. For these subjects, the *fist-to-nose* was predictive of an unpleasant consequence; a harsh door buzzer, concrete drill, or food blender sounds accompanied by rapid movements of the object. The specific cue-response-consequence ($S^d \rightarrow R \rightarrow S^r$) relationship was reversed for the remaining children.

The results showed that children learned to use the mother's cue as a discriminative stimulus for reaching, depending on the consequences associated with the cue. That is, children showed greater reaching than baseline rates when the *palms-to-both-cheeks* cue was associated with the pleasant consequence, and less reaching when it was associated with the aversive consequence.

Thus, the experimenters showed that any arbitrary stimulus could come to function as a discriminative stimulus whose function is much like that of the mother's facial expression in social referencing. Gewirtz and Pelaez-Nogueras,

(1992) argued that this is a laboratory metaphor for the way social referencing develops in the child's interactions with the parents. That is, the child learns through operant conditioning that the caretaker's facial expression becomes reliably associated with specific consequences that the child experiences.

Sibling Rivalry

An example of how peers are entangled in a system involving themselves and their parents is in sibling jealousy or "sibling rivalry". A common experience of parents (just ask them) with more than one child is the setting event of a telephone call or a neighbor coming to the front door. Suddenly, two children begin to act up, argue with each other and make enough noise that the parent can't continue with the phone call or conversation. Conventional wisdom is that this is worse with twins for whom the sibling rivalry is greatest. Because "sibling jealousy" or "sibling rivalry" are descriptive terms, they do not constitute true explanations of behavior. That is, to say that twins are acting up because they are jealous is tantamount to saying "They're acting up because they're acting up"; a circular explanation.

Instead, to explain this behavior, it may be better to ask, "Under what conditions does the acting-up occur?" In a laboratory analog of real-life jealousy, Roth and Gewirtz (1995) did exactly that. They reasoned that jealous behavior occurs in triadic (i.e., three-person) social contexts or setting events where the mother's attention elsewhere becomes a discriminative stimulus for emitting jealous behaviors. Depending on the child's interactional history, the class of jealous behavior may take the form of crying, fussing, whining, screaming, whimpering, calling for the mother, hitting, punching, proximity seeking, reaching out to be picked-up, staring, frowning, pouting, stiffening the body, placing the body between the mother and the other child, or even imitating the behavior of the rival (Roth and Gewirtz, 1995). As an operant, the development of jealous behavior is under the control of its consequences. Regardless of topography, the functional class of jealous responses is aversive to the mother and she is negatively reinforced for attending to them since when she does, the aversive jealous behavior stops. At the same time, mother's attention positively reinforces that child's jealous behaviors. A further problem with jealous behavior is that the rival observes the reinforcing consequences received by the other child which makes that more likely to engage in jealous behavior herself/himself.

In the study, Roth and Gewirtz worked with three sets of twins and their own mothers. One of each set was put in playpens placed 1.4 meters apart. Their mother sat on a chair about a meter in front and equal distance between the playpens. The mother wore an earphone so that she could hear instructions from the experimenter. Two conditions, CRF (Continuous ReinForcement of jealous behavior) and DRO (Differential Reinforcement of Other than jealous behavior) were alternated between each twin over a total of three phases. In the first phase, after a brief period facing forward, the mother was asked to turn toward and speak to Twin 1 and thus reinforce this twin's non-jealous behaviors (DRO). When Twin 2 emitted a jealous behavior the mother was instructed to turn to that infant and interact with that infant. In essence that reinforced Twin 2's jealous behavior (CRF). When Twin 1 showed non-jealous behavior, the DRO procedure was used and that behavior reinforced. The initial length of time with no protests required for Twin 1 to receive reinforcement was started at 2 seconds and was lengthened to 10 seconds. Thus the DRO procedure also included shaping of a longer period of non-jealous behavior. In phase 2, the contingencies were reversed and in phase 3 the contingencies were reversed again so that they were the same as phase 1.

The contingencies of reinforcement determined the amount of jealous behavior shown by the twins. Under CRF conditions for jealous behavior, jealous protest behavior was high. When behavior other than jealous protests were reinforced, jealous behavior decreased. The study suggests that we look may look at social behaviors, such as jealousy, as a class of operants reinforced by dynamical interactions in the family system rather than as individual traits.

Social Behaviors in the Preschool Years

Altruism

Altruism is defined as the principle or practice of unselfish concern for or devotion to the welfare of others (Random House, 1973). Thus, the development of altruism concerns how we engage in behaviors that directly benefit others, not ourselves.

A number of prominent theorists have asserted that infants are incapable of altruistic behavior. For example, Freud maintained that from birth to one year (the oral stage) a child obeys the *pleasure principle* by selfishly behaving in ways which will orally gratify the sex instinct. The child continues to obey the pleasure principle, according to Freud, from one to three years of age (the anal stage) when the focus of his pleasure-seeking behavior shifts from the mouth to the anal region. It is not until three to six years of age (the phallic stage) that the child exhibits altruistic behavior. During this stage the child develops a superego by internalizing his parents moral values, including altruism. Once the superego is formed, altruistic behavior is possible.

Similarly, Piaget held that from birth to six years of age (i.e., during the first stage and most of the second stage of cognitive development) the child's behavior serves her selfish interests. Indeed, Piaget theorized that the preoperational child reasons egocentricly and thus, behaves in a self-centered manner. However, during the last year of child's second stage of *cognitive* development, the child enters his first stage of *moral* development. Specifically, Piaget asserted that at six years of age a child begins to observe socially defined rules, including those requiring or encouraging acts of altruism.

As we have seen, both Freud and Piaget claimed that altruism appears rather late in childhood. There are some data to support the claim that infants are non-altruists. For example, 6 to 12 month old infants show little response when others are in distress (Hay, Nash, & Pedersen, 1981; Zahn-Waxler & Radke-Yarrow, 1982).

However, there is considerable evidence that at approximately one year of age children begin displaying altruistic behaviors. In surveying the literature, Eisenberg and Mussen (1989) found evidence that 12 to 18 month olds often respond to another's distress with agitation or prolonged attention (Kiselica & Levin, 1987), 18 month olds often respond to another's suffering by trying to comfort them, and that by two years of age, children will frequently try to help someone in distress by bringing them an object, verbally comforting them, or offering suggestions (Radke-Yarrow, Zahn-Waxler, & Chapman, 1983).

There is also evidence that altruism in children increases with age. For example, the value of anonymous gifts given to those in need usually increases with the age of the gift giver (Radke-Yarrow et al., 1983). Furthermore, there is a small increase in helping behavior with age (e.g., Underwood and Moore, 1982). In their survey of the literature, Eisenberg and Mussen (1984) concluded that, despite some evidence to the contrary (e.g., Gottman & Parkhurst, 1980; Ekholm, 1984), as the child ages there is generally an increase in prosocial behavior.

Causes of Altruistic Behavior

Phylogenic Factors

In presenting his theory of evolution by natural selection, Darwin (1859) characterized the daily life of individual organisms as a "struggle for existence." Each individual must fend off predators, compete for limited life-sustaining resources, and struggle against other threats to its existence. As a result of variations between individuals, some are better fit than others for this struggle. Those better fit are more likely to survive and reproduce; those less fit are less likely to live long enough to produce offspring. As a result of this differential reproduction, the environment selects favorable, genetically controlled variations to be passed on to succeeding generations while unfavorable, genetically controlled variations tend to die out. Borrowing a phrase from Herbert Spencer, Darwin came to characterize this process of natural selection as the "survival of the fittest."

The principle of natural selection presents a problem for genetically-based accounts of altruistic behavior. Individuals who inherit genes for altruistic behavior are likely to act in ways that decrease their own chances of surviving and reproducing. Thus, according to the principle of natural selection, genes for altruistic behavior should become quite rare over the history of a species. How, then can one successfully argue that altruistic behavior is the product of genetic inheritance? As E. O. Wilson (1975) succinctly phrased the question, "how can altruism, which by definition reduces personal fitness, possibly evolve by natural selection?" One suggested mechanism is selection by the group, rather than the individual.

Group Selection

Wynne-Edwards (1962) argued that animals generally refrain from over exploiting the resources of their environment, especially the available food supply. He asserted that they avoid this over exploitation by practicing reproductive restraint.

As he theorized it, animals engage in genetically determined behaviors called ***epideictic displays*** which allow the members of a given species living in close proximity, to judge their numbers in relation to the available resources. Examples of epideictic displays include the pre-dawn howling of monkeys and the evening flight of flocks of birds. According to Wynne-Edwards, if such displays indicate that a species numbers within a region exceed the available resources, the species members living within that region will restrict their rate of reproduction.

For example, consider the female English great tit (a bird). Although it sometimes produces a clutch with as many as thirteen eggs, on average these birds produce only nine or ten eggs per clutch (Lack, Gibb, & Owen, 1957; Barash, 1982). Thus the English great tit typically produces a smaller number of offspring than she is capable of producing. It would appear that she is behaving altruistically by suppressing her reproductive rate. How can we explain this apparently altruistic behavior in Darwinian terms? Doesn't the principle of natural selection suggest that the frequency of genes for producing larger clutches would have greatly increased over evolutionary time, resulting in larger clutch sizes as the rule instead of the exception? Wynne-Edwards' theory suggests that, in response to some level of epideictic display, the English tit restricts its reproductive behavior.

In proposing his theory of the altruistic behavior of reproductive restraint, Wynne-Edwards began by noting that animals form into discrete groups which compete against each other. Next, he argued that any group which, as a whole, is better fit to survive than its competitors has a reproductive advantage and will be selected as a group by the environment. Any group which is less fit is likely to reproduce in smaller numbers and die out. Classical Darwinian theory postulated that natural selection operates on individual organisms. However, Wynne-Edwards' theory utilizes the mechanism of group selection to explain the alleged evolution of behavior which is detrimental to the survival of a given individual but which promotes the survival of the group.

Group selection theory has not been limited to explaining apparent reproductive restraint. For example, Campbell (1965) has invoked this theoretical approach as part of his explanation of self -sacrificial behavior in humans. History is replete with examples of individuals who have sacrificed their lives to help others or in defense of ideologies. An individual pushes a stranger out of the way of an oncoming car and in so doing is struck down himself. Others go off to war and die in defense of abstractions like freedom, Christianity, or the American way. As Campbell observed, if self-sacrifice is not universal, it is at least ubiquitous. Campbell concluded that self-sacrificial behavior is caused, in part, by genes which have survived and proliferated because they promote the survival of groups.

Recently, David Sloan Wilson and Elliott Sober (1994) have supported the group selection view. They argue that groups function as higher order organisms in selection. That is, the level of organism, individual, or group, is irrelevant. Selectionism can occur on the group, in much the same was as for the individual. Groups or individuals are merely "vehicles" for selection.

In sum, the phylogenic view suggests that behavior, such as altruism, which is detrimental to the individual, but adaptive for the group may be selected by natural consequences. However, the consequences must select group-wise, rather than for the individual's behavior.

Chapter 12

Development of Antisocial Behaviors

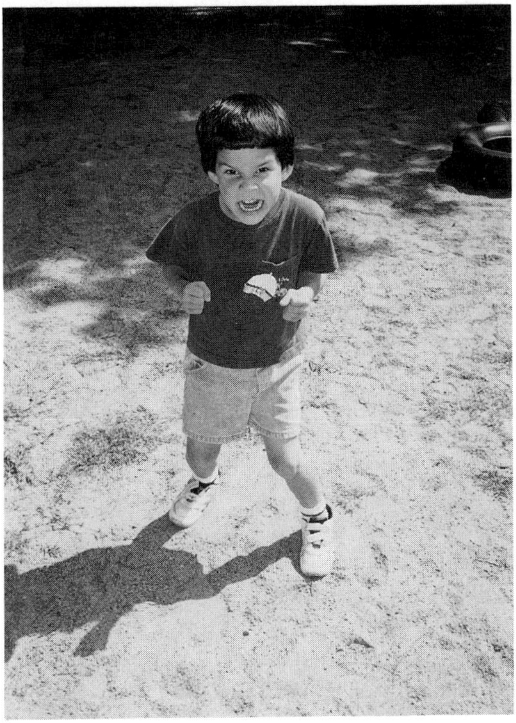

Antisocial Interactions

One of the most important issues facing society is the problem of antisocial behavior, or aggression. Crime is one of the top issues in public opinion polls. Violence intrudes into more lives each year. We all experience the effects vicariously from virtually every local news broadcast or newspaper front page. Increasingly antisocial behavior is becoming more violent. The U.S. Justice Department (1994) reported that there were nearly one million crimes involving handguns in 1992, resulting in over 13,200 homicides. All told, there were more than 23, 000 murders in the U.S. in 1992. From 1991 to 1993, more than 11,000 children in California were wounded or murdered by firearms (McLeod, 1995). California children have become more likely to die from gunshots than from automobile accidents. In 1993, more than 61,000 juveniles were arrested in the U. S. for weapons crimes, more than double the number in 1985 (Sniffen, 1995)

Homicides and violent crimes are the most dramatic cases, but the development of antisocial behaviors begins early and effects extend well through adulthood. More children are referred for psychological treatment for behavior disorders than any other condition. People fail to hold jobs, maintain marriages, and run into trouble with the law because of the antisocial behaviors they commit. This chapter looks at antisocial interactions as a developmental process.

What are antisocial interactions?

Most people would equate antisocial behavior with aggression. However, the term aggression is a social, not a psychological one. Two characteristics are normally present when society deems an act aggressive. First the behavior must be at a high intensity or rate. Hitting, biting, kicking, and hair-pulling are high magnitude behaviors in children. Verbal aggression and "passive" aggression (refusing to comply) are also intense behaviors.

Second, society requires that for an act to be aggressive, it must be intentional. Accidents are not considered aggressive. We infer intentionality from the aggressor's behavior, including facial expression and verbalizations. Our jury system acknowledges the importance of intention in sentencing a person for killing another: manslaughter is the verdict if the act was an accident; murder if the act was intentional (First degree for premeditated).

Psychologists have difficulty objectively studying ***intentionality***, since it must be inferred, rather than directly observed. However, its presence seems crucial in a socially valid definition of aggression. According to the traditional mentalistic account, an intentional act is one which is preceded and caused by a specific mental act. For example, a gunman's thought about shooting an adversary causes him to pull the trigger.

On the other hand, for the behaviorist an intentional act is one which occurs because it has been reinforced. Johnny hits his younger brother Bill because the latter then gives up his candy. However, this is not a complete behavioral account. Johnny is also likely to have been punished in the past for hitting his brother. For example, his parents might have grounded him for a night, resulting in his aggressive behavior decreasing dramatically for some time. In short, aggressive behaviors have participated in conflicting contingencies of reinforcement and punishment. How then does the behaviorist explain why, at one moment, Johnny intentionally aggresses and at another moment intentionally behaves nonaggressively?

There are many explanations possible. Johnny, though effectively punished in the past, may again aggress against his brother when the punishing agents (his parents) are out of the room. Or he may aggress when his parents are in the room because the reinforcing consequences (his brother has Johnny's favorite candy) outweigh the punishing consequences (being grounded for the night).

Let us consider how transactional development affects intentional acts of aggression. Active genotype/environment interactions may mean that Johnny may seek environments which reinforce aggressive behaviors. That is, Johnny may select situations in which his active behavior is reinforced by "weenie" children who cry, whimper, give him their candy, and then rat on him to his teacher. While this may be facilitated by the genetic contributions to his large bodily build, as his genotype reciprocally interacts with his selected environment, these characteristics shift from being genotype/environment to person/environment interactions (see Chapter 10).

The Functions of Aggression

The Ethological Perspective

Ethologists view aggression as behaviors which evolved in species because of natural selection. In this view, aggression has adaptive significance for maintaining the species. Moyers (1967) identified seven types of aggression observed in the animal kingdom. He suggested that humans exhibit many of these behaviors as well. As you read these types of aggression, see if you can apply them to human behavior too.

- Predatory - Animals attack others that they will eat.
- Intermale, spontaneous - Two male animals will fight to establish dominance. There is often a threat display preceding the aggression.
- Terror-induced - Animals that are cornered and under intense arousal will respond with violence.
- Irritable - Animals respond with aggressive acts to eliminate an irritating stimulus.
- Territorial Defense - Some animals mark their "turf" and respond with aggression when their turf is invaded.
- Defense of the young - (Mostly female) animals respond violently when their offspring are threatened.
- Instrumental - Animals aggress to get something from their environment.

The Control of Aggression

An eminent ethologist, Konrad Lorenz (1966) argued that in addition to aggressive instincts, animals have also evolved unlearned mechanisms to inhibit aggression within their own species. Lorenz argued that intermale, spontaneous aggression would have evolved through natural selection for survival of the fittest and therefore, improvement of the species. However, taken to the extreme, uncontrolled intraspecies aggression would result in elimination of much of the population, thus threatening the species. Natural inhibitors of aggression would have, then, adaptive significance for a species.

Lorenz suggested that there exist in species innate releasing mechanisms (or unconditioned stimuli) which elicit aggression inhibition. For example, timber wolves are very aggressive defenders of their turf against other timber wolves. Their fights are vicious and bloody, but not always lethal. There comes a point in the fight when there is a clear victor atop his victim. Just as he is about to use his fangs to slash open the throat of his beaten foe a strange thing happens. The victim, rather than protecting his vulnerable jugular, instead bears it to the top dog. A second strange thing happens, rather than slashing this exposed throat, he lets his victim go off, perhaps to heal. Why should such strange events happen?

Lorenz argues that the unique white patch on the throat of the wolf serves as the innate elicitor of an aggression inhibition response. Do other animals, including humans, respond to unlearned aggression response stimuli?

A Dynamical Systems Approach

Now let us consider a dynamical systems approach to aggression and other forms of antisocial behavior. In this approach, aggressive transactions develop because of reciprocal interactions between the person and the environment. Thus developmental outcomes of aggressive behavior are a function of organismic and environmental transactions. First among the organismic factors, we consider the phylogenic ones: genetic make-up.

The Role of Genetic Make-up

Some biological theories of aggression suggest direct genetic causation. One such theory focused on men who had an extra Y chromosome making them XYY. Some studies reported that XYY men were more likely than XY men to engage in aggressive behavior and were over represented in the prison population. These "supermen" were also described as being physically large and active. Subsequent research has brought into question the strength of the relationship between XYY chromosomes and aggression. Because of the small number of XYY men available for study, the studies are inconclusive. However, we know that most individuals who are incarcerated for aggressive crimes have no known genetic or chromosomal cause.

Yet, genetic make-up could contribute to the development of aggressive behavior, perhaps indirectly. Again we return to the idea of genotype/environment interactions. Some children may inherit characteristics, including physical ones (e.g. size, muscles) which react to a physically stimulating environment. Eysenck (1964) reported that individuals we now call sociopaths inherit a characteristic (i.e., psychotocism – See Chapter 10) which produces unresponsiveness to pain. This is based on research which suggests that compared to normal individuals, sociopaths do not learn paired associates when shock is used as a negative reinforcer. A genetic lack of responsiveness to pain is a passive genotype/environment interaction since individuals with this genotype would not react to aversive stimuli in their environments.

Inherited physical and behavioral characteristics also serve evocative roles. A big, robust, strong infant will evoke (and reinforce) rough and tumble play behavior from the parents. These same characteristics will likely reinforce more aggressive behavior. Children with certain genotypes actively seek environments that evoke and reinforce aggressive behavior. Thus, active genotype/environment interactions may also play a role in the development of aggressive behavior.

However, the role of genotype in aggression, as with other human behaviors, is not simple. Lore and Schultz (1993) have argued that while aggression occurs in most species, so too does control of aggression. Furthermore, they make a point for cultural determination for the control (or lack of control) of aggression. They point out, for example, that the risk of being murdered in the United states is 7 to 10 times greater than it is in most European countries. Among the crucial determining processes of the culture is the way parents control early aggressive behavior which builds up a history of interactions between the child and the social environment.

The Role of Interactional History

Recall that in Horowitz's model (see Chapter 2), once the child has learned something as a function of environmental interactions, that which is learned becomes part of the organismic dimension. That is, our history of interactions become part of us. Early interactional histories then form the basis for later transactions. Thus, development involves ever-changing, dynamical interactions of the person and the environment. This is certainly true of the development of aggression.

Patterson, Littman, and Bricker (1967) described the development of aggression in the preschool environment. They found that the typical preschool provides many opportunities for the development of aggression. Children who interacted with their peers at a high frequency and magnitude were most likely to be reinforced for aggressive behavior. Children who were aggressive toward other children were likely to be reinforced by victims who cried, gave up their toys, or were passive. If a child aggressed against another and the victim successfully counter-aggressed (i.e., retaliated or told the teacher) the aggressor changed victims. Rather than reinforcing the aggressor's behavior, this punished the behavior so that the aggressor switched victims. The aggressors tried another victim because they had learned that in the past, other victims have reinforced the aggression.

Not only are those who initially aggress against others more likely to aggress again because of reinforcement, but the victims who successfully use counter aggression are also more likely to aggress in the future. The pattern that Patterson, et. al, found was (a) unassertive children were frequently the focus of aggression; (b) when a child successfully counter-aggressed and terminated the aggressive behavior the counter-aggressive behavior was strengthened through negative reinforcement (i.e., it terminated the behavior of the aggressor); (c) the result of this dynamic transaction was that the formerly unassertive victim not only counter-aggressed when attacked, but also learned to initiate attacks on others.

The Role of Current Physiological Conditions

Physiological arousal is a powerful contributor to aggression. Emotional arousal is elicited by unconditioned stimuli, such as pain. Emotional arousal may also be elicited by conditioned stimuli, too. For example, someone may call the child a negative name (e.g., "You're a real jerk.") which serves as a CS for arousal. The arousal response includes increased heart-rate, muscle tension, pupil dilation, a flush feeling in the face, and internal changes, such as a release of adrenaline. This complex system of unconditioned or conditioned responses is called the ***activation syndrome***. Some have termed this the ***fight or flight reaction*** since the bodily reactions facilitate vigorous action. Which operant behaviors are established by the emotion arousal will depend on the situation. For example, the terror induced aggression of a cornered animal (human or non-human) produces fight when the flight option is impossible. A history in which aggression has been reinforced and current environmental conditions will help determine which behaviors are "fueled' by the "hot-blooded" arousal. Azrin, Hutchinson , and Hake (1966) found that aggression (in the form of severe biting) was the common response to an unconditioned electric shock. We shall see that physiological arousal plays a key role in escalating coercive family interactions and in changing physical punishment into physical abuse.

Current Environmental Condition Effects

Environmental conditions may serve as discriminative stimuli, consequences, or setting events for antisocial behavior. A person's behavior or possession may function as a cue for aggressive responses in hostile and instrumental aggression. Likewise, there is ample evidence that aggression, just as with other behavior, is reinforced. In the case of hostile aggression, it may be reinforced by inflicting injury or pain on the target of hostility. Victims who cry easily are good targets for such reinforcement. Children who give up their possessions also positively reinforce antisocial behavior. Adults and others who attend to antisocial behaviors also positively reinforce the behaviors.

Much antisocial behavior is negatively reinforced. That is, it terminates or removes aversive stimuli. For example, hitting is likely to occur if hitting another child may get them to stop calling you names. Threats are likely to be frequent if they get the other person to back off. Since aversive stimuli also produce emotional arousal, we are likely to see an interaction between respondents and operants. For instance, name calling may elicit the respondent emotional arousal we call anger; the operant aggressive act may be reinforced by terminating the same aversive stimulus.

Finally, consider the role of setting events or establishing operations as current environmental stimuli in aggression. Mood may make some operant contingencies more or less likely to occur. That is, a child who is in a good mood may respond to the name calling by laughing. In a foul mood, the same child may lash out.

There are some common setting events for antisocial behaviors in children. Consider the supermarket as a setting event for a preschooler's tantrumming. One frequent setting event for child misbehavior is the presence of an adult. Besevegis and Lore (1983) observed pairs of children playing together under two different setting events: adult present and adult absent. The frequency of fighting and disagreements was higher with the adult present then when not. The presence of the adult increases

Figure 12.1
A Developmental Progression for Antisocial Behavior
After Patterson, Debaryshe, & Ramsey, 1989; Patterson, Reid, & Dishion, 1992

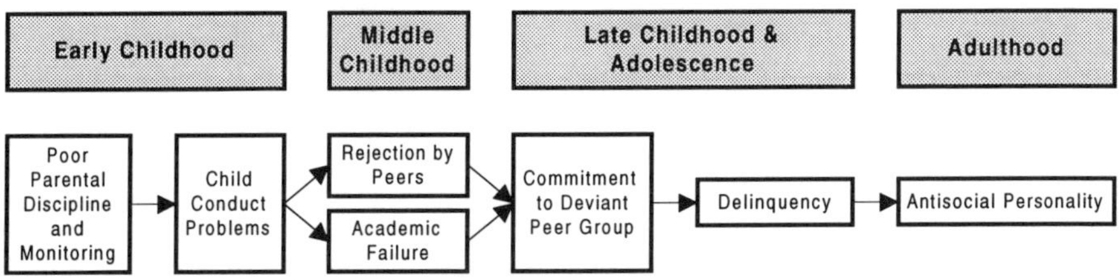

the likelihood of reinforcement with attention for aggression. In many families, one of the surest setting events for child misbehavior is the presence of mom talking on the phone. It seems that most children figure out these environmental conditions.

Before we examine the details of the contingencies affecting child-parent interactions, we will take a look at the long-term development of antisocial behavior.

The Development of Aggression (Patterson, DeBaryshe, & Ramsey, 1989)

Patterson, DeBaryshe, and Ramsey (1989) describe a sequence of steps leading to delinquency in adolescence (see Figure 12.1). Using data from a series of observational studies, Gerald Patterson has constructed a number of ***structural equation models*** which show the relationship between variables and the direction of influence over time (Patterson, Reid, & Dishion, 1992). They found that aggression, like charity, begins at home.

Aggression in Early Childhood – Basic Training in the home

Patterson, et al., (1989) found that aggression starts in early childhood. The source of child conduct problems in early childhood are inept parental discipline methods and monitoring of their children. Patterson (1980, 1982) described the transactions that develop between the mother and aggressive children as a ***coercive family process***. This process has several important features (shown in Figure 12.2) and described below:

Figure 12.2
The Coercive Family Process (Patterson, 1980)

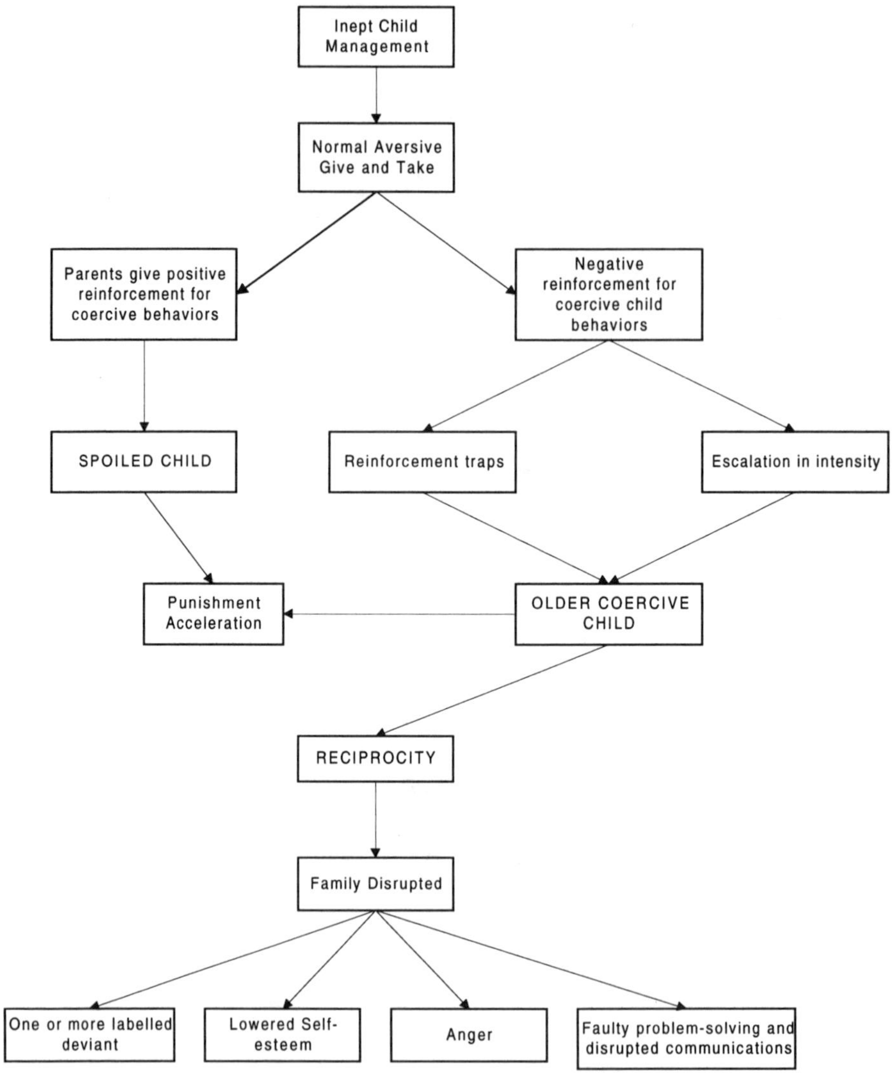

Coercive Family Process (Patterson, 1980)

1) Constitutional Differences Among Children and Parents

The development of the coercive family process begins at the upper right of Figure 12.2. Genetic make-up and interactional history produce differences in temperaments and personality characteristics between children and their parents. Some mismatches may occur.

2) Inept Child Management

Parents of aggressive children have poor child management skills. They tend to be inconsistent, use many commands, threats, and may use delayed physical punishment. Mothers of aggressive children may be less likely to identify obnoxious behavior than mothers of normal children.

3) Normal Aversive Give and Take

Patterson (1980) has shown that in normal homes there is a high level of aversive interactions. Minor aversives include whining, noncompliance, verbal negatives and others. On average there is a minor coercive exchange about once every three minutes. Major aversive exchanges may occur up to three times an hour. In families with aggressive children, the numbers increase to one minor event every three-quarters of a minute. There are increases in major events as well.

4) Negative Reinforcement for Coercive Child Behavior

Child coercive behaviors such as whining, yelling, and hitting are aversive stimuli for the parent. Parents are likely to drop their demands and terminate their own coercive behavior directed at the child. This increases the child's coercive behavior through negative reinforcement.

5) Reinforcement Traps

The naturally occurring negative reinforcement of both child and parent coercive behavior constitutes a ***reinforcement trap***. The participants trapped by negative reinforcement will likely emit these behaviors toward each other in the future.

6) Escalation of Response Intensity

Listen to the following coercive transaction between mom and her six-year-old son, Attila:

Mom: "Atty, pick up your socks."
Attila: (Whining) "I'm busy."
Mom: "Atty, this is the last time I'm going to tell you: Pick Them Up!"
Attila: "NO, YOU DO IT!"
Mom: "I SAID THAT'S THE LAST TIME I'M GONNA TELL YOU – PICK THEM UP!!!"
Attila: **"NO! PICK THEM UP YOURSELF!! "I'M NOT GOING TO!!!"**
Mom: **"THAT DOES IT. WAIT TILL YOUR FATHER GETS HOME."**
(At this point Mom picks up the socks).

Notice the escalation of the coercion both in terms of threats and intensity of the voices. Patterson (1980) has observed that the child escalates his/her aversive behaviors faster and to a higher level than the mother. This increases the probability that it is the mother who will give in before the child does.

7) Older Coercive Child

The outcome of the above steps is an interactional history of coercion. When we return to Patterson, et al.'s developmental model (Figure 12.1), we shall see the role this plays in later development.

8) Reciprocity

Patterson points out that the parents and children reciprocate, coercing against each other. This reciprocity of aversive attacks lead to family disruption in four ways.

9) Family Disruption

a) One or more family members are labeled as "deviant." The child may be labeled as "aggressive," a "behavior problem," or "hyperactive." Siblings and/or parents may be labeled as well.
b) Lowered self-esteem. Members of the family develop negative self-statements about themselves. Children acquire self-labels ("you're a real brat") from parents; parents may acquire labels ("you're a lousy parent", "you're mean") from children. Patterson (1980) reported that raising normal children produces ***dysphoria*** (negative mood states) in mothers. The amount of dysphoria increases in rearing aggressive children.
c) *Anger.* Anger in the above exchange should be apparent.
d) Faulty problem solving and disrupted family communications. Not only does anger fuel the coercive transactions, but it may have long lasting effects that disrupt the family relationships. Family members become aversive stimuli who are to be avoided.

Modeling of Aggressive Behaviors

Aggressive models may be present in the form of an aggressive or abusive parent. Aggressive models may also be present from television, movies, and videos. Preschoolers may have aggressive playmates who serve as models as well.

Remember, it is not only the presence of models, but the observed consequences of their behaviors that is important. Seeing an aggressive model leads to aggressive behavior if the child has a history of being reinforced for imitation of the model or observes the model's aggressive behavior being reinforced.

Middle Childhood – Rejection & School Failure

Returning to Figure 12.1, poor parental discipline and monitoring leads to child conduct problems (i.e., aggression, coercion, noncompliance) in early childhood. This takes us to the period of middle childhood.

Antisocial children do poorly in school (Hawkins & Lishner, 1987; Wilson & Herrnstein, 1985). Why is this? Patterson cites studies which suggest that the child's behavior problems, particularly noncompliance and under-controlled behavior, directly interfere with learning. Furthermore, the aversive behavior of the child leads to rejection by the teacher.

Concurrent with school failure is rejection by the normal peer group. Normal peers dislike and avoid coercive children. Their behaviors are aversive to normal peers who do not invite them to participate in their social activities.

Late Childhood and Adolescence – Deviant Peer Group Membership

School failure and rejection by normal peers mean that the opportunities to succeed academically and socially in school are minimal. These children become involved in a group of similarly failing and rejected peers. Membership in this deviant peer group is a nonfacilitative environment that has ominous effects of later development. Patterson, et al. (1989) suggest that this deviant group serves as a source of modeling and reinforcement for the development of delinquent behaviors. Specifically, the deviant group shapes attitudes, motivation, and rationalizations for antisocial behavior. The group also provides opportunities to emit specific antisocial behaviors. Buehler, Patterson, & Furniss (1966) showed that such peer groups positively reinforce deviant behaviors and punish conforming ones.

The final steps in this developmental progression of antisocial behaviors are delinquency and the development of an organized pattern of an antisocial personality. The outcomes of this deviant developmental path is a legacy of school dropout, substance abuse, employment problems, marital problems, multiple offenses, incarceration, and institutionalization (Patterson, et al., 1989; Caspi, Elder, & Bem, 1987; Huesmann, Eron, Lefkowitz, & Walder, 1984; Robins & Ratcliff, 1979). Let us now turn to one further legacy of this developmental history, child abuse.

A Dynamical Systems View of Physical Child Abuse

Child abuse is a form of antisocial behavior directed at children. It takes many forms, including physical abuse, psychological abuse, sexual abuse, and neglect. Many have focused on a history of being abused as a child as a significant determinant of later abusiveness as an adult. However, most abused children grow to adulthood without becoming abusive to their children. The development of abusiveness is a complex developmental process. Ross Vasta offered a model for physical child abuse which incorporates many of the processes relevant to a dynamical systems approach to development.

Although, in fact, his model has multiple components, Vasta calls his a ***"dual-component" model*** of child abuse in the sense that emphasizes the significance of **(1) operant and (2) respondent behaviors**. He also incorporates many of the known genetic, historical and environmental contributors to abuse. Figure 12.3 shows Vasta's model. It is arranged into (a) predisposing factors, (b) precipitating conditions (c) mediating responses, (d) behavioral responses, and (e) behavioral consequences. As shown in Figure 12.3, these factors are consistent with the four-term contingency.

Figure 12.3
Connections Among Coercion Concepts
Adapted from Vasta's Dual Component Model
of Physical Child Abuse, 1982

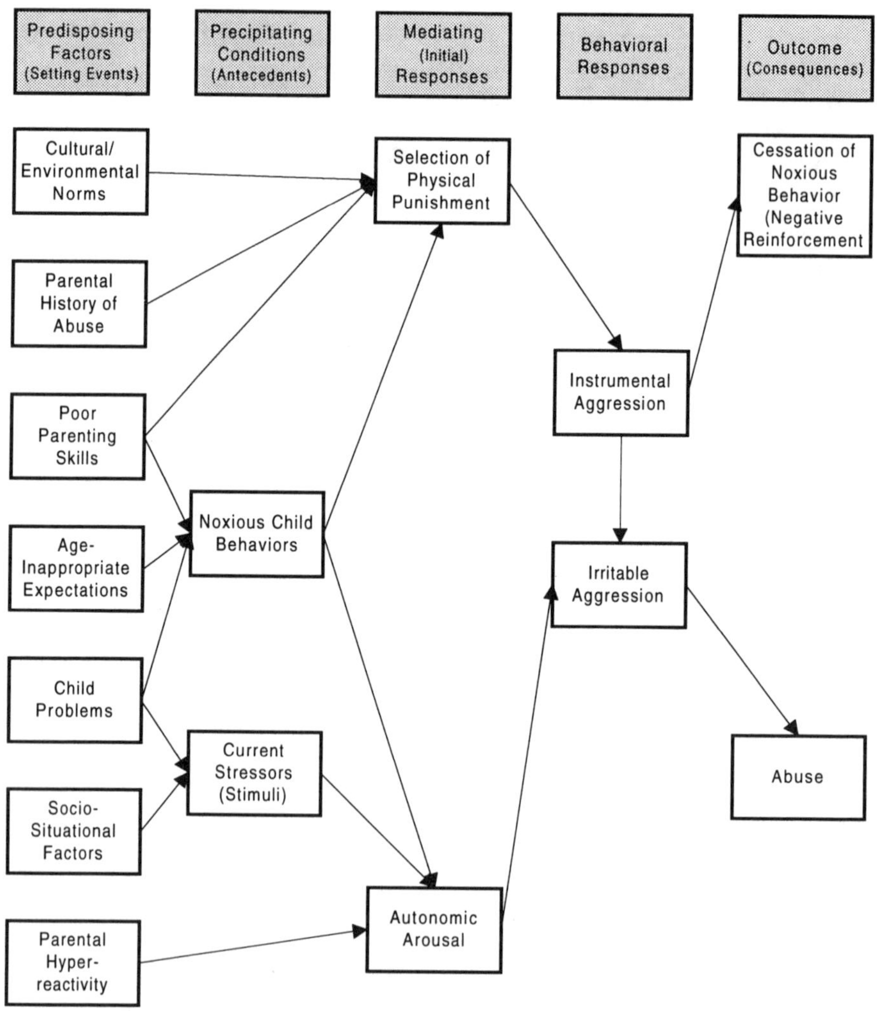

Predisposing Factors

These are characteristics of the parent or characteristics of the child which may function as setting events. Various combination of genetic make-up and histories of transactions produce these factors that make abuse more likely to occur.

(1) *Cultural/Environmental Norms.* Some cultures emphasize physical punishment (e.g., "spare the rod, spoil the child") as a way of disciplining children. On the other hand, the Tasaday people of Mindinao of the Philippines, do not.

(2) *Parental History of Abuse.* One of the most replicated findings in the literature on child abuse (e.g., Curtis, 1963; Spinetta & Rigler, 1972) is that abusive parents frequently have a history of being abused as children.

(3) *Poor Parenting Skills.* Unskilled and insensitive parents are likely to have difficulty in controlling undesirable behavior in their children.

(4) *Inappropriate Age Expectations by Parent.* Some abusive parents have been found to lack knowledge of the sequence and timing of the development of their children (Blumberg, 1974). When this happens they may expect a young child to behave in ways that the child is as yet incapable of doing. An example would be expecting a 5-month-old to be potty trained.

(5) *Child Behavior Problems.* Children who have a history of being difficult to control, are aggressive, or otherwise present problems are more likely to be the focus of abuse.

(6) *Socio-situational Factors.* This includes factors such as unemployment, socioeconomic status, and physical medical problems in the family. For example, in a study looking at 13,000 cases of abuse, Gil (1971) found that half of the fathers were out of work in the year immediately preceding the child abuse incident.

(7) *Parental Hyper-reactivity.* Because of their own transactional histories, some individuals are more sensitive to irritating stimuli than others. In addition, their reactions may be more intense than others. When child noxious behaviors occur, these parents over-react and will be more likely to abuse than parents whose sensitivity is less.

Precipitating Conditions

These include both setting events (e.g., some current stressors) and discriminative stimuli. These are acute events which, when they occur, make it more likely that abuse will happen.

(1) *Current Stressors.* Among stressors, the loss of a job, marital problems, and death of a family member are a few of the majors.

(2) *Noxious Child Behaviors.* These would include the whining, nagging, non-compliant, and oppositional behaviors identified by Patterson (1980). For example, under various setting events, a child's crying or whining may be a stimulus for abuse.

Mediating Responses

These are the initial behaviors of the abuser that are part of the chain leading to the abuse. These may be overt behaviors or private events such as autonomic arousal or cognitive behavior.

(1) *Selection of Physical Punishment as Response.* Note the arrows in Figure 12.3 which lead from specific setting events to noxious child behavior. Cultural norms (i.e., whether the culture or subculture encourages corporal punishment or not), history of abuse of the parent, and poor parenting skills (see Patterson, 1980) increase the likelihood that the parent will select physical punishment as the response to the child's noxious behavior.

(2) *Autonomic Arousal.* Vasta noted that the consequences of physical acts against others that characterize abuse are far beyond that of simple negative reinforcement. If only negative reinforcement were involved then abusers should terminate their attacks when the victim gives up. Vasta suggests the fuel for the violence of abuse comes from autonomic arousal (including increased heart rate and breathing, perspiration, the feeling of heat from blood rushing into the face, and other physiological responses). The child's noxious behavior elicits the arousal. Some of these noxious behaviors may be unconditioned stimuli for arousal. Others, such as the child's voice, may acquire the role of conditioned aversive stimuli.

Behavioral Responses

There are two components that make this a dual-component model. One is an operant component (i.e., instrumental aggression) and the other, a respondent component (irritable aggression).

(1) *Instrumental Aggression.* This aggressive behavior is operant because it is reinforced by terminating the child's noxious behavior (negative reinforcement). For example, the parent slaps the child and the child stops crying.

(2) *Irritable Aggression.* This is respondent behavior. It is *elicited* by the child's noxious behavior. Both increased noxious child behaviors (crying, screaming, name-calling) and the abuser's own aggressive responses can elicit even more irritable aggression. The result may be described as rage.

Behavioral Outcomes (Consequences)

Each component (operant and respondent) has certain outcomes which Vasta refers to as "consequences" – however, in the technical sense they are really only consequences for the operant component (see Chapter 7).

(1) *Cessation of the Child's Noxious Behavior (Negative Reinforcement).* This negative reinforcement is a consequence which strengthens the abuser's abusive behavior. Notice the child's noxious behaviors serve as both antecedent and consequence (negative reinforcer).

(2) *Physical Abuse.* The result of the respondent component is that the operant behaviors are delivered with an increased intensity beyond what would occur without it. We deem these behaviors and their effects "abuse".

Vasta's model shows the complexity of the child abuse process. It involves the reciprocal interactions between the child and the parent. Both transact based on their own unique genetic, historical, and current factors. When their paths of development collide, the developmental outcomes are poor.

Box 12

A DMZ in the Food Wars

One situation which frequently serves as a setting event for the coercive family process is meal time. Move the setting to a public area, such as Thanksgiving at Grandma's house or to a restaurant, and the conditions for even more disruptive behavior is substantially increased. Indeed, many families have given up all together the very idea of eating out with the kids until it's time for their wedding rehearsal dinner. In an attempt to arm parents with effective strategies for taking children out to dinner, Bauman, Reiss, Rogers, and Bailey (1983) developed an advice package for parents.

This package included ten steps which parents should employ. What is of interest is that these steps cover all aspects of the four-term contingency, especially setting events and antecedents. The use of these procedures is designed to preempt child misbehavior by anticipating conditions that are likely to lead to misbehavior, and to avoid these conditions from occurring in the first place. The steps are:

1) Decide upon what is appropriate behavior for the children in the restaurant and let them know what is expected of them. This specifies appropriate behavior to the children and to the parents, and prevents on-the spot debates and arbitrariness.

2) Find a table away from other people. This ensures a setting in which they will get little attention from others.

3) Seat the children on the inside, next to the wall. This will limit the child's ability to interact with outsiders and get attention. The child will have to crawl over the parent to get into things.

4) If there is more than one child, separate them. This makes it more difficult for children to get each other going by hitting, pinching, etc.

5) Bring along some crackers or other item as a premeal snack for the children. Even adults can get "antsy" waiting for their food to come.

Don't expect children to be any better.

6) Order food that the child likes. Parent's are expecting their waiting behavior to be reinforced. They should make sure the children are reinforced by the food, too.

7) Provide small interesting toys for the children to play with while waiting for the food. Parents may enjoy conversing with each other to pass the time. Don't expect children to be saints and just sit there.

8) While waiting for the food to come, remove the eating utensils from the children's reach. These are not toys – well, they're not supposed to be toys – so remove them before they become toys.

9) Remove the toys and return the utensils when the food comes. This makes it clear that food is the reinforcer and that eating, not playing, is the desired response.

10) Periodically praise the children for their good behavior. Don't expect the restaurant ritual to be as reinforcing to the children as it is to you – catch them being good.

Bauman, et al. (1983) found this package to successfully reduce children's disruptive behavior in restaurants. Furthermore, they found that these procedures could be learned easily by parents, even by those reading a pamphlet provided on the table. Parents were observed as providing more praise and less disapproval of child behavior following their use of the advice package. Most families observed reported that the package was easy to use, made the restaurant experience more pleasant, and said that they would probably use the steps in the future.

Many parents find fast-food restaurants are the only refuges for eating out with their children. Interestingly, most fast-food places provide some of the conditions outlined above. For example, they often have special kids meals which include toys and food which appeals to the little one's palette. Since the food is served almost instantaneously, there is little waiting time to cause problems. As a last resort, parents can avoid all the problems associated with eating in public with their children by using the drive through window. The package outlined above has been shown to provide the parent with skills that can broaden their culinary pleasures and their family ones as well.

Chapter 13

The Family System

Families as the Mediators of Society and Culture

In the human species, the family is the primary context in which a child develops. With some variation across cultures, the child will be raised in this family context for approximately twenty years. Yet, the family influence is not likely to end when the child leaves home, but, rather, it changes. The adult is likely to create his or her own family context in which the original roles continue to be influential to some degree.

This illustrates the dominance of the family system for understanding human development. How shall we view the family? Modern developmental psychology treats the family as one system among many in which the child is embedded (Bronfenbrenner, 1979). Bronfenbrenner has identified three levels of systems: the Microsystems, mesosystems, and macrosystems. The ***microsystems*** are the smallest units functioning as complete systems. In Bronfenbrenners's view, the family, the school, and the child's peer group are three examples of microsystems.

The ***mesosystems*** are the intermediate system levels. The combined contexts of the family, school, and peer groups, as well as any other microsystems that the child finds herself embedded in are collectively a mesosystem. These contexts plus outside systems (Bronfenbrenner calls these exosystems–including communicty organiations, mass media, neighbors and other outside influences) make up the child's culture and society. Bronfenbrenner calls this level of system, the ***macrosystem***.

The child is just one of the individuals who collectively make up the family microsystem. Family systems have their own dynamics that emerge from the dynamic reciprocal transactions of the individuals that constitute it. At System Level IV we are concerned with systems of systems. When analyzing at the level of the family (System Level IV), we see characteristics that are not present at the level of the individual (System Level II) or at the level of transactions between individuals (System Level III).

The Universal Functions of Parenting

LeVine (1974) has noted that all families, regardless of the culture from which they come, have the same three basic goals and perform the same three basic functions of child development. The functions are (1) survival, (2) economic, and (3) self-actualization. Furthermore, these functions are arranged in a hierarchy, in which the more fundamental functions must be taken care of before higher level ones can be accomplished. We can conceptualize these universal functions of families as a pyramid in which the survival functions form the base upon which economic functions and finally, self-actualization functions may be built.[1] Until the more foundation functions are fulfilled, it may be impossible for the family to focus on higher-level goals.

Consider a family in war-ravaged Bosnia-Herzogovenia. Neither self-actualization functions, such as promoting the study of music and literature, nor economic goals, such as basic education, may occur within the family. Instead, it is likely that all family functions will be concerned with survival goals, such as food, shelter, and safety. Ironically, ten years ago, that same family, in what was a relatively prosperous Yugoslavia may have had few concerns about survival, and even economic needs. Instead they may have functioned more to promote self-actualization of its members.

The Social and Cultural Context of Families

One of the most important functions of the family (as is true with the schools, media, and peers) is to serve as a context for the transmission of societal and cultural influences. The societal and cultural influences are mediated by ***values***. Values are the explicit and implicit contingencies specified by the culture. Explicit values may be moral or religious tenets such as "Honor thy father and thy mother," "Do unto others as you would have others do unto you." Other values, such as a work ethic or having a large (or small) family may be promoted by modeling (e.g., a hard working parent), or by prompting (e.g., "So when are you going to have another child?") the desired behavior, and then reinforcing the valued behavior when it occurs (e.g., "That makes us very happy, you're such a good son/daughter"). Family configuration (i.e., two parent nuclear family, single parent family, etc.) is, in large part, a function of society and culture.

In 1994, the United Nations sponsored a conference in Cairo, Egypt, concerning world population growth. According to the United Nations, the entire world population in 1950 was 2.4 billion. By 1994, the world population had reached 5.6 billion people. With an annual increase in world population, estimated to be 94 million people per year, it is estimated that by the year 2020, there will be an additional 2.4 billion above the 1994 level. That is, in a 70 year span, the world's population will have more than tripled!

Many of the concerns raised at the Cairo conference focused on family planning issues. The controversies emerged from differences in values resulting from different cultural views of the family systems. Although religious values played significant roles in controversies over restricting family size through sex education, birth control and abortion, other cultural values, including economic ones pitted culture against culture.

Coinciding with the Cairo conference in 1994 were renewed interest shown by politicians in the United States about family values (spoofed in the 1993 film, *Adams*

Family Values). Both President Clinton and former Vice-President Quayle gave highly publicized speeches, within days of each other, on the importance of the traditional family system for raising children in America.

Family Structure

In modern American families, the traditional family, the ***nuclear family***, consisting of a mother, father and one or more children, is the dominant family structure. Yet, in recent years, there has been an increase in other types of families in the United States. One of the largest recent increases is in the number of ***single-parent headed families***. In a single-parent family, the custodial parent provides the roles, or functions that both parents provide in a nuclear family.

In ***extended families***, grandparents or other adults are present and provide child caretaking functions. Extended families may exist for a variety of societal and cultural reasons, many of which are economic. These are very common in farm based cultures where it is an economic advantage to have different people available to work. If the mother is required to do farm chores, the grandparents may take over child care functions. Wilson (1989) has noted the historical, marital, interpersonal, and socioeconomic factors that have made extended families a prominent part of African-American culture. In this culture, uncles, aunts, cousins, grandfathers, and particularly grandmothers, frequently provide support needed in low income or single-parent families.

Yet another family structure is the, so-called ***Nontraditional family***. Nontraditional families consist of gay or lesbian partners and children. Finally, we may have a ***reconstituted*** or ***blended family*** consisting of children and parents from two previous family systems who spent time as single-parent families. Now they are combined into a new family with step-parents and step-brothers and sisters. While all family systems are complex, the series of transitions in which members of reconstituted families have experienced different roles, makes this one of the most complex and interesting developmental contexts.

The Family as a System of Systems

It is common among psychologists to view the family as a system, whether functional or dysfunctional. Perhaps it would be better to view the family as a system of systems. That is, what emerges as a family is the interrelationship between more basic wife-husband, mother-child, father-child, and child-child relationships. Thus, at systems Level IV, we are analyzing development at the level of systems of systems.

Therefore, the family is a complex relationship built upon other relationships. An example of this is the tremendous effect the arrival of a child has on the husband-wife relationship. The changes in interactions necessitated by redirecting attention to the needs of the baby pervades nearly every aspect of the spousal relationship, from eating meals, to sleeping through the night. Years later, when left with an "empty nest," the spousal relationship may have to go through a period of readjustment to a new family system.

Indeed, the development of the family system is dynamical, and may best be characterized by what Hetherington (1989) called "transitions". As family circumstances change, gradual adjustments or ***transitions*** occur in the family system. Some of these changing circumstances may be dramatic, such as divorce, death of a parent, or loss of family income. Other changed circumstances may be less impactful, such as moving to a new town. Nevertheless, changes in conditions bring about changes within the family system that may initially be dramatic, but eventually, the family system adapts to the changes.

From a dynamical systems view, the idea of transitions is an especially attractive notion. The family, from this perspective, is itself a dynamical system composed of the smaller systems of transactions between pairs of family members. The family patterns of transaction emerge as the results of reinforcement contingencies affect the members of the family. That is, the family system coalesces as the results of individual and two-way transactions are assembled by the contingencies.

Clarke-Stewart (1978) provided a good example of this. In her research, the she found that a baby's cry might not directly be the antecedent for the mother to react to the baby. Instead, the baby's cry is more likely to bother the father who in turn requests the mother to respond to the baby, which she does. Thus, in family systems, transactions are not simply two-way transactions, but involve multi-way transactions between members of the family system. Changes in to one part of the family may have subtle effects on all others, just as throwing a stone into a still pond produces ripples throughout.

Since the effect of the contingencies may require time to shape new behavior, the initial period following a dramatic change in conditions may be a period in which many previously reinforced behaviors are met with extinction and resulting frustration. This is a period of disruption in the interaction between individuals. Individual roles and functions may be unclear. Hetherington (1989) calls this a period of crisis. However, in dynamical systems approach, this is an example of a phase shift. Initially, changes in the system perturb the existing dynamic attractors (i.e., patterns of interaction). Eventually, the contingencies will gradually shape the individual interactions to a point at which the family system coalesces into a new one. At that point, the individuals in the family system will again be functioning to produce mutually reinforcing consequences.

Functional and Dysfunctional Families

Family systems theorists, such as Minuchin (Minuchin, Baker, Rosman, Liebman, Milman, & Todd, 1975) draw a distinction between functional and dysfunctional families. Dysfunctional families are ones in which individuals support the maladaptive behavior of one family member. For example, Minuchin and his colleagues (Liebman, Minuchin, & Baker, 1974; Minuchin, Rosman, & Baker, 1974) see such dysfunctional systems as maintaining the eating disorder, ***anorexia nervosa***, in teenage daughters. Since the severe loss of weight and other aspects of anorexia are maladaptive, families who receive reinforcement for reinforcing anorexic behavior are deemed dysfunctional.

Note, however, that as individuals, the members of a dysfunctional family system are functioning exactly as they should given the contingencies in effect. In the last chapter, Atilia and his mother were clearly dysfunctional. That is, from the view of an outside observer, their behavior was maladaptive: they treated each other badly and were angry at each other. Yet, as a system, this maladaptive behavior has come together, organized by natural contingencies of positive, but especially, negative reinforcement. These contingencies shaped the "dysfunctional" system. Therefore, in the value judgment of an outside observer, this is a dysfunctional family system. However, as a system itself, it is perfectly functional, matching behavior to its consequences.

In family systems therapy it is common to view the maladaptive behavior of the family member as ***dependent***. That is, much like in the case of addiction, the person with the problem is seen as dependent on other family members to maintain the maladaptive behavior. In turn, those whose behaviors are reinforced by maintaining the maladaptive behavior of the one seen as having the original problem are themselves viewed as having maladaptive behavior and are called ***codependent***. It is most likely that a therapist would view Atilia's behavior as maladaptive and dependent. His mother's behavior would then be seen as codependent.

From a dynamical systems view, the interaction between family members produce behaviors that are dynamic attractors. That is, there are characteristic patterns of interaction that are loosely assembled by the contingencies. The family is functioning as it should given the conditions in effect. Remember, these conditions include genetic make-up of the individuals, a long history of interactions between family members, and current physiological and environmental conditions. The results are many behavioral traps in which maladaptive, as well as adaptive behaviors are reinforced by naturally occurring, but unintentional consequences of reinforcement.

The Functions of Family Members

Mothers, fathers, and siblings provide different functions in family life. Society and culture largely determine what these functions should be either through verbal rules or the shaping process called socialization. When we attach the functions to a specific person, we call the functions ***roles***. When these roles are clearly defined and widely accepted by society, we have ***role stereotypes***. Although roles are continually changing, in traditional nuclear families, of our society, mothers, fathers, and siblings have distinct roles. Roles are the expected functions of the family member; that is, what the family member prompts, models, and reinforces.

Let's test your views of traditional family roles. On a piece of paper, make columns titled "Mother", "Father", "Sister", and "Brother". Under each title, write down the words that describe the roles or functions provided by that family member.

The Mother -
The Father -
Siblings -

Levels of Systems: How Society Influences Child Development

At this point, it is necessary to summarize the big picture of how society & culture exert their influences on the child. At System Level IV, society promotes values through mass media, local institutions (such as church and school), and family history. These values are modeled and the behavior of family members that is consistent with societal values is reinforced. Thus, looking from the perspective of System Level III, mothers, fathers, and siblings have been shaped to behave in accord with societal values by members of their society and culture. Among the behaviors they have developed are the teaching of socially appropriate behaviors to the child. Thus, mothers, fathers, and siblings model, prompt, and reinforce socially appropriate behaviors in the process called ***socialization***.

At System Level II, we view the child as developing appropriate (prosocial), or inappropriate (antisocial) behaviors. Finally, at System Level 1, we focus on the functions of basic process, especially operant learning, in the development of individual responses, some of which are social in nature. Just as the dots of paint construct the big picture, so too do basic learning processes bring societal and cultural values to fruition.

What Happens When the Role is Absent or Changed?

In traditional (i.e., nuclear) families, individual members may have distinctive roles. What happens in families in which traditional roles change? What happens if one or more of the family members are absent, as in a single parent-headed family? Changes in family systems, such as (changing the "bread-winner" role), are increasingly more common in American families. Such changes may include those occurring through economic necessity or through personal decisions. An important change is frequently the absence of one of the family members because of divorce, death, or abandonment. What are the effects on the family system and the child when roles change or are missing?

Maternal Employment

A common stereotype of the American family is the father as "bread-winner." Reruns of TV shows from the fifties and sixties, starting with "Ozzie and Harriet", through " The Honeymooners", "Father Knows Best", "Leave it to Beaver" , and ending with "The Partridge Family", and "All in the Family" provide evidence for the "father-as-bread-winner" role in year's past. Perhaps, this role is best summed up in Ricky's famous greeting to Lucy: "Honey, I'm home!"

The role of the father as sole provider for the family has become an exception, rather than the rule. By 1989 (Hoffman, 1989), most mothers, too, were wage earners. In 1990, 71% of two-parent American families, mothers were employed outside the home compared with only 43% in 1960. The U. S. Bureau of Labor

Statistics (1991) reported that 52% of mothers with children under two-years of age and 75% of mothers whose youngest child was of school age were in the labor force. Until the mid 1980's mothers of children under two-years old in two-parent families where both parents worked were less likely to work than mothers who were the sole parent of an infant. By 1990 that had reversed, and the dual wage earning families were more likely to have the mother employed outside the home (U. S. Department of Labor, 1991).

The change in the parental roles that has resulted from the increased likelihood of mother working has been examined by Lois Wladis Hoffman (1989). Hoffman has looked at the effects on several components of the family system: the child, the father, the marital relationship, and on the mother herself. As a part of a dynamical family system, the effects on individuals are ultimately determined by the combination of many factors. Simple effects that are true in all family situations should not be expected. Rather, the effects of maternal employment depend on complex interaction among many variables, including the cultural, economic, and social contexts in which the family is embedded. We first look at the effects of maternal employment on the mother.

Effects of Maternal Employment on the Mother

Hoffman (1989) found two major effects of maternal employment on the mother. First, for some mothers, outside employment serves as a "morale booster." Patterson (1980) found that the child rearing role for some mothers brought on increased feelings of ***dysphoria***. Mothers of difficult children seemed to be particularly helped by the "relief" of outside employment (Dinestag, 1986). Hoffman (1989) concluded that women who were able to gain employment because of lessened homemaking responsibilities or increased educational levels expressed higher levels of self-satisfaction than non-employed mothers. Increased satisfaction was expressed by both professional (Birnbaum, 1975) and blue-collar women workers (Feree, 1976).

Not all mothers receive a morale boost from outside employment. While mothers' who wanted to work outside the home did not show higher depression and stress scores (Hock & DeMeis, 1990), for some mothers, outside employment is just one more stressor in life. For these mothers, the demanding role of employee is added to the already demanding roles of mother, housemaker, and wife. For these mothers, work is one more role to assume.

The Effects of Maternal Employment on the Father

Although influenced by the extent to which parents share household and caretaking responsibilities (Hoffman, 1989), the effects of the mother's employment on the father's life seem to be influenced by social-cultural factors. For some fathers, the increased economic and social benefits of maternal employment have positive effects. However, for fathers holding traditional role values, maternal employment tends to have more negative reactions. Specifically, fathers' self-esteem in blue-collar families is negatively affected because these fathers are more likely to feel they have failed in the bread-winner role that they value most highly (Staines, Pottick, & Fudge, 1986).

The Effects of Maternal Employment on the Marital Relationship

These effects, too, are complex and dependent on the many specific factors in action in a particular family. Hoffman (1986) found positive effects on the relationships in dual-career families where both spouses value work. This was especially true in well-educated or middle-class families where the mother wants to work and the work is part-time. In these families, the mother's report of satisfaction with the relationship tends to be higher than the father's judgments of the marriage.

In contrast, maternal employment tends to influence negative judgments of the marriage in other family situations. The factors associated with negative marital satisfaction include families where the spouses have more traditional sex role values, in lower-class families, and in situations where either spouse resents the maternal employment.

The Effects of Maternal Employment on the Child

In her review of available studies examining the long-term effects of maternal employment of child development, Hoffman (1989) concludes that mother's employment has little lasting effect. The best documented effect seems to be positive effects on daughters of working mothers. Daughters of working mothers seem to benefit from a working role model and are more likely to have higher self-esteem and reject traditional values of the limitations of women in the work force. Furthermore, daughters seem to benefit from additional independence training that working mothers provide. Mothers who work have less time to dote on and make their children dependent.

Does the Mother's Work Role Change Her Role at Home?

Looking at maternal employment is a good place to see how a change in one part of the family system (i.e. the mother) changes interactions throughout the entire family system. Because, in most American families, mothers perform many if not most of the child-rearing and house-keeping functions, her removal from the home to work outside means that (a) someone else must assume these functions, (b) the functions must change, (c) the mother must perform work and home functions, or (d) the functions will not be performed at all. The result of this change in function is a transition period, in which the relationships among family members are disrupted. Relationships stabilize and become assembled again in some reorganized pattern in which roles are changed.

In general, studies show that there is a "modest" increase in father participation in household and child-rearing tasks when mother goes to work (Hoffman, 1986). However, because this increase is the result of necessity, rather than the father seeking out increased participation because of a genuine interest in housework or child care, this situation may lead to lower satisfaction with the marriage by the father (Hoffman, 1989).

One of the benefits of increased father participation in child care is that increased father involvement leads to higher academic and social development skills for both sons and daughters (Gottfried, Gottfried, & Bathurst, 1988). Apparently, father participation widens the range of skills and values that are taught to the children.

The children of working mothers spend more time in child care outside the home. Unfortunately, in most families, when the mother enters the work-force, the increase in paternal involvement or outside care does not entirely compensate for the mother's absence. In many cases, this means that the mother plays significant roles both at work and at home. Interestingly, the effects of the mother's outside work on the child are not linear. Part-time work seems to have more advantages for the family than a non-working mother. Negative effects on the children are generally not seen until the mother works more than a normal forty hour work week outside the home.

Paternal Job Loss

There has been a downward trend in *paternal* employment that has coincided with the increase in maternal employment seen in American society. This trend, which began in the 1980's (McLoyd, 1989), has continued into the 90's and may reflect a dramatic structural change in the U.S. economy.

Economic loss also includes reduction in wages, as many fathers who are laid off from well-paying manufacturing jobs take jobs at reduced pay, when they can find work. Work-force reductions in manufacturing have disproportionately involved men. Furthermore, as a group, African-American men have experienced proportionately more of the economic losses in jobs and wages (McLoyd, 1989).

McLoyd (1989) has proposed a model for the way in which paternal economic loss affects children. The model is consistent with a dynamical systems approach. It involves three sources of effects: (1) effects on the father, (2) effects on the child, and subsequently, the relationship between father and child.

Effects on the Father

Unemployment is sometimes the result of individual choices. However, people sometimes lose jobs for reasons beyond their own control. Conditions in society leading to "downsizing" of the work-force may lead to termination of employment or underemployment. Based on research conducted during the Great Depression of the 1930s and also in the 1980 recessions, there is evidence that economic loss has clear effects on the head of the household. These effects may be positive or negative, depending on the circumstances surrounding the job loss and family configuration. Significantly, the appraisal of the cause of job loss affects the personality of the father.

Effects on the Father's Personality

Besides defining the father's role as breadwinner, the father's job helps structure his personality. To a large extent, the job environment determines who he is and how he acts. It is not surprising, therefore, that job loss may have a major impact on a father's identity. This effect is magnified in homes where there are dependent children because of the increased pressure that the financial stress applies (Scholzman & Verba, 1978).

Effects on the Child

McLoyd (1989) has focused on three areas of child development affected by the father's loss of employment (1) socioemotional functioning, (2) the child's aspirations and expectations, and (3) physical health. These are mediated by (1) the loss of family income and (2) the effect that paternal job loss has on the interactions between father and child.

Socioemotional Effects

Paternal job loss and the resulting loss in economic status and embarrassment affects the personality and social interactions of the child. Children are likely to withdraw from existing social relationships because of embarrassment or because they no longer have the spending money to participate in social activities. McLoyd (1989) cites studies that associate paternal job loss with mental health problems (Werner & Smith, 1982), including loneliness and depression (Lempers, Clark-Lempers, & Simons, 1989). These effects seem to be enhanced by the reaction of the parents, which often is decreased monitoring and increased punishment (Lempers, et. al, 1989).

Child Aspirations and Expectations

With job loss there is lower family income. This drop of income increases parental pessimism about the child's future. The parental responsibility to help with the child's career development and/or higher educational goals becomes an area of stress. The effect of such a change in a family's configuration results in lower aspirations of college and career for the child. Girl's college and career expectations are particularly adversely affected by the father's pessimism (McLoyd, 1989).

Physical Health

Because job loss is often associated with loss of health insurance, reduced medical care, and poorer quality diets due to reduced income, children suffer physically. Margolis and Farran (1981) found a number of illnesses to increase when a parent looses a job.

Maternal Job Loss

In American society, the psychological effects are likely to impact most strongly the father who looses a job. These effects are due to the high reinforcement value placed upon the breadwinner role of the father. However, as noted above, there are increasingly more mothers who contribute to the economic well-being of the family through the work-force. Thus there are increasingly more mother-headed families where the breadwinner role provides both critical economic and psychological reinforcers for the family. Thus, maternal job loss is likely to have similar significant effects on the child that paternal job loss does.

Loss of A Parent

One of the most stressful events in a family system is the loss of one of its members. Children are particularly upset by the loss of a parent. Loss of a parent can occur suddenly, as with a death. Frequently, loss of a parent in a family system occurs through divorce and the process may be a long one. One estimate is that a majority of children born in the late 1970's and 1980's will experience divorce. Because 75% of divorced mothers and 80% of divorced fathers remarry (Hetherington, Stanley-Hagan, & Anderson, 1989), children of divorce experience a series of reorganizations of the family systems. In a sense, then, the members of the family go through a series of transitions. A family system that is disrupted by divorce experiences a period during which the new family functions coalesce into a new family system. In this new system, the child is likely living in a single-parent family and further disruption may follow in remarriage by the joining into a new reconstituted family system.

It has been assumed that divorce has a negative impact on all children. The work of Mavis Hetherington and her associates have shown that some children are more vulnerable to the effects of family disruption than others. Some children may even have a better developmental outcome as a result of the divorce. Hetherington and her colleagues have identified which factors influence the effects of divorce on children. Three main areas stand out, (1) characteristics of the child, (2) characteristics of the family, and (3) factors (extrafamilial) outside the family such as school and friends. Below we look at how these factors exacerbate or moderate the effects of family disruption.

The Effects of Divorce – Determining Factors

Child Characteristics

Each individual child's characteristics, the result of the coalescence of a history of interactions, may help determine the effects that divorce may have. Among those characteristics identified by Hetherington and her associates (Hetherington, 1989; Hetherington, et al., 1989) are:

1. The cumulative amount of stress the child has been under .

Factors such as the amount of conflict in the home and economic conditions are likely to influence the child's reaction to divorce. Emery (1982) has concluded that divorce may have beneficial effects when the pre-divorce environment was hostile and parents engaged in fighting and other conflicts. Divorce, in these cases, actually reduced the amount of conflict the child was exposed to and had a beneficial effect. Likewise, divorced parents who cooperate on child rearing issues and financial support are likely to reduce stress and have a positive impact on the child.

2. The child's temperament and personality.

Recall the characteristics of the difficult child. Hetherington (1990) has found difficult children react more negatively to the stress of divorce than do easy tempered children. Furthermore, the difficult child may elicit more negatives and place more stress on the custodial parent. Likewise, aggressive and noncompliant children with behavior problems may be a contributing factor to the divorce itself.

3. The child's developmental status.
The child's level of understanding of divorce may influence the reaction to it. Young children seem to react most negatively at first. They are more likely to blame themselves for being abandoned by a parent. However, with time, they seem to recover from the effects more fully. It is as if their limited level of understanding allows them to adapt better to the new circumstances. Older children may be better able to disengage from the turmoil of divorce, relying more heavily on peers and other support systems outside the home.

4. The child's gender.
Boys and girls react differently to divorce. This gender effect is in part due to the fact that 90% of divorced children live with the mother. Under these conditions, boys react more negatively than girls, showing higher incidence of behavior disorders and problems at home and in school. Effects continue longer for boys, with non-compliance being a problem even three years later (Hetherington, Cox, & Cox, 1982; 1985); but with most girls little effect is seen after two years. The effects on girls are likely to take the form of personality disorders like anxiety and depression (Emery & O'Leary, 1982).

As part of a family system, girls are in a very different position in relation to the mother. Hetherington (1990) reports that very often, girls adapt to the divorce by taking on the role of "friend" to the mother. The result is that the mother may treat the daughter as more of a peer as she relies on the daughter's help. Thus, daughters may have more difficulty with a remarriage than sons who are getting a new father. For girls, the men her mother dates may interfere with their new role as "friend". Hetherington reports daughters who stay up late waiting for their mothers to come home from a date, experiencing a kind of role reversal. When remarriages do occur, the daughter-stepfather relationship may be a particularly difficult one in our society. Neither daughter-stepfather nor stepfather-daughter behaviors are well defined. Hetherington's research (1990) suggests the consequence of this is that stepfathers are likely to withdraw from active interaction with the stepdaughters.

Family Characteristics

As mentioned, the amount of conflict present in the home prior to the divorce is a factor determining the effects on the child. Where there are high levels of conflict and fighting, divorce may actually benefit children. Since divorce almost always results in a lower economic standard for the custodial parent, this too affects the child. In many cases the custodial mother returns to the work-force for economic reasons and the mother-child relationship changes dramatically. Hetherington (1989) finds typically that lowered economic conditions are also associated with the following: dependence on welfare, poorer quality of housing, neighborhoods, schools, and child care. In addition, the economic problems may lead to less stability that results in the family living with the consequence of loss of social support from accustomed friends, neighbors, and teachers.

When a custodial parent enters the work-force, the effects will, in part, depend on the mother's reactions to the new role. High maternal satisfaction with work may influence the children positively.

Remarriages significantly enhance the economic situation of the family. While conflict over how to spend new resources may emerge, the effects of increased income have clear benefits on both parents and children (Hetherington, 1989).

One other area of concern in a divorcing family system is a period of reduced child monitoring by both parents (Hetherington, 1990). This may be the result of many factors, including resentment toward the other parent, the parents requiring more time for their own adjustments, the belief that the other parent is paying attention to the child's behavior, or time spent filling other roles. In essence, the child is at risk of falling through the cracks. The effect of this lack of discipline on the child, as suggested by Patterson and his colleagues (Patterson, et al., 1989), is subsequent behavior problems.

Finally, the presence or absence of grandparents in extended families may exert a positive influence on the child. The engaged grandparent may take over some of the roles left absent by the missing parent (Hetherington, 1990). Grandparents can provide financial, emotional, and caretaking support. Crockenberg (1981) found that a responsive and sensitive grandmother can moderate the influences of an insensitive mother. Wilson (1989), found that the grandmother plays a particularly prominent role in African-American single mother-headed extended families.

Extrafamilial Factors

Finally, factors outside of the home can influence the effects a divorce will have on the child. Hetherington (1990) found two key factors: peers and the school.

Peers

Having a friend that the child can confide in seems to moderate negative effects of divorce. The intimacy of the friendship seems to be even more important than the number of acquaintances the child has.

Schools

Hetherington found structured schools had a moderating effect on the impact of divorce on children. Schools that provided consistency and predictability in personnel and routines were better than unstructured schools.

The effective extrafamilial factors seem to moderate divorce effects by providing a consistency in the child's environment when the family system is in transition. This consistency and predictability enables the child to maintain a constancy in person/environment relationships no longer provided in the home. When contingencies are forming in the newly structured home, the already organized behavior patterns with friends and the school maintain some level of behavioral stability. The extent to which the transition period in the home affects the child is, of course, also dependent upon the required change needed to stabilize the system. For example, a drastic change in parenting styles (discussed below) may have more of an effect than just a change of residence.

Patterns of Family Discipline

Donna Baumrind (1966) identified three distinct styles of parental discipline: ***authoritarian, permissive,*** and ***authoritative***. Each of these differed along two identified dimensions of parental styles: warmth versus hostility, and responsiveness vs. demandedness (Greenberger & Goldberg, 1989). These two dimensions form independent continuums along which parents may vary. Authoritarian, permissive, and authoritative styles fall on different quadrants of these dimensions.

The authoritarian parent is characterized by low warmth and high control. They strongly value virtue and favor punishment and negative reinforcement to control the child's behaviors not in accord with the authoritarian parent's strict views. The child is treated as submissive and to be kept in his/her place. Order and traditional values are reinforced, individualism, and non-conventional behavior is punished. The child's views are not solicited and not considered. Right and wrong are viewed as absolute and originating from the laws of God. The authoritarian parent is high on demandedness and generally low on warmth.

The permissive parents are accepting of the child's behavior without attempting to modify it. They present themselves as resources for the child to use, providing the child with information and support, but they do not direct the child's behavior. Unconditional positive reinforcement, where reinforcement is non-contingent upon any desired behavior, is characteristic of permissive parents. They are low on demandedness, and generally, high on warmth.

Authoritative (not to be confused with authorit*arian*) parents are more reasoning. They consider the child's viewpoints and value them, but remain in control. They view the child's behavior in relation to the context in which it happens, not in absolute terms. They are more directing than permissive parents. Authoritative parents use mostly positive reinforcement with some negative reinforcement, and only seldom do they punish. They tend more toward the responsive end of the continuum, but less so than permissive parents. They may range along the entire warmth-hostility dimension, although hostility in authoritative parents is rare.

What are implications of differing parental styles? As mentioned above, they parental styles likely to (a) be involved in different kinds of four-term contingency relationships with their children, and, as a result (b) differentially reinforce different kinds of behavior in daily interactions which in turn influence the probability of these behaviors becoming organized behavioral systems.

Differing Contingencies in Parental Styles

Setting Events

The overall home environments established by parents with different child discipline styles are distinctive. These setting events provide different contexts that influence nearly all the discriminative stimulus-behavior and behavior consequence relationships between parents and child. That is, an overall tone pervades nearly all interactions between the child and parent. Consider the differences in how the overall context affects the child in a home with two permissive parents versus a home in which both parents are strongly authoritarian. For example, take a phrase "My, don't you look handsome." In a permissive home, this compliment may be ineffectual because the child is satiated by parental approval. On the other hand, the same compliment coming from an authoritarian parent may be so unusual, that its effect is very powerful. Unfortunately, in that context, it may be so unusual as to be taken as sarcasm that can result in the punishing rather than strengthening behavior. Thus, the overall different setting events prevalent in different styles of parenting may influence specific environment/behavior relationships.

Differences in Antecedents and Consequences

Authoritarian, permissive, and authoritative parents are likely to differ in the type of antecedents or discriminative stimuli they provide. Authoritarian parents, because they are more demanding are more likely to give commands. Permissive parents are least likely to give commands to children, but when they do, their commands are followed by fewer and less effective consequences. Instead, permissive parents are likely to tolerate more deviant behavior until a point at which they can no longer do so. Then, they are likely to consequate the behavior ineffectively as is typical in Patterson's coercive family process (Chapter 12).

Authoritative parents tolerate more freedom of child behavior than do authoritarian parents. In contrast to permissive parents, authoritative parents set limits that are clear to the child from both verbal statements and past actions. Thus, authoritative parents provide the conditions for the development of rule governed behavior by specifying the contingencies and consequating them in a consistent manner. As in Patterson's examples of effective parenting practices, authoritative parents tend to ignore minor child irritations, but are clear about what is acceptable and consequate immediately and effectively. Authoritative parents are more likely to use verbal rationales and non-physical consequences, such as time out, or loss of privileges. Authoritarian parents are more likely to spank or paddle, while permissive parents are likely to try to reason with the child but not to use effective consequences.

Parents Differ in The Behaviors They Shape

Studies of Baumrind's three distinct parental discipline styles show that they have different effects on child behavior. The different effects occur immediately in the response of the child to the parent's behavior. These effects also follow a dynamical systems approach by building cumulatively over a long history of parent-child interactions. The results show clear long run effects in the child's cognitive as well as social and emotional development.

Baumrind (1967) summarized the typical characteristics of children raised under different parenting styles. Authoritarian parents tended to have children who were: fearful, apprehensive, moody, unhappy, easily annoyed, passively hostile, aimless, vulnerable to stress, sulky, and unfriendly. Permissive parents had children who were typically rebellious, low in self-reliance and control, impulsive, aggressive, domineering, aimless, and low in achievement. Finally, authoritative parents were likely to have children who turned out to be self-reliant, self-controlled, cheerful and friendly, able to cope with stress, cooperative, curious, showing purpose, and achievement oriented.

By middle childhood (age 8 to 9) the parenting style children received tended to affect their cognitive and social skills. As summarized by Baumrind (1977), the daughters of authoritarian parents had average social and cognitive abilities while their sons had average social and low cognitive skills. Permissive parents were likely to have daughters who were low in cognitive and social skills and sons who were *very* low in cognitive and low in social abilities. Finally, the real winners were the daughters and sons of authoritative parents. Daughters of authoritative parents had very high cognitive and social abilities and sons had high abilities in both domains.

These effects continue into adolescence. Dornbusch, Ritter, Leiderman, Roberts, and Fraleigh (1987) administered a questionnaire to high school students concerning their parents' discipline styles. The authors then correlated the three discipline styles to the students' high school grades. They found that an authoritarian parenting style was negatively correlated with grades whereas the authoritative style was positively correlated. No relationship was found between a permissive style and high school grades.

Other investigators (Buri, Louiselle, Misukanis, and Mueller, 1988) looked at the self-esteem of adolescents and the perceived parental style of their parents. Children who reported their parents had an authoritarian style had the lowest self-esteem while those reporting being raised by authoritative parents had high self-esteem. Permissive parenting was unrelated to the self-esteem measure.

Clearly authoritative parenting produces the most desirable outcomes in children. Authoritative parents allow the child to choose and participate within clear guidelines, use effective, but not strongly aversive consequences, and encourage the development of achievement and self-reliant behavior.

Do parents change their style as the child develops? Apparently not. McNally, Eisenberg, and Harris (1991) administered the Child-Rearing Practices Report to a group of parents starting when their children were 7-or 8-years old, and for the last time when the children were 15-16-years old. They found a great deal of consistency in parenting behaviors across the eight year period. Among the changes found was an increase in maternal control when the children hit mid-adolescence, and a decrease in positive and increase in negative affect from the mothers as the children got older. Also, there were changes in specific discipline techniques as the child got older with the use of isolation decreasing and deprivation of privileges being used more. Finally, as the children got older, mothers placed more emphasis on the child's achievement. However, the study suggests that, overall, the result of constant mother/child interaction maintained the mothers' parenting style throughout childhood and even into adolescence.

Children In the Context of Poverty

There are many contexts in which the family system is embedded. One of the most pervasive and increasingly common is poverty. The lack of money for the family means that survival goals become important. Along with the lack of money come many setting factors that play havoc with the prospects of the child's development within the family. Horowitz (1989) would consider poverty, along with other general conditions, such as race, a ***social address***. By this she means that poverty is a general condition that influences a child somewhere on the developmental path. As such, we may view it as a setting event – a context. Where that child winds up is not the direct result of poverty, but rather the kind of transactions that result from "residing" in poverty. Below, we explore some of the specific causal factors associated with poverty and their resulting effects.

The Extent of the Problem

The latest census of the United States lists 21.9% of U.S. children living in families below the poverty line. (U.S. Bureaus of the Census, 1992). This is a greater rate than Chile, Colombia, Jamaica, Costa Rica, and Cuba (Pollitt, 1994). The U.S. rate is about two times higher than most other industrialized nations (Huston, 1994). The National Center for Children in Poverty estimated that 6 million children under age 6 live in poverty (Associated Press, 1995). However, many more children's families live near that line. Poverty is not spread uniformly over ethnic groups. While the majority of children living in poverty are of European descent, 47% of African-American and 40% of Hispanic children are living at this income level (U.S. Bureaus of the Census, 1992).

Huston, identifies three reasons for these high numbers. First, structural changes in the U.S. economy have led to the loss of many well paying industrial jobs for lower skilled workers. These workers and their families have suffered serious income loss. Second, the percentage of children living with single-parent mothers has increased dramatically. There is a high rate of poverty among these families. Third, government benefits have declined during the 1970's and 1980's. Recent changes in Congress further threaten what has been called a safety net, which may result in letting more children fall into poverty.

The Effects of Poverty on Children

Many disadvantageous conditions are associated with poverty. These include poor health care, inadequate housing (including, at its extreme, homelessness), environmental toxins such as lead poisoning, and neighborhoods that are violent or provide little support (Huston, McLoyd, Garcia, & Coll, 1994). Furthermore, there may be the effects of parental job loss described above. Because the conditions of poverty may affect organismic conditions (through lack of prenatal care and poor health care) they render the child impaired and vulnerable. Since the effects of these organismic conditions are likely to be exaggerated by a nonfacilitative environment, poverty puts the child "double jeopardy" for poor developmental outcome (Parker, Greer, & Zuckerman, 1988).

Poverty and Nutrition

Nutrition is an example of how one variable may serve as a setting event influencing developmental contingencies. Studying a naturally occurring severe food shortage in Kenya that lasted several months, McDonald, Sigman, Espinosa, and Neumann (1994) found major effects on school-age children. Toddlers, whose food energy intake did not decline, did not exhibit the same effects. School-age children showed less time spent in high-activity play, less positive peer interaction, less general activity, and poorer in-class attention. Their social and cognitive behavior were not affected during this famine. Thus, for the children whose food intake was reduced, lower energy levels reduced certain types of play and school interactions. In an interesting example of the complexity of family dynamics, toddlers were spared most of the effects of the famine by their families who made sure the toddlers were nourished. As a result, toddlers' behaviors were unaffected. Nutrition is just one disadvantageous setting event of poverty.

Poverty and Parental Discipline

Poverty also directly affects environmental conditions such as parental discipline. Sampson and Laub (1994) compared data collected on delinquent and nondelinquent adolescents during the Great Depression. They found that family processes were responsible for about two-thirds of the effects of poverty on delinquency. Poverty seems to inhibit effective informal parental control (what Patterson would consider "ept" parenting – monitoring and effective discipline) over adolescents. Indeed, delinquency increased directly in proportion to the amount of harsh and erratic discipline employed by parents. Furthermore, 83% of the adolescents in families showing low supervision or monitoring were delinquent. In contrast, only 10% of adolescents in families with good supervision were delinquent.

As suggested by Patterson's coercive family process (See Chapter 12), the influences are complex and multidirectional. That is, not only is the child's delinquency affected by the parents' poor monitoring and discipline, but the parents are affected by the child's coercive behavior as well. Sampson and Laub (1994) found that the child's difficult and antisocial behavior disrupts effective parenting. Children who were difficult, showed misbehavior early in life, and had frequent violent tantrums led, as might be expected, to lower levels of maternal supervision when adolescents. It is no surprise that these adolescents also had less attachment to their mothers (Sampson & Laub, 1994). Thus this research supports a dynamical systems view in which both the child and parents reciprocal transactions determine development.

This view is also supported by Conger, Ge, Elder, Lorenz, and Simmons (1994). These authors studied families going through financial distress due to economic difficulties occurring in the Midwest. Conger, et al., proposed a model for how poverty works. The model predicts that adverse economic conditions places economic pressure on the parents which in turn leads to depressive moods and resulting marital conflict. In this model, it is the economic pressure and marital conflict that leads to parent-child coercion over economics and to parent hostility toward the adolescent. The result of this is a coercive family process with two outcomes: (1) either the child withdraws or (2) the child acts out problem behaviors. Thus again, poverty may bee seen as a setting event for poor developmental outcome. Poverty is an important variable that sets the conditions that make these types of behavioral transactions more likely.

Variability in Reactions to Poverty

As evidenced in the famine study described above (McDonald, et al., 1994), not all children show negative effects of poverty conditions. Poverty may make certain conditions more likely, but its effects ultimately depends on the interaction of genetics, interactional history, current physiological conditions, and current environmental conditions, as described in Chapter 2. A study by Bradley, Whiteside, Mundfrom, Casey, Kelleher, and Pope (1994) illustrates this. The authors found that of 243 premature, low-birthweight children living in poverty, 26 were in the normal range for cognitive, social, health, and growth measures. This is not a high number. Yet, it suggests that there may be some resiliency possible even under conditions of impairment and vulnerability. What facilitative environmental conditions produced these more favorable outcomes? The authors found that a responsive, accepting, stimulating and organized environment "protected" these children. That is specific parent behaviors that encourage interaction between the child and the environment prevents many negative effects of poverty.

Preventing Poverty's Effects

What happens when home environments are non-protective or non-facilitative? Intervention programs, including early childhood education, may lead to better developmental outcome. Some programs may focus on early intervention. For example, Granthan-Mc Gregor, Powell, Walker, Chang, and Fletcher (1994) showed that even effects of early malnutrition can be overcome by teaching the mother to be more interactive, sensitive, and teach cognitive skills. Indeed, 14 years later, the malnourished children whose mothers received the training had children who were not significantly different from normal nutrition controls on IQ and school achievement. However, a group of malnourished infants whose mothers were not trained in interaction skills showed significant deficits in IQ and school achievement throughout school.

However, not all schools may be equally functional at overcoming the effects of poverty (See chapter 14). Phillips, Voran, Kisker, Howes, and Whitebook (1994) found that centers serving predominately low-income children were of lower overall quality than found in Head Start and public school funded programs. Thus, children living in poverty may have access to less facilitative programs than they need.

Fortunately, many studies (e.g., Lazar & Darlington, 1982; Weisberg, 1992, 1994; Johnson & Layng, 1994; Campbell & Ramey, 1994) have demonstrated that effective early intervention and education can moderate the effects of organismic vulnerability and nonfacilitative environments. For example, Howard, Williams and McLaughlin (1994) cite at least 18 studies that have successfully changed behavior problems of children prenatally exposed to drugs. These authors prescribe how the four-term contingency may be effectively used with these children who not only

Box 13

Using Behavioral Systems to Prevent Child Abuse

Families living in poverty confront many problems. Solutions based on solving just one or two of these provide Band-Aid approaches to the family system. An alternative approach is a multifactorial approach to the problems of child abuse in low income families. John Lutzker and his associates have taken such an approach in two well documented programs, Project 12-Ways (Lutzker, 1984) and Project Ecosystems (Lutzker & Campbell, 1994). Both these programs have developed a systems of comprehensive services to families to prevent child abuse and neglect. These projects use what Lutzker calls an "ecobehavioral:" approach (Lutzker & Campbell, 1994). The term ecobehavioral reflects the importance of changing behaviors in the real-world environments in which children and parents live.

Project 12-Ways was developed in 1979 at the University of Southern Illinois at Carbondale to provide services to rural families in 10 Southern Illinois counties. Adopting a systems approach, it's primary focus is to teach children and their parents the skills necessary to get along together without abuse and neglect. It attempts to do this by reducing stressors and providing skills for family members. The comprehensiveness of this approach can be seen in the 12 ways in which these goals are approached.:

Parent-Child Training:
Assertiveness Training:
Basic Skills:
Health Maintenance and Nutrition:
Job Finding:
Family Activities:
Problem Solving:
Money Management:
Multiple Setting Behavior Management:
Prevention (Single Parents):

Self-Control:
Stress Reduction:

In Los Angeles, Lutzker developed a new systems approach for the prevention of child abuse in the families of developmentally delayed children called Project Ecosystems. There are six components of Project Ecosystems. These are:

Parent/Child Relationship Training. There are two major components of the parent training. The first is compliance training. Compliance training emphasizes the use of antecedents, particularly instructions called alpha commands. Parents are taught to give these simple commands which can be carried out by the child within a few seconds, rather than beta commands.

A second important component of parent training is planned activities training developed by Sanders and Dadds (1982). PAT teaches parents how to provide structured activities and good interaction skills to prevent misbehavior. By teaching parents to provide a reinforcing environment, much child misbehavior, which serves as an antecedent for abuse, can be avoided.

Basic Skills Training. Since many developmentally disabled children lack basic skills such self-feeding, self-dressing, safety, and hygiene, counselors may train children directly. These counselors, who are college students, use basic behavioral methods to accomplish this and then the control over the procedures is gradually faded into the mothers' control.

Behavioral Pediatrics. This program is designed to train parents in managing the often complicated medical procedures of developmentally disabled children. For example, a reinforcement system might be taught to the parent for increasing the child's taking of asthma medicine.

Stress Reduction. As noted in Vasta's dual component model, child problems, such as developmental disabilities can be a setting event or antecedent for abuse because it leads to a stressful household. Stress reduction methods, including relaxation techniques are taught to the parents to make the household less stressful.

Problem Solving. Parents of developmentally disabled children in our society are confronted with frequent problems in child care and in obtaining the best services from agencies. Project Ecosystems has a training manual for the development of specific and general problem solving skills to enhance the life of the parent and child.

Assessment. Like its predecessor, Project Ecosystems stresses ongoing assessment and evaluation of its own effectiveness. Individual, as well as project-wide programs are evaluated for effectiveness and improvements are made to ensure effectiveness.

Many published studies have demonstrated the effectiveness of these ecobehavioral approaches to preventing child abuse. (cf., Lutzker, Campbell, Newman, & Harrold, 1989). Despite the fact that the parents treated in Project 12-Ways were known abusers, during treatment there was an overall abuse rate of 2% versus a rate of 11% in a comparison group. A year after treatment, the Project 12-Ways rate was 10% compared with 21% for the comparison group. Among the first 75 families served by Project Ecosystems, only one case of abuse or neglect was reported (Lutzker, Campbell, Newman, & Harrold, 1989). Thus, treating child abuse by treating the family systems has proven to be effective.

were impaired and vulnerable, but provided with a nonfacilitative environment by a drug abusing parent.

Many of the educational issues will be discussed in the next chapter. We end this chapter with a look at two comprehensive approaches to dealing with the multifactor problem that is poverty and its effects on development.

Footnotes

[1]Students of other fields of psychology may take note that LeVine's hierarchy is similar to Abraham Maslow's hierarchy of individual needs.

Chapter 14

Schools

The Schools As Agents of Society & Culture

In the last chapter, we saw how societal and cultural values are transmitted through the actions of individuals in the family system. As mentioned, schools are an important source of societal transmission. While the family continues to be a major source of influence, entry into the educational system exposes the child to extrafamilial values. Schools tend to promote the values of the mainstream culture and the society in which the child lives. It provides us with a common culture.

The Functions of Education

Schools developed out of society's need to extend the economic and self-actualizing goals of families beyond the home. In some societies, schooling continues in the home throughout childhood. Even in societies where there is public education, the child's first teachers are still the parents. Nevertheless, there are two main reasons for the development of extrafamilial schooling. One reason is the extended knowledge and abilities of specialized teachers and educators. This provides the child with more educational expertise than would be available from the parents alone. The second reason for the development of schools is largely economic: sending the child to school enables both parents to work. A system with one teacher and 35 children is economically more efficient than one with one teacher (a parent) and one or two (or a few more) children.

However for many reasons, children may still be home-taught. One increasingly popular reason is that some parents believe that they can do a better job meeting their children's' individual economic and self-actualization goals than can the public schools.

The demand for early childhood education outside the home has increased in the recent years due to the increase in two-income families. In former decades American society encouraged mothers to stay home until the children were of school age. This is no longer the case. In 1991, 58% of mothers who had children under six years of age were in the work force. This is more than three times as many as were in the labor force 30 years earlier (Committee for Economic Development, 1993). Finding child care that is reasonably priced and environmentally enriching for a child is a taxing problem. Thus, a push for improved and affordable public child care (through early education) has come under recent political discussion.

If the purpose of schools is to provide for the economic and self-actualization goals for children, a primary function of education must be to increase the cognitive development of children. As you recall from Chapter 8, cognitive skills are knowledge (i.e., knowing about things), abilities (knowing how to do things), and problem solving. These skills also are the cognitive functions of education. A second, and often implicit, function is to promote the social development of children. Social development includes social knowledge, social abilities, and social problem solving. These social skills are generally considered the socialization function of education.

Type S and Type F Systems

Schools are one of many organizations in society. Some, such as business organizations, are concerned with private matters and may have the interests of individuals, such as shareholders, as their major priorities. Others, such as the military, the congress, police, and the schools are public institutions. These are organizations that are concerned with "the common good" and exist for the purpose of furthering society's values. These organizations are medium to large scale systems that have been organized for some original function. Sometimes the organization formed because of some specific act of society, such as the formation of a three branch government by a constitutional convention. Mostly, organizational systems have emerged because of the coalescence of factors driven by a goal or need to perform a function, such as the coming together of a Continental Congress to proclaim independence. As in our own nation's history, often more formal principles of organization follow the emergence of a system that has been assembled by the task at hand.

Schools are organizations that exist to further the society's values for the education of its citizens, especially children. Schools exist to further the family's (and society's) economic and self-actualization goals. Private and public schools emerged out of these societal needs. Once schools emerged, structure was imposed upon them with the purpose of enhancing their ability to meet their goals. Individual schools became part of school systems with administrators assigned to enhance the function of the schools. However the central question remains: "How good a job are schools doing of achieving their economic and self-actualization goals?"

In recent years there has been great public debate on this question. Most of the conclusions drawn from the data show the educational system failing to meet society's goals. As part of the complex system of development there are, of course many factors that determine the effectiveness of schools, including the teachers, the curriculum, societal values, and the child. One interesting view of the role of the schools-as-systems was presented by Pennypacker (1994).

Organizations, such as school systems, corporations, and governments, emerge due to the natural contingencies that exist in society. They coalesce around a task (e.g., education, profit, public services). Contingencies shape the formation and evolution of systems into their emergent characteristics. In Pennypacker's view, organizations can be classified into two types: Type S (or static) and Type F (or functional).

Type S (Static) Organizations

The original contingencies for either system may have been to solve a societal need. However, Type S organizations are under contingencies which shape and maintain the organization's survival, without regard for the organization's effect on the societal needs upon which it may have been founded. For example, a government organization, such as Congress, would be considered a Type S organization if the contingencies determining the behavior of its members were to maintain their position (i.e., get re-elected) rather than serve the public. In Pennypacker's analysis, the self-survival contingencies in effect for Type S organizations select for certain characteristics that maintain the organization's status quo.

There are several characteristics of Type S organizations. First, the behavior of the organization is primarily controlled by avoidance contingencies (negative reinforcement). This means that the organization reacts to crises and meets deadlines to avoid aversive consequences. For example, Congress may pass a bill on crime in order to avoid appearing weak and being voted out of office. Likewise, a school system may bring in a new curriculum in order to show that it is doing something about increasingly lower test scores.

A second result of the self-survival consequences affecting Type S organizations is that they will do nothing that makes changes that might lead to their elimination, even if it means that it will solve the problems that they were organized to solve. For example, let us say, that giving classroom teachers total judgment over curriculum leads to better test score results. A Type S school system would not allow this, because it threatens the existence of the organization even though it furthers the purposes for which the organization was founded. The failure to enact campaign reform in Congress, and the failure to control violence in media are examples of survival contingencies selecting the status quo.

A third characteristic of Type S organizations is that the selection by survival and avoidance contingencies produces reliance on the knowledge of "experts." This is what Pennypacker (1994) calls ***invented wisdom***. In order to maintain themselves, organizations depend on experts to state whether what the organization is doing is correct and effective. Such experts may rely on other experts (e.g., theorists, philosophers) and generate statistics or anecdotes to "prove" their point about what is being done or what further needs to be done. For example, the government may receive a report from a task force on crime, or a school system may adopt a curriculum for mathematics instruction based on a theory of cognitive development. By behaving in accordance with this invented wisdom of the experts, the organization can justify its existence. In this regard, Type S organizations are more rule governed than they are contingency shaped.

A fourth Type S characteristic is the development of a bureaucratic structure (indeed, Type S could stand for "structure" as well as "static"). A bureaucracy usually has a top-heavy layer of administration to generate the rules. A bureaucracy can create a web of rules and regulations (based on invented wisdom) which requires more bureaucracy for maintenance. This is the ultimate formula for self-survival and leads to the fifth and defining characteristic of Type S organizations: lack of variability and change.

Change threatens Type S organizations because it might lead to their demise. Solving a problem might lead to the elimination of personnel or other resources. This is a threat to survival that the Type S organization will react to avoid. The result is the status quo with little effective change in the practices of the organization. It is unlikely that Type S organizations will bring about effective changes to real problems.

Type F (Functional) Organizations

In contrast to Type S organizations, Type F organizations are controlled by the effects their actions have on the environment rather than by social control. Type F organizations are functional, in the sense that they are controlled by contingencies associated with the problems that produced their emergence. Thus, a Type F government actually reduces crime, a Type F business actually makes a profit, and a Type F school system actually educates its students. In each case, the Type F organization does whatever is necessary to reach its goals. This may mean going against the collective invented wisdom in order to do something that works. What are the other characteristics of Type F organizations? According to Pennypacker (1994) there are five.

First, Type F organizations place a high value on the discovery of new knowledge that can be empirically verified. That is, Type F organizations constantly seek new technologies and methods, but they base these new developments on ***discovered knowledge*** that must be shown to be effective. In contrast, a Type S organization will implement methods based on the invented wisdom of experts, and will rely on the testimony of experts about effectiveness.

Second, the contingencies maintaining the Type F organization are based on the cost versus the benefits of actions. Such cost/benefits contingencies involve both positive (producing benefits) and negative (avoiding societal costs) contingencies. Sensitivity to both cost and benefit contingencies means that Type F organizations place emphasis on positive reinforcing consequences where change and variability are likely to occur.

Because they are sensitive to contingencies that produce societal benefits rather than self-maintaining ones, if Type F organizations are successful, they will flourish. If they are very successful and solve the problems that led to their emergence, they will no longer be necessary and will go out of existence. So for example, if the curriculum experts in a school system were to develop and implement a highly successful curriculum that maximized student learning, they would no longer be needed.

Finally, Type F organizations reinforce variability, not the *status quo*. Variability means that organizations will try out many things in order to find which ones work. Effective governmental, corporate, or educational practices will be selected by cost/benefit contingencies.

Clearly, the characteristics of Type F organizations are more beneficial to society. Unfortunately, all too often, self-maintaining Type S organizations gain a foothold, and by their nature, flourish to the detriment of the people they are supposed to serve. Much of today's cynicism toward our political and educational institutions may be traced to the public's frustrations with Type S organizations.

Cathy Watkins (1988) presents an example of the reluctance of educational organizations to change, even in the face of discovered knowledge. Her example is concerned with Project Follow Through, an educational experiment intended to study various curricula designed to maintain gains achieved by minority children in the preschool Head Start program. Project Follow Through became the most expensive experiment in education ever funded by the federal government, with costs totaling nearly one billion dollars (Watkins, 1988).

Researchers had shown that within three years, gains in IQ and preacademic skills acquired in Head Start were lost, leaving these minority children again below average. By following through with additional years of compensatory educational programs, educators hoped that these gains could be permanently maintained. The federal government paid to have more than a dozen curriculum models implemented in sites across the nation, and to have the effectiveness of these models evaluated by independent agencies. These agencies (Stanford Research Institute collected the data and ABT Associates analyzed them) evaluated the programs in three areas:

Basic skills: Word knowledge, spelling, language, and math computation.

Cognitive/conceptual skills: Reading comprehension, math concepts, and math problem solving.

Affective measures: Self-concept.

When the results were in, one curriculum model stood out: Direct Instruction, which was developed at the University of Oregon. It produced significant positive effects in all three areas. Two others, the Behavior Analysis developed by the University of Kansas and the Florida Parent Education models produced smaller, but still positive effects. Other than one positive significant effect, the remaining projects produced either no effect or actually produced effects that were even worse than the control condition of doing nothing.

Did this lead to the adaptation of Direct Instruction model for the implementation of Project Follow Through? It did not. The Office of Education ignored the data, and instead, averaged the results across all programs, which led to the conclusion that none of the programs worked. Instead of funding the programs that produced the best results, the government funded the programs that produced the worst results. Why would they do this? Watkins (1988) concluded that the programs that were demonstrated to be the most effective were also the ones that clashed with the views and opinions of the educational establishment...the experts. Thus, this is a case of invented wisdom, and not discovered knowledge, guiding educational practice. Unfortunately, this is another case where taxpayers invested their educational dollars in the least effective schooling, when demonstrably more effective alternatives were available. As Watkins concluded: "The educational establishment's vested interests have effectively prevented the largest experiment in history on instructional methods (costing almost one billion dollars) from having the impact on daily classroom practice that its results clearly warranted" (Watkins, 1988, page 10).

Many educators reject behavioral approaches to education, because they see them as promoting academic achievement at the expense of social emotional development. For example, DeVries and her associates (DeVries, Haney, & Zan, 1991; DeVries, Reese-Learned, & Morgan, 1991) compared observations of child-teacher and child-child interactions in kindergarten classrooms representing three types of instruction: Direct Instruction, Constructivist, and Eclectic. Their observations led to the conclusions that the direct instruction teacher was more authoritarian and academically oriented.

The Constructivist teacher (whose program was based on Piagetian principles and more likely to let the children determine what they did) was least authoritarian, least academically oriented, and most likely to encourage cooperation and reasoning. DeVries, Reese-Learned, and Morgan (1991), also found that in interacting with their peers, kindergartners in the direct instruction class used lower level negotiating strategies while those in the constructivist classroom more often used higher level strategies. Two questions arise concerning these observed differences. First, are the differences real? Hatano (1991) and Gersten (1991) believe that these observations on interpersonal understanding are too narrowly focused. This type of focus resulted in a bias against the direct instruction classroom, which had different goals than the constructivist classroom. As Hatano (1991) notes, it would be possible to provide a program for the enhancement of interpersonal skills in a direct instruction program, if that were a goal that was deemed important.

Enhanced educational achievement is one goal shared by most educators. Gersten (1991) pointed out, that the data presented on academic skills by DeVries and her colleague finds clear superiority for the direct-instruction classroom. The eclectic class was listed next for academic success and closely followed the direct instruction class in style (DeVries, Haney, & Zan, 1991).The constructivist classroom showed the least improvement on academic skills. Thus, we should view the effects of educational programs on several dimensions, but always taking the stated goals of the curriculum into account.

Indeed, the evaluation of Project Follow Through is evidence for goal stated assessment. Based on its stated goals, each of the curriculum models was placed into one of three model categories. Both the Direct Instruction and Behavior Analysis models were placed into the Basic Skill model category. Other model categories were called Cognitive-Conceptual or Affective-Cognitive. An example of the latter, was the Bank Street model developed by the Bank Street College of Education. Its primary emphasis was the development of positive self-image, creativity, and using language to express ideas. Contrary to the invented wisdom of the experts, all three of the basic skills models and one of the cognitive-conceptual models produced increases on the affective outcome measures. All of the other models, including all of the affective-cognitive programs, had significant negative effects on self-image. Apparently, providing children with useful basic academic skills, has a much more positive effect on self-image and other affective measures, than does a program focusing on building self-esteem without teaching basic academic skills.

Other researchers have supported the findings of positive outcomes in direct instruction and other behavioral programs. Weisberg (1988; 1994) has presented positive data on a preschool for poverty-level children that used direct instruction for reading.

If direct instruction and other behavioral methods have superior academic, cognitive, and affective outcome, why are they not more widely adopted by an educational system in search or more effective methods? One important reason for the rejection of behavior analysis in mainstream education, is a difference in worldviews regarding the nature of children and the role of teachers. Watkins (1988) suggested that the educational establishment has a vested interest in the status quo much as Pennypacker's Type S institutions do.

"Developmentalism" and Behavior Analysis

John Stone, a dean of education, identified a worldview he called "developmentalism." Stone defined developmentalism as "a theoretical perspective," which overemphasizes three points: (1) that a natural inclination in all children is sufficient, (2) that the limits posed by biological and environmental constraints on learning are too strong to overcome, and (3) instruction is tailored to the learners' attributes and inclinations and not on data provided by others, including the teacher, in areas that they believe the student must know (Stone, 1994).

In Stone's view, developmentalism has become the dominant viewpoint of most members of the educational profession to the detriment of the children they are supposed to educate. In Stone's eyes, educators with this worldview are more concerned with the edict; "Do no harm," than in meeting society's imposed economic needs for children. According to Stone, the dominant worldview of developmentalism has led to many of the failures of American education. Specifically, he cites a curriculum that de-emphasizes achievement through hard work, overemphasizes maturational "readiness," and fails to use successful teaching methods, as reasons for the failure of an educational system made ineffective by the stranglehold of developmentalism's worldview.

As you recall from Chapter 6, learning is the relatively permanent change in behavior that is due to experience. By this definition, learning is a change in the behavior of a person, the student; but learning is a function of experience.

Experience is the action of the environment on the student that produces the change. Experience is the action of the teacher on the student.

Learning and teaching

Structural Approach

In a structural analysis of teaching, teaching is anything that the teacher does to the student. Thus, giving a lecture, assigning homework, giving praise, even showing a film are defined as teaching. Teaching simply is what the teacher does.

Functional Approach

A functional analysis of teaching looks a the function, or outcome of what the teacher does. That is, the effect it has on the student – learning. In this view, the teacher has taught when the student has learned. Therefore, teaching can be defined as creating conditions (that is, experiences) which bring about the relatively permanent changes in behavior, which we call learning. Thus, in a functional approach, lecturing, showing a film, assigning homework, etc. are considered teaching if, and only if, they have the function of changing the child's behavior.

Teaching as Applied Developmental Psychology

If we define teaching as the act of providing conditions that produce relatively permanent changes in behavior, we see the importance of understanding learning principles in education. From a developmental psychology viewpoint, teaching involves providing conditions that promote progressive changes in the interactions between the child and the environment. In both cases, teaching is producing changes, not just providing a stimulating environment.

From this viewpoint, teachers are actually applied developmental psychologists. Aided by the knowledge of both developmental and learning processes, they arrange conditions to bring about development in their students.

As applied developmental psychologists, teachers must be concerned with the two main questions of development: "*What?*" and "*How?*"

The Developmental Questions: "What?" and "How?".

Recall the two key questions in developmental psychology: (1) What? – or What develops? and (2) How? – or How does development occur? You may, also, recall that a better way of asking the "How?" question is "Under what conditions does development occur?"

In viewing teaching as applied developmental psychology, the two same questions are relevant. The "What?" question is: "What should be taught?" This is curriculum. The "How?" question is: "How should it be taught?" This is the question about the appropriate educational practices or methods. Both are important questions in teaching. We turn first to the question of "What?".

Worldviews and the Curriculum

How do we determine what should be taught to our students? Mostly, what is taught reflects the values of a society. What is taught reflects the current worldview of what society believes will best provide the child with the knowledge and abilities necessary for economic independence and personal development. The specifics of curriculum reflect the society's worldview of what is necessary to fulfill these goals. For example, in contemporary technologically advanced and developing countries, computer literacy has become as important a part of the curriculum as reading. In agrarian cultures, computer knowledge and skills may be of little value and absent from the curriculum.

Who Determines Curriculum?

Curriculum development is largely influenced by the coming together of many social and political factors. For example, parents may want sex education changed to reflect a society's worldviews on what children should know about sex (e.g., teaching condom use to prevent HIV infection, or emphasizing abstinence). Society's views, as reflected in the words and actions of parents, politicians (including school board members), and the media, are put into action by the individual teachers and local school administrators who interact with the children. We call such this implicit or ***emergent curriculum***. New lesson plans are implemented or discontinued as a society's implicit worldviews are reflected in teacher behavior.

There is also curriculum that is developed by institutions specifically to address societal needs. This is called explicit or ***formal curriculum***. Formal curriculum may be developed by both Type S or Type F institutions. When developed by Type S institutions, formal curriculum is likely to reflect a structural approach to what is taught. Type F institutions are likely to develop functional approaches to curriculum.

What Makes for Effective Teaching

As suggested by the principle of equifinality (see Chapter 2), effective teaching practice will vary from situation to situation based on the interactions between the child and teacher. However, some general statements can be made regarding effective teachers. Walberg (1990) generalized findings from over 7,000 studies of educational practices from the U.S. and elsewhere. Walberg's findings show that practices which share many principles common with dynamical systems and behavior analysis approaches are effective in educational settings. In fact, many findings are consistent with the four-term contingency (c. f. Good & Weinstein, 1986).

Walberg titled the significant aspects of the teaching process as "cues, engagement, and reinforcement (Walberg, 1990, page 471); he went on to state that the importance of these three terms is "enormous." You may recognize these as antecedent (cue), behavior (engagement of the reader into action) and consequences (reinforcement). While he did not note setting events, Walberg does list some factors which function as the fourth term. Let us see what the educational research summarized by Walberg says about the importance of learning contingencies.

Effective Teaching and the Four-Term Contingency

Walberg found that the crux of the four-term contingency, the antecedent, response, and consequence relationship, were central to effective teaching. Greer (1994) has gone on to identify this contingency, which he calls a ***learn unit***, as the most important measure of teacher performance. Using data collected on six different schools over a seven year period, Greer (1992) found that the achievement of objectives was directly predicted by the number of three-term contingency learn units that the teachers provided and subsequently, that the students performed.

Antecedents or "Cues"

The function of cues or antecedents in teaching is to show the child what is to be learned. For example, the letter "d" is a cue for the sound "ddd" (which sounds similar to "duh"). Other cues include instructions, directions, and prompts. According to Walberg, research shows that the effectiveness of cues is determined by their clarity and salience. Examples of effective cues given by Walberg include the following:

> **Advance Organizers**: Brief overviews that review old learning and relate it to what is to come.
>
> **Adjunct Questions**: Provide the students with key questions that are most central to what is studied. These are particularly effective when they relate to similar, although not necessarily identical questions on the posttest.
>
> **Goal Setting**: These are specific objectives, methods, and standards that are made explicit. Like adjunct questions, these explicit objectives tell the students what they are supposed to know and what the standards are.
>
> **Learning Hierarchies**: Presentations are structured along a hierarchical sequence based on logical or functional task analysis.
>
> **Pretests**: Not only do pretests allow the teacher to adjust instruction to the level of the student, but according to Walberg (1990) research shows that pretest information serves as cues to the child about what he knows and needs to know.

Active Responding or "Engagement"

The key term of effective teaching does not differ from the key term of the four-term contingency. It is, as Skinner stated, all behavior. Behavior analysts (e.g., Greenwood, Delquardri, & Hall, 1984, Greenwood, Hart, Walker, and Risley, 1994) have emphasized the importance of the teacher providing extensive student ***opportunities to respond.*** Walberg labeled this behavior "engagement" of the student and found it to be central to effective teaching. As he summarized: "A high degree of engagement is indicated by an absence of irrelevant behavior and by concentration on tasks, enthusiastic contributions to group discussion, and lengthy study"

(Walberg, 1990, page 471)". Heward (1994) found three benefits of active student responding:

1) Active student responding generates more learning than a passive lesson of equal length.
2) Active student responding provides important feedback to the teacher.
3) Active student responding is related to more on-task and less off-task behavior. This means students are more attentive, less disruptive and more pleasing to teachers.

Among the methods found to successfully enhance student learning though active engagement are (Walberg, 1990):

Frequent testing: Tests stimulate greater effort and require studying responses by students. The effectiveness of smaller, more frequent quizzes is greater than that for final exams.

Questioning: Teacher questions encourage student thinking and verbal responding. Furthermore, giving students time to think rather than requiring immediate responding, may be most effective.

One problem with questioning in medium to large classes is that other students may be unengaged with only one student answering a question. We probably have all sighed with relief and stopped listening when the person next to us was called on to answer a tough question. At least two procedures have been devised to increase the active responding to questions of students in large classes. The first is ***choral responding*** (Heward, 1994). There are six key elements in choral responding:

1) The teacher provides clear directions and models one or two practice trials.
2) The teacher provides a pause for student thinking. Generally the length of the pause is based on the complexity of the task and the students' level of skill.
3) The teacher uses a clear, consistent cue to signal students to respond. This might be a word like "Class!" or "Now!" and may be helped with a visual prompt like a hand signal or touching the chalkboard.
4) The teacher provides feedback for the majority's response. Praise when nearly all students are correct; and repeating the answer provides reinforcement for correct responses. When a significant portion of students gives the wrong answer, a correction procedure such as giving the correct answer and then repeating the learning trial is used.
5) The teacher should occasionally call on a random individual student. This variable ratio schedule is employed to prevent individuals from hiding behind the responding of others, such as the student who has the right answer but is two milliseconds slow.
6) The teacher should maintain a lively pace by preparing the materials ahead of time. This keeps the session moving and interesting. Choral responding can be fun, but only if the teacher keeps it moving. Choral responding is a key element in direct instruction (e.g., Englemann & Brunner, 1988; Carnine, 1976) and other behavioral teaching methods.

A second solution to encouraging responding in large classes is the use of ***response cards*** (Heward, 1994). Response cards are items such as cards, signs, or objects that students hold up on cue to indicate their understanding of a question. They are used like an instantaneous multiple choice or true-false test. For example, students may be given a green card with the word "true" on it an a red one with "false" written on it. Students are taught the procedure that involves holding up one of the cards when given the appropriate cue. Then during lecture a teacher may get feedback on the students' understanding of a concept by posing a question and looking at the number of correct cards held up by students. As with other forms of active responding this (1) enhances the likelihood that students will actively respond to the material, (2) provides feedback to the teacher about whether to go on or repeat material, and (3) keeps students on task. Similarly multiple choice answers, and even pictures or words (e.g., "Hold up the word 'elephant'") can be used as response cards. Again, this requires advance teacher preparation, but according to research summarized by Heward (1994) the procedure can be very successfully used for all grades. Mallott and his colleagues have even used response cards with college students.

The two active responding methods described above work well with groups, but are best limited to material that has short answers (although response cards could have complex answers on them). Heward suggested a third active responding method: ***guided notes*** (Heward, 1994) or ***framed outlines*** (Horton & Lovitt, 1989; Bergerud, Lovitt, & Horton, 1988). Heward cites research (Baker & Lombardi, 1985; Carrier, 1983) showing that accurate note taking and studying of these notes leads to better test scores than those who just read a textbook and passively listen to lecture. Unfortunately, not all students are effective note takers. However, with guided notes, students are provided with handouts from the lecture in which key elements are left blank. There is space for students to complete the notes.

Greenwood and his associates (Greenwood, et al., 1994) have identified seven components of active student responding. These components consist of writing, academic game play, reading aloud, silent reading, academic talk, answering questions, and asking questions. Taken together, these measures are associated with increased achievement test scores (Greenwood, Delquadri, Stanley, Sasso, Whorton, & Schute, 1981). This study compared the time spent in active engagement of inner-city fourth-grade children who were lower in IQ and standardized achievement to a group of suburban children. Greenwood and his associates (Greenwood, et al., 1984) found the inner-city children actively engaging in academic tasks twelve minutes per day less. While this may sound inconsequential, the twelve minutes per day comes to the equivalent of 1.6 additional school months when figured for the entire school year. Given the correlation of opportunity to respond, is it any wonder that the inner-city sample was behind intellectually and academically?

Consequences: Reinforcement and Corrective Feedback

Consequences are crucial since they strengthen some responses and weaken others. Without a strong and immediate consequence, behavior is not changed, and learning does not occur. Teaching therefore involves the planned application of consequences. In many cases, teachers may be able to arrange for the delivery of natural or logical consequences. For example, a wide variety of textures may naturally reinforce exploratory behavior of objects or the plot of a story may reinforce reading. However, natural consequences may not always be possible or practical. In these cases it is the teacher's role to provide consequences so that correct responses are strengthened and incorrect ones are weakened. Walberg (1990) identified two types of consequences that produced effective instruction: corrective feedback and praise.

According to Walberg, corrective feedback has moderate effects because it remedies errors by reteaching. Behaviorally, corrective feedback seems to serve two functions. First, it punishes the incorrect response. Second, it models the correct response. Englemann and Carnine (1992) have developed several correction procedures that maximize the effectiveness of corrective feedback.

Praise is a common form of positive reinforcement. As with all reinforcement, praise is only positive reinforcement if it contingently strengthens behavior. Walberg finds praise to have a small positive effect on teaching effectiveness, possibly because it is used inappropriately. That is, praise may be used excessively and produce satiation. Furthermore, the praise from some teachers may be aversive or non-reinforcing because they have never established their praise as a secondary reinforcer. Finally, and surprisingly often, praise is used too infrequently by many teachers, thus not consequating many behaviors.

Good and Brophy (1984) have provided the following guidelines for the use of effective praise:

- Praise should be simple and direct.
- Use straightforward, declarative sentences, not "gushy" statements like "Wow!" (Although even Good and Brophy might find "Cool!", cool).
- Specify the particular accomplishment being praised and any effort, care or perseverance the child shows (e.g., "That's really good. I like how you finished the whole thing").
- Vary your statements and the way you deliver praise.
- Have your non-verbal communication back-up your vocal praise.
- Avoid ambiguous statements (e.g., "You were really great today"). Statements like these do not reinforce specific behaviors.
- In sum, be sincere, be enthusiastic and be contingent. Finally, remember, praise is a reinforcer *only if it strengthens behavior*.

Bill Hopkins (1994) related many of his experiences and ultimately, his frustrations, in making changes in the schools in Lawrence, Kansas, (where he is a professor at the University of Kansas). He began as a consultant and found that getting teachers to provide frequent immediate positive reinforcement, such as: "Good work, Mary," or "Great job, Johnny" had significant effects on the children's schoolwork. Teachers increased their praise and children increased their knowledge. Hopkins, as would most of us, thought that once teachers discovered the effective-

Box 14-1

A Model for Schooling

One comprehensive approach to education using dynamical systems and behavior analysis principles is seen in the Morningside Academy in Seattle Washington. (Johnson & Layng, 1994). The Morningside Academy started out as a broad series of programs for learners of all ages. Today it is primarily a year-round school program for children with learning and attention problems who are below grade levels in academic achievement. One of the most unusual aspects about the Morningside Academy is its two academic money-back guarantees. For children who are two or more years behind in school and would generally be classified as "learning disabled," the guarantee is that they will gain at least two grade levels per year or receive a tuition refund proportionate to the shortfall. The second guarantee is for children with problems such as distractibility, hyperactivity, and poor study skills who might generally be classified as "attention deficit disorder" (ADD) children. For these children, the guarantee is that they will increase their ability to stay on task (generally from their typical starting 1-3 minute attention span to 20 minutes or more) and increase their learning level to the 65th percentile nationally. In its history of offering guarantees (now more than seven years), Morningside has never had to pay off on these guarantees! How has this remarkable feat been accomplished when most of the educational system is in crisis? The answer is in the use of behavioral and dynamical systems principles in its curriculum and methods.

Curriculum (What is Taught)

The Morningside Academy approach to education follows a skills learning approach (See Chapter 8) to the development of intellectual behavior. What to teach is identified by task analysis. Conceptual behavior, which is defined as the behavior of identifying instances of events and things forms the basic skills of the curriculum. Conceptual behavior is taught primarily through discrimination training in which a series of positive and negative examples of the concept is introduced, and active responding is prompted. Correct responses are reinforced, incorrect responses are corrected, and discrimination training trials are prompted again. Once basic concepts are learned, exercises that are designed to produce generalization through relating and combining simple concepts into complex ones. Consistent with the hierarchy of skills learning approaches (See Chapter 8), the development of questioning and writing skills are further methods for producing complex conceptual behavior. The development of generalized and complex conceptual skills is planned, rather than left to chance.

There is extensive use of the four-term contingency. Aside from providing motivation and facilitation through appropriate setting events, the Morningside Academy emphasizes three-term learn units. Responses are prompted by materials and teachers and responses are consequated. Extensive use of natural contingencies and automatic reinforcement as well as teacher provided reinforcement occur.

Two key elements of the Morningside Academy approach are its emphasis on learning rate and fluency. Arguing that if slow learners continue at the same rate of academic development, that they will continue to fall farther and farther behind (the so-called "cumulative deficit"), Johnson and Layng (1994) focused on accelerating learning. By continually collecting data on each student, teachers could set goals and monitor the progress of individual students, effectively using the 3C/ROD principle. Thus, Morningside is able to correct instruction that is not working for its students.

Fluency is defined as behaviors which satisfy five criteria: retention, endurance, application, performance, and stability (REAPS). The REAPS criteria were discovered by teachers using a method called Precision Teaching and has been shown to produce long-lasting and powerful learning. It means that learning of a concept must occur until the REAPS criteria are obtained, rather than just to simple acquisition. For example, a child who only has learned to spell C-A-T is cat to a single picture of a cat has not met the REAPS criteria. Research shows that that child is less likely to be able to spell the word for other pictures, prompts, or over the long-term. Meeting the REAPS criteria requires extended practice at a high level of proficiency and in many situations. However, once the REAPS criteria have been met, fluency in a skill has been obtained.

For example consider your own language skills. You are likely fluent in at least one language (let us say English). In addition, you may have studied another. At some point, while you were studying that language, you were probably able to demonstrate some accurate skills but not to the extent to meet the definition of fluency specified by REAPS. Perhaps you were able to pronounce vocabulary or even carry out a formal greeting. Most students of a language have had the experience wherethey are able to use their acquired skills well enough to function within the confines of their class room, but fall completely apart the first time they have to talk to a native speaker in a real-life context. This difference in the ability of one who is fluent in a skill with one who is not, is why the Morningside Academy emphasizes fluency.

Early on it was discovered by teaching to fluency, nonlinear phase shifts in skills often occurred. These "curriculum leaps" began to occur when fluent learners were challenged. This sudden combination of component skills has been called "contingency adduction" (Andronis 1983; Johnson & Layng, 1992) because the qualitatively different skill is assembled or adduced by the contingencies of reinforcement. As suggested by Skinner's writings on creativity, new behaviors may emerge under conditions in which the person is reinforced for unique combinations of existing knowledge and skills repertoires. You may recognize this as the same as the principle of coalescent organization introduced in Chapter 21.

Because of the discovery that teaching skill fluency leads to emergent behaviors and acceleration of learning, the Morningside Academy curriculum emphasizes the fluency building of relatively few skills compared to the superficial learning of many concepts. Thus, while traditional schools may spend 70% in establishing skills and only 20% in practicing these, it is the reverse at Morningside. Here, 70% of student time is in practicing the skills to fluency and only 20% of the time is devoted to new skills. Because of the power of skills developed to the REAPS criteria, many new skills emerge without the need (and time!) to teach them directly.

Methods (How it is Taught)

As already mentioned, most of the establishment of conceptual behavior is accomplished through discrimination training. Once a skill is acquired, practice sessions are used to establish fluency of the skills. Thus, unlike in other programs, much more time is spent on fluency building than on establishing skills. In order to accomplish fluency, a number of principles are followed . These steps are listed below:

- Identify the component elements of instructional objectives. This is accomplished through task analysis and analysis of sequences of skills. For example reading has prerequisite pointing, decoding, and scanning skills.
- Measure their frequency until true mastery (as identified by REAPS) of these behaviors is achieved. Accomplished by initial pretesting and continual pretesting. Records of progress toward skill mastery are posted in public.
- Establish a component behavior through highly interactive, contingent exchanges between learner and teacher. Accomplished by small group (12 or less) instruction. Direct instruction , programmed instruction (including computer programs), and the system of

personalized instruction (PSI) are used. Instruction class size can be kept small by instructing only those deficient in the skills (based on pretesting) with those already possessing the skill engaged in practice rather than instruction. Once the skills are established, coaches interact with students to increase the student's speed on the skill in a method called "sprinting".

- Build the component skills to fluency so as to ensure remembering. Once the skill is firmly established and strengthened, activities, such as worksheets are used to bring the skill to fluency by practice on the basic skills and their combinations.
- Build the endurance of component skills that are repeated in succession en masse in the real world. Once basic skills are fluent, composites are practiced to the REAPS criteria by extended worksheets and activities.
- Include application activities that allow multiple component skills to combine in ways that define the higher-level complex activities of an expert in a field. This is accomplished through activities, simulations, and games designed to strengthen composite skills and generalize them to new environments. Joe Layng has applied the Morningside model to college students at Malcom X. College in Chicago who are lacking in necessary academic skills. For their final project in an art class, students must build a portfolio that will be accepted by and displayed by the curator of an art museum! (Layng, 1995).
- Alter the procedures according to the data collected. A basic assumption of the Morningside model is that teaching is applied science and has a self-correcting mechanism built in. As with 3C/ROD, constant contact with the relevant outcome data will lead to the abandonment of ineffective practices and their replacement by effective ones.

ness a little more frequent and a little more direct praise provided, they would be reinforced by the children's' responses and increase their reinforcing behavior. This was not the case, and once the consultants returned after a month-long absence, the level of praise had declined, and so had student achievement.

Hopkins felt the solution would be to train the school principal in the procedure. He worked with the principal, who in turn supervised his teachers in the effective use of positive reinforcement. Results showed an increase in the teacher's level of praise as well as an increase in academic performance. However, weeks later, when Hopkins returned, neither the principal nor the teachers had maintained their

Under what conditions are teachers and principals likely to adopt effective teaching strategies? One is to teach them how to evaluate the effectiveness of their work with children and to encourage them to monitor their students' progress. Bushell and Baer (1994) believe that *close, continual contact with relevant outcome data* or ***3C/ROD*** (pronounced "three-cee-rod") would work. 3C/ROD means that teachers and administrators would determine objectives for each child and continually measure progress toward these goals. The kinds of measures that they suggest are not very difficult to collect.

As an example, they had a teacher identify, at the beginning of the year, how many pages of reading and what level of accuracy (say, 80% accuracy) should be reached over a specified amount of time. Suppose 360 pages of reading in a 40 week school year was the goal. Each ten pages would be a step. They had the teacher record the number of students who were reading at each step and then they graphed this. The graph provided a clear picture of class progress. As they summarized:

"The teachers always knew where they were in relation to the objectives, and in relation to where they had been last week and last month. Their teaching had been brought into close, continual contact with its most relevant consequences. If you behaviors. Finally, Hopkins ran for, and was elected to the school board, in order to be able to apply some contingencies to the larger system.

Hopkins' experience points out the fact that even simple procedures which work, may not work in the long run if they are not reinforcing to the person who must use them. Teaching, particularly with more than thirty children in a classroom is hard work. Under the conditions in which most teachers work, praise may not come naturally, and finding the time and the opportunity to praise every child frequently may not occur. Hopkins admitted that he was somewhat naively expecting the use of praise to be a positive reinforcement trap in which the teacher would use praise because it's use was strengthened by its natural consequences of increasing student performance. In fact, while praise did increase the children's' performance, those effects were not sufficient to maintain the teachers' use of contingent praise.
asked *those* teachers if it had been a good week, and how it compared to the previous week, they could answer exactly" (Bushell & Baer, 1994, page 6).

It is likely that there are extremely rare classroom teachers who actually do this on their own. It is rarely a part of the training teachers receive in their credentialling programs. However, the consequences for teachers are positive. The charts took about twenty minutes a week to prepare. For this, the charts evoked a great deal of positive comment from the principal and other teachers. This led to the teachers preparing charts for individual students. These progress charts were sent home so parents could see the progress of their children. Bushell and Baer suggest that older children (their study was done with first-graders) could be taught to graph their own progress. What function did the charts have apart from the positive reinforcement for teacher charting behavior? Coming into close, continual contact with relevant data means that a teacher knows what is and is not working, and can make changes in the methods. She knows which children are succeeding and which need further attention. This is truly a functional approach to teaching.

Training teachers to measure their effectiveness may be one way to provide them with positive reinforcement for effective teaching. Stokes, Fowler, and Baer (1978) found an unusual and less obvious way. They taught preschoolers social skills which got adults to praise them. In an even simpler demonstration of the bidirectional power of praise, when children complete a school unit, Don Bushell gives students a card to wear around their necks. The card has something written on it such as "I can count to 20!" This generally has one or two effects on adults. Either they praise the child's behavior, or else they ask the child to engage in the behavior and then praise it. Either way, Bushell reports that this has led to increased academic performance (and happy children and adults).

The role of natural (or intrinsic versus contrived consequences is at the heart of the debate for those who take the "do no harm!" approach to education. In the view of these educators, pushing the child too soon will destroy the child's intrinsic motivation and her love of learning.

The issue of intrinsic versus contrived consequences was discussed in some detail in Chapter 7. As you may recall, it was suggested that contrived consequences, be used only when intrinsic ones are absent. Unfortunately, in learning some things, intrinsic reinforcers *are* absent or very delayed. What is to be done in this case? Some suggest doing nothing – when the child is ready to learn he will. Others suggest that *not* using contrived reinforcers and other effective educational practices is a form of educational malpractice. One group (the Association for Behavior Analysis, Task Force on the Right to Effective Education) believes it is the right of every child to receive effective education (Barrett, Beck, Binder, Cook, Engelmann, Greer, Kyrklund, Johnson, Maloney, McCorkle, Vargas, & Watkins; 1990). Their points are summarized in Box 14.2.

From a developmental view, it is desirable to encourage the establishment of positive reinforcers and generalized positive reinforcers appropriate for the child's developmental history. For some, this may be accomplished by allowing the child to experience the "joy" of learning. In many cases it involves the pairing of learning with praise and other effective positive reinforcers. In other cases, it may require the development of an effective teaching system in which intrinsic and contrived reinforcers both are effectively used.

In addition, it is important to avoid making schooling aversive. Setting up conditions that lead to constant failure and the use of ridicule or other coercive behaviors, are likely to punish learning rather than reinforce it.

In summary, praise and corrective feedback can change behavior. As Bushell and Baer (1994) state, "criticism does not improve the outcome data nearly as well as praise reserved for good performance" (page 8).

Box 14-2
The Association for Behavior Analysis
Position Statement on Students' Rights to Effective Education
November, 1990

The current crisis in American education and the destructive consequences of its failure for the economic, social, and cultural future of our country are receiving national publicity. At the same time, research findings are repeatedly demonstrating the superiority of specific instructional approaches and methods based on well-researched scientifically valid principles continue to be ignored. As a result, students are denied access to the most effective educational practices.

The Association for Behavior Analysis therefore issues the following position statement setting forth elements shown to maximize students gains throughout the course of their education.

Based on principles that have been demonstrated to improve student learning and performance, the following are recommended educational entitlements for all students in the nation's schools:

1. The student's overall educational context should include:

- social and physical school environments that encourage and maintain academic achievement and progress, and discourage socially deviant or unacceptable behavior.
- schools that treat students with care and individual attention, comparable to that offered by a caring family
- school programs that provide support and training for parents in parenting and teaching skills, and
- consequences and attention at home that encourage and maintain success at school.

2. Curriculum and instructional objectives should:

- be based on empirically validated hierarchies or sequences of instructional objectives and measurable performance criteria that are demonstrated to promote cumulative mastery and that are of long-term value in the culture
- include mastery criteria that specify both the accuracy and speed dimensions of fluent performance
- include instructional objectives that promote both long-term and short-term personal and vocational success, and that, once mastered, will

be maintained by natural consequences in everyday living, and

- include long-term retention and maintenance of skills and knowledge as explicitly measured instructional objectives.

3. **Assessment and Student Placement should involve:**

- assessment and reporting methods that are sufficiently criterion-referenced to promote useful decision-making based on actual levels of skills and knowledge rather than on categorical labels such as "emotionally disturbed" or "learning disabled", and
- placement based on correspondence between measured entering skills and skills required as prerequisites for a given level in a hierarchically sequenced curriculum.

4. **Instructional methods should:**

- allow students to master instructional objectives at their own pace and to respond as rapidly and as frequently as they are able during at least some self-paced instructional sessions each day
- provide sufficient practice opportunities to enable students to truly master skills and knowledge at each step in the curriculum
- provide consequences designed to correct errors and/or to increase frequency of responding and that are adjusted to individual performance until they enable students to achieve desired outcomes
- adjust in response to measures of individual learning and performance, including use of individualized instruction when group instruction fails to produce desired outcome
- regularly employ the most advanced equipment to promote skill mastery via programs incorporating validated features described in this document, and
- be applied by teachers who receive performance-based training, administrative and supervisory support, and evaluation in the use of measurably effective, scientifically validated instructional procedures, programs and materials.

5. **Measurement and Summative Evaluation should entail:**

- decision-making via objective curriculum-based measures of performance, and
- reports of objectively measured individual achievement and progress rather than subjective ratings, norm-referenced comparisons, or letter grading.

6. **Assumption of Responsibility for Success should be such that:**

- financial and operational consequences for school personnel, should depend on objective measures of student achievement

- teachers, administrators, and the general educational program should assume responsibility for student success, and change programs until students achieve desired learning outcomes, and
- students and parents should be allowed and encouraged to change schools or school programs until their educational needs are met.

The above statement is an abbreviated version of a report by the Association for Behavior Analysis, Task Force on the Right to Effective Education (members: B. H. Barrett [Chair], R. Beck, C. Binder, D. A. Cook, S. Engelmann, R. D. Greer, S. J. Kyrklund, K. R. Johnson, M. Maloney, N. McCorkle, J. S. Vargas, C. L. Watkins). Ogden R. Lindsley was the original Council Liaison. He was followed in this capacity by Julie S. Vargas and Kennon A. Lattal. This report was accepted by the ABA Executive Council, however it does not necessarily reflect the view of the majority of ABA members nor does it constitute official ABA policy. The complete report will be published in an upcoming issue of *The Behavior Analyst*, which can be ordered from The Association for Behavior Analysis, Western Michigan University, 258 Wood Hall, Kalamazoo, MI 49008-5052 (cost $2.00).

The Fourth Term: Setting Events or Establishing Operations

Although many writers have specified the importance of the first three terms of the operant contingency, many educators have also focused on setting events or establishing operations. Recall, these are events that affect the contingency either by influencing the discriminative stimulus-response or the response-consequence relationship. General conditions such as the physical setting (e.g. whether a school room is bright and open or dark and in need of repair), the time of day (e.g., contingencies for difficult subjects may be more favorable early in the day than just before going home), and school breakfast programs (e.g., hungry children may have increased difficulty doing school work) affect learning. These are just a small set of the many conditions that influence the child's interactions with teachers, peers and academic tasks. Together, the four-term contingency is a powerful determinant for learning. Effective teachers make maximum use of it.

What & How to Teach: Final Comments

We end this final chapter on developmental psychology by turning to comments by B.F. Skinner (1984). In his advice, Skinner outlined several basic points that apply to teaching at all levels. These are:

- Be clear about what is to be taught.

- Teach first things first.
- Stop making all students advance at essentially the same time.
- Program the subject matter. How do these points relate to dynamical systems and behavior analysis?
- Be clear about what is to be taught: By specifying the problem, you are specifying
- Teach first things first: More complex behaviors are built upon more basic ones. As suggested by Fischer's Skill Theory of cognitive development, complex cognitive skills emerge from the transformation of basic skills. This principle also relates, in general, to the principle of shaping or reinforcing successive approximations. By starting with simple responses that can be reinforced, teachers can gradually increase the standard for reinforcement to shape complex behavior.
- Stop making all students advance at essentially the same time. As individuals with unique genetics, interactional histories, and environments, students may require unique conditions for learning. Traditional education employs a group approach that is moderately effective for most students. However, not all fourth-graders are equal. Group teaching is poor for optimizing the development and learning of each individual. Under group teaching conditions, most children will learn something, a few will learn much, and some will learn very little, or not at all. Accepting the normal curve as the standard for teaching seems an admission that our educational approach is weak. After all, why should we be satisfied that teaching should produce the same kind of curve that can be found in nature without any special treatment? Shouldn't effective teaching produce better performance than that? Finding ways to individualize instruction, a difficult task with limited economic resources, should be a goal of educators.
- Program instruction: Teaching can be made more effective if what is to be taught, and how it is to be taught can be programmed. Programming instruction means that what is to be taught is arranged in the most effective sequence so that basic concepts are taught first and form the foundation for complex ones. Furthermore, programmed instruction means the use of technology to present material clearly, provide individual pacing, and provide immediate consequences. This technology may be high tech, in the form of multimedia computers, or low tech, as in programmed textbooks.

References

Acredolo, L. P., & Goodwyn, S. W. (1985). Symbolic gesturing in language development: A Case Study. *Human Development, 28*, 40-49.

Acredolo, L. P., & Goodwyn, S. W. (1988). Symbolic gesturing in normal infants. *Child Development, 59*, 450-466.

Acredolo, L. P., & Goodwyn, S. W. (1990). Sign language in babies: The significance of symbolic gesturing for understanding language development. In R. Vasta (Ed.), *Annals of Child Development* (Vol. 7, pp. 1-42). London: Jessica Kingsley Publishers.

Aherne, W., & Dunnill, M. S. (1966). Morphometry of the human placenta. *British Medical Bulletin, 22*, 5-8.

Ainsworth, M., Bell, S., & Stayton, D. (1972). Individual differences in the strange situation behavior of 1-year-olds. In H. R. Schaffer (Ed.), *The origins of human social relations*. New York: Academic Press.

American Medical Association (1991). Use of folic acid for the prevention of spina bifida and other neural tube defects - 1993-1991 (Morbibity and mortality weekly reports). *Journal of the American Medical Association, 266*, 1190-1191.

Anastasi, A. (1958). Heredity, environment, and the question "How?". *Psychological Review, 65*, 197-208-208.

Andronis, P. T. (1983). *Symbolic aggression by pigeons: Contingency coadduction*. Unpublished doctoral dissertation, The University of Chicago.

Anisfeld, M. (1991). Neonatal Imitation. *Developmental Review, 11*, 60-97.

Anslin, R. N. (1987). Visual and auditory development in infancy. In J. D. Osofsky (Ed.), *Handbook of infant development* (Second ed., pp. 5-97). New York, NY: Wiley.

Ashmead, D. H., DeFord, L. D., Whalen, T., & Odom, R. D. (1991). Sound localization and sensitivity to interaural time differences in human development. *Child Development, 62*, 1211-1226.

Azrin, N. H., Hutchinson, R. R., & Hake, D. F. (1966). Extinction-induced agression. *Journal of the Experimental Analysis of Behavior, 9*, 191-204.

Baer, D. M. (1976). The organism as host. *Human Development, 19*, 87-98.

Baer, D. M., & Rosales, J. (1994, May). Behavioral cusps: An organizing concept for a developmental behavior analysis. Paper presented at the 20th international meeting of the Association for Behavior Analysis, Atlanta, GA.

Baer, D. M., & Sherman, J. A. (1964). Reinforcement control of generalized imitation in young children. *Journal of Experimental Child Psychology, 1*, 37-49.

Baker, L., & Lombardi, B. R. (1985). Students' lecture notes and their relation to test performance. *Teaching of Psychology, 12*, 28-32.

Baltes, M., & Reese, H. W. (1977). Operant research in violation of the operant paradigm? In B. C. Etzel, J. M. LeBlanc, & D. J. Baer (Eds.), *New developments in behavioral research: theory, method and application* (pp. 11-30). Hillsdale, NJ: Lawrence Erlbaum Associates.

Bandura, A. (1965). Influence of models' reinforcement contingencies on the acquisition of imitative responses. *Journal of Personality and Social Psychology, 1*, 589-595.

Bandura, A. (1969). *Principles of behavior modification*. New York: Holt, Rinehart & Winston.

Bandura, A. (1977a). Self-efficacy: Toward a unifying theory of behavioral change. *Psychological Review, 84*, 191-215.

Bandura, A. (1977b). *Social Learning Theory*. Englewood Cliffs, NJ: Prentice-Hall.

Bandura, A., & Walter, R. (1963). *Social learning and personality development*. New York: Holt, Rinehart and Winston.

Bandura, A., Ross, D., & Ross, S. A. (1963). Imitation of film-mediated aggressive models. *Journal of Abnormal and Social Psychology, 67*, 527-534.

Barash, D. P. (1982). The fitness of categories and vice versa. *Neuroscience & Biobehavioral Reviews*, *6*, 95-104.

Barrett, B. H., Beck, R., Binder, C., Cook, D. A., Engelmann, S., Greer, R. D., Kyrklund, S. J., Johnson, K. R., Maloney, M., McCorkle, N., Vargas, J. S., & Watkins, C. L. (1990, November). The Association for Behavior Analysis position statement on students' rights to effective education.

Barrett-Goldfarb, M. S., & Whitehurst, G. J. (1972). Infant vocalizations as a function of parental voice selection. *Developmental Psychology*, *8*, 273-276.

Barton, S. (1994). Chaos, self-Organization, and psychology. *American Psychologist*, *49*, 5-14.

Bauman, K. E., Reiss, M. L. Rogers, R. W., & Bailey, J. S. (1983). Dining out with children: Effectiveness of a parent advice package on pre-meal inappropriate behavior. *Journal of Applied Behavior Analysis*, *18*, 55-68.

Baumrind, D. (1966). Effects of authoritative parental control on child behavior. *Child Development*, *37*, 887-907.

Baumrind, D. (1967). Child care practices anteceding three patterns of preschool behavior. *Genetic Psychology Monographs*, *75*, 43-88.

Baumrind, D. (1977, March). Socialization determinants of personal agency. Paper presented at the biennial meeting of the Society for Research in Child Development, New Orleans.

Bayer, R. (1994). Ethical challenges posed by zidovudine treatment to reduce vertical transmission of HIV. *The New England Journal of Medicine*, *331*, 1223-1225.

Belin, H. (1989). Piagetian theory. In R. Vasta (Ed.), *Annals of Child Development* (Vol. 6). Greenwich, CT: JAI Press.

Bell, S. (1903). The significance of activity in child life. *Independent*, *55*, 911-914.

Bem, S. L. (1974). The measurement of psychological andrognyny. *Journal of Consulting and Clinical Psychology*, *42*, 155-162.

Bem, S. L. (1975). Sex-role adaptability: One consequence of psychological androgyny. *Journal of Personality and Social Psychology*, *31*, 634-643.

Bem, S. L. (1978). Beyond androgyny: Some presumptuous prescriptions for a liberated sexual identity. In J. A. Sherman & F. L. Denmark (Eds.), *The psychology of women: Future dimensions in research*. New York: Psychological Dimensions.

Bem, S. L. (1981). Gender schema theory: A cognitive account of sex typing. *Psychological Review*, *88*, 354-364.

Berger, S. M. (1962). Conditioning through vicarious instigation. *Psychological Review*, *69*, 450-466.

Bergerud, D., Lovitt, T. C., & Horton, S. (1988). The effectiveness of textbook adaptations to life science for high school students with learning disabilities. *Journal of Leering Disabilities*, *21*, 70-76.

Berko, J. (1958). The child's learning of English morphology. Word, *14*, 150-177.

Besevegis, E., & Lore, R. K. (1983). Effects of an adult's presence on the social behavior of preschool children. *Aggressive Behavior*, *9*, 243-252.

Best, D. L., Williams, J. E., Cloud, J. M., Davis, W. S., Robertson, L. S., Edwards, S. R., Giles, H., & Fowles, J. (1977). Development of sex-trait stereotypes among young children in the United States, England, and Ireland. *Child Development*, *48*, 1373-1384.

Bijou, S. W. (1975). Development in the preschool years: A functional analysis. *American Psychologist*, *30*, 829-837. (N)

Bijou, S. W. (1992). Early childhood and parent education. In R. P. West & L. A. Hamerlynck (Eds.), *Designs for excellence in education: The legacy of B.F. Skinner* (pp. 163-185). Longmont, CO: Sopris West.

Bijou, S. W., & Baer, D. M. (1961). *Child development I: A systematic and empirical theory* (Vol. 1). New York: Appleton-Century-Crofts.
Bijou, S. W., & Baer, D. M. (1965). *Child development: Universal stage of infancy* (Vol. 2). New York: Appleton-Century-Crofts.
Bijou, S. W., & Baer, D. M. (1978). *Behavior analysis of child development.* Englewood Cliffs, NJ: Prentice-Hall.
Birnbaum, J. A. (1975). Life patterns and self-esteem in gifted family-oriented and career-committed women. In M. S. Mednick, S. S. Tangri, & L. W. Hoffman (Eds.), *Women and achievement* (pp. 396-410). Washington, DC: Hemisphere.
Bjorklund, D. F. (1987). A note on neonatal imitation. *Developmental Review, 7,* 86-92.
Bjorklund, D. F. (1989). *Children's thinking: Developmental function and individual differences.* Belmont, CA: Brooks/Cole.
Blaich, C. F., Miller, D. B., & Hicinbothom, G. (1989). Alarm call responsivity of mallard ducklings: Vii. Interaction between developmental history and behavioral context. *Developmental Psychobiology, 22,* 203-210.
Blumberg, M. (1974). Psychopathology of the abusing parent. *American Journal of Psychotherapy, 28,* 21-29.
Bornstein, M. H. (1981). Psychological studies of color perception in human infants: Habituation, discrimination and categorization, recognition, and conceptualization. In L. P. Lipsitt & C. K. Rovee-Collier (Eds.), *Advances in infancy research* (Vol. 1, pp. 1-40). Norwood, NJ: Ablex.
Bower, T. G. R. (1977). *A primer of infant development.* San Francisco: Freeman.
Bowlby, J. (1960). Separation anxiety. *International Journal of Psychoanalysis, 41,* 89-113.
Bowlby, J. (1969). *Attachment and Loss* (Vol. 1: Attachment). New York: Basic Books.
Bowlby, J. (1973). *Attachment and loss* (Vol. 2: Loss). New York: Basic Books.
Bowlby, J. (1980). *Attachment and loss* (Vol. 3 Separation: Anxiety and Anger). New York: Basic Books.
Boyer, P. J., Dillon, M., Navaie, M. Deveikis, A. Keller, M. O'Rourke, S., & Bryson, Y. J. (1994). Factors predictive of maternal-fetal transmission of HIV-1: Preliminary analysis of zidovudine given during pregnancy and/or delivery. *Journal of the American Medical Association, 271,* 1925-1930.
Bradley, R. H., Whiteside, L., Mundfrom, D. J., Casey, P. H., Kelleher, K. J., & Pope, S. K. (1994). Early indications of resilience and their relation to experience in the home environments of low birthweight, premature children living in poverty. *Child Development, 65,* 346-360.
Brandenburg, G. C., & Brandenburg, J. (1919). Language development during the fourth year: The conversation. *Pedagogical Seminary, 26,* 27-40.
Branscum, E., & Novak, G. (1995, May). The importance of compound stimulus presentation in language acquisition through dialogic reading sessions. Paper presented at the 21st annual convention of the Association for Behavior Analysis, Washington, D.C.
Bretherton, I. (1987). New perspectives on attachment relations: Security, communication, and internal working models. In J. D. Osofsky (Ed.), *Handbook of Infant Development* (Second ed., pp. 1061-1100). New York: Wiley.
Bridger, W. H. (1961). Sensory habituation and discrimination in the human neonate. *American Journal of Psychiatry, 117,* 991-996.
Bronfenbrenner, U. (1979). *The Ecology of Human Development.* Cambridge, MA: Harvard University Press.
Bronfenbrenner, U., & Crouter, A. C. (1983). The evolution of environmental models in developmental research. In P. H. Mussen (Ed.), *Handbook of child psychology* (Vol. 4th ed., Vol. 1, pp. 357-414). New York: Wiley.

Bronshtein, A. I., & Petrova, E. P. (1967). The auditory analyzer in young infants. In Y. Brackbill & G. C. Thompson (Eds.), *Behavior in infancy and early childhood* (pp. 163-172). New York: Free Press.

Brophy, J. (1986). Teacher influences on student achievement. *American Psychologist, 41,* 1069-1077.

Brown, R. (1973). *A first language: The early stages.* Cambridge, MA: Harvard University Press.

Brown, R., & Hanlon, C. (1970). Derivational complexity and order of acquisition. In J. R. Hayes (Ed.), *Cognition and the development of language* (pp. 11-53). New York: Wiley.

Brown, R., Cazden, C., & Bellugi, U. (1969). The child's grammar from I to III. In J. P. Hill (Ed.), *Minnesota Symposium on Child Psychology* (Vol. 2). Minneapolis, MN: University of Minnesota Press.

Bruner, J. S. (1964). The course of cognitive growth. *American Psychologist, 19,* 1-15.

Bryan,, J. W., & Luria, Z. (1978). Sex role learning: A test of the selective attention hypothesis. *Child Development, 49,* 13-23.

Buehler, R. E., Patterson, G. R., & Furniss, J. M. (1966). The reinforcement of behavior in institutional settings. *Behavior Research and Therapy, 4,* 157-167.

Buri, J. R., Louiselle, P. A., Misukanis, T. M., & Mueller, R. A. (1988). Effects of parental authoritarianism and authoritativeness on self-esteem. *Personality and Social Psychology Bulletin, 14,* 271-282.

Bushell, D., & Baer, D. M. (1994). Measurably superior instruction means close, continual contact with the relevant outcome data. Revolutionary! In R. Gardner, D. M. Sainato, J. O. Cooper, T. E. Heron, W. L. Heward, J. Eshleman, & T. A. Grossi (Eds.), *Behavior analysis in education: Focus on measurably superior instruction* (pp. 3-10). Pacific Grove, CA: Brooks-Cole.

Cairns, R. B. (1991). Multiple metaphors for a singular idea. *Developmental Psychology, 27,* 23-26.

Caldwell, D. F., & Werboff, J. (1962). Classical conditioning in newborn rats. *Science, 136,* 1118-1119.

Campbell, D. T. (1965). Ethnocentric and other altruistic motives. In D. LeVine (Ed.), *Nebraska symposium on motivation* (Vol. vol. 13). Lincoln, NB: University of Nebraska Press.

Campbell, F. A., & Ramey, C. T. (1994). Effects of early intervention on intellectual and academic achievement: A follow-up study of children from low-income families. *Child Development, 65,* 684-698.

Campos, J. J., Langer, A., & Krowitz, A. (1970). Cardiac responses on the visual cliff in prelocomotor human infants. *Science, 170,* 196-197.

Carnine, D. W. (1976). Effects of two teacher presentation rates on off-task behavior, answering correctly, and participation. *Journal of Applied Behavior Analysis, 9,* 199-206.

Carrier, C. A. (1983). Notetaking research: Implications for the classroom. *Journal of Instructional Development, 6,* 19=29.

Caspi, A., Elder, G. H., & Bem, D. J. (1987). Moving against the world: Life course patterns of explosive children. *Developmental Psychology, 23,* 308-313.

Cernoch, J. M., & Porter, R. H. (1985). Recognition of maternal axillary odors by infants. *Child Development, 56,* 1593-1598.

Chomsky, N. (1959). Review of B. F. Skinner's Verbal Behavior. *Language, 35,* 26-58.

Chomsky, N. (1972). *Language and mind (2nd Ed.).* New York: Harcourt.

Clarke-Stewart, K. A. (1978). And daddy makes three: The father's impact on mother and young child. *Child Development, 49,* 466-478.

Cohn, J. F., Campbell, S. B., Matias, R., & Hopkins, J. (1990). Face-to-face interactions of postpartum and nondepressed mother-infant pairs at two months. *Developmental Psychology, 26*, 185-193.

Commons, M. L. (1991). A comparison and synthesis of Kohlberg's cognitive-developmental and Gewirtz's learning-developmental attachment theories. In J. L. Gewirtz & W. M. Kurtines (Eds.), *Intersection with attachment*. Hillsdale, NJ: Erlbaum.

Commons, M. L., & Rodriguez, J. A. (1993). The development of hierarchically complex equivalence classes. *Psychological Record, 43*, 667-695.

Conger, R. D., Ge, X., Elder, G. H., Lorenz, F. O., & Simmons, R. L. (1994). Economic stress, coercive family process, and developmental problems of adolescents. *Child Development, 65*, 541-561.

Cooper, J.O., Heron, T. E., & Heward, W. L. (1987). *Applied Behavior Analysis*. Columbus, OH: Merrill.

Cowley, G. (1994, March 7). Locking HIV out of the womb. *Newsweek, 123*, 53.

Crampton, G., & Lucot, J. B. (1991). Habituation of motion sickness in the cat. *Aviation, Space, and Environmental Medicine, 62*, 212-215.

Crockenberg, S. B. (1981). Infant irritability, mother responsiveness, and social support influences on the security of infant-mother attachment. *Child Development, 52*, 857-865.

Curtis, G. (1963). Violence breeds violence. *American Journal of Psychiatry, 120*, 386-387.

Darwin, C. R. (1872/1965). *The expression of emotions in man and animals*. London: John Murray (Chicago, University of Chicago Press).

DeCasper, A. J., & Fifer, W. P. (1980). Of human bonding: Newborns prefer their mothers' voices. *Science, 208*, 1174-1176.

DeCasper, A. J., & Sigafoos, A. D. (1983). The intrauterine heartbeat: A potent reinforcer for newborns. *Infant Behavior & Development, 6*, 19-25.

DeCasper, A. J., & Spence, M. J. (1986). Prenatal maternal speech influences newborns' perception of speech sounds. *Infant Behavior & Development, 9*, 133-150.

DeVries, R., Haney, J. P., & Zan, B. (1991). Sociomoral atmosphere in direct-instruction, eclectic, and constructivist kindergartens: A study of teachers' enacted interpersonal understanding. *Early Childhood Research Quarterly, 6*, 449-471.

Dickinson, A. M. (1989). The detrimental effects of extrinsic reinforcement of "intrinsic motivation. *The Behavior Analyst, 12*, 1-16.

Dienstag, E. L. (1986 (August)). The transition to parenthood in working and non-working pariparous mothers. 1986 (August). Paper presented at the meeting of the American Psychological Association, Washington, DC.

Dobson, V., & Teller, D. Y. (1978). Visual acuity in human infants: a review and comparison of behavioral and electrophysiological studies. *Vision Research, 18*, 1469-1483.

Doernberger, C., & Zigler, E. (1993). Project Follow Through: Intent and reality. In E. Zigler & S. J. Styfco (Eds.), *Head Start and Beyond: A National Plan for Extended Childhood Intervention* (pp. 43-72). New Haven: Yale University Press.

Dolan, L. J., Kellam, S. G., Brown, C. H., Werthamer-Larrson, L., Rebok, G. W., Mayer, L. S., Laudolff, J., Turkkan, J. S., Ford, C., & Wheeler, L. (1993). The short-term impact of two classroom-based preventative interventions on aggressive and shy behaviors and poor achievement. *Journal of Applied Developmental Psychology, 14*, 317-345.

Dolgin, K. G., & Azmitia, M. (1985). The development of the ability to interpret emotional signals–What is and is not known. In G. Zivin (Ed.), *The development of expressive behavior: Biology-environment interactions*. Orlando, FL: Academic.

Donahoe, J. W., & Palmer, D. C. (1994). *Learning and Complex Behavior*. Needham Heights, MA: Allyn and Bacon.

Donahoe, J. W., Burgos, J. E., & Palmer, D. C. (1993). A selectionist approach to reinforcement. *Journal of the Experimental Analysis of Behavior, 60*, 17-40.

Dornbusch, S. M., Ritter, P. L., Leiderman, P., Roberts, D. F., & Fraleigh, M. J. (1987). The relation of parenting style to adolescent school performance. *Child Development, 58*, 1244-1257.

Dunn, J., & Plomin, R. (1990). *Separate lives: Why siblings are so different*. New York: Basic Books.

Dusek, J. B., & Flaherty, J. F. (1981). The development of the self-concept during the adolescent years. *Monographs of the society for research in child development, 46.*

Eichorn, D. (1970). Physiological development. In P. H. Mussen (Ed.), *Carmichael's Manual of Child Development* (pp. 157-283). New York: Wiley.

Eimas, P. D., Siqueland, E. R., Jusczyk, P., & Vigorito, J. (1971). Speech perception in early infancy. *Science, 171*, 303-306.

Eisenberg, N., & Mussen, P. H. (1989). *The roots of prosocial behavior in children*. New York: Cambridge University Press.

Eisenberg-Berg, N., Boothby, R., & Matson, T. (1979). Correlates of preschool girls' feminine and masculine toy preferences. *Developmental Psychology, 15*, 354-355.

Ekholm, M. (1984). Readiness to help others and tolerance: Attitude development during the school years and a ten-year comparison. *Scandinavian Journal of Educational Research, 28,* 71-86.

Emde, R. N., Gaensbauer, T. J., & Harmon, R. J. (1976). *Emotional expression in infancy: A biobehavioral study*. New York: International Universities Press.

Emde, R. N., Harmon, R. J., & Gaensbauer, T. J. (1976). Emotional expression in infancy: A biobehavioral study. *Psychological Issues*, 1976, 10 (whole no. 1).

Emery, R. E. (1982). Interpersonal conflict and the children of discord and divorce. *Psychological Bulletin, 92*, 310-330.

Emery, R., & O'Leary, K. (1982). Children's perception of marital discord and behavior problems of boys and girls. *Journal of Abnormal Child Psychology, 10*, 11-24.

Engelmann, S., & Bruner, E. C. (1988). *Reading mastery: Fast cycle (DISTAR)*. Chicago: Science Research Associates.

Engen, T., Lipsitt, L. P., & Kaye, H. (1963). Olfactory responses and adaptation in the human neonate. *Journal of Comparative and Physiological Psychology, 56*, 73-77.

Eyesenck, H. J. (1993). Comment on Goldberg. *American Psychologist*, 1299-1300.

Fantino, E., & Logan, C. A. (1979). *The experimental analysis of behavior: An experimental perspective*. San Francisco: W. H. Freeman.

Fantz, R. (1958). Pattern vision in young infants. *Psychological Record, 8*, 43-47. (Child Development)

Fantz, R. (1961). The origin of form perception. *Science, 204*, 66-72.

Feree, M. (1976). Working-class jobs: Housework and paid work as sources of satisfaction. *Social Problems, 23*, 431-441.

Ferster, C. B., & Culbertson, S. A. (1982). *Behavior Principles* (3rd ed.). Englewood Cliffs: Prentice-Hall.

Field, T., Heay, B., Goldstein, S., Perry, S., Bendell, D., Schanberg, S., Zimmermann, E. A., & Kuhn, C. (1988). Infants of depressed mothers show "depressed" behavior even with nondepressed adults. Child Development, 59, 1569-1579.

Field, T., Healy, B., Goldstein, S., & Guthertz, M. (1990). Behavior state matching in mother-infant interactions of nondepressed versus depressed mother-infant dyads. *Developmental Psychology, 26*, 7-14.

Fields, L. (1993). Foreword: Special issue on stimulus equivalence. *Psychological Record, 43*, 543-546.

Fischer, K. W. (1980). A theory of cognitive development: The control and construction of hierarchies of skills. *Psychological Review, 87*, 477-531.

Fischer, K. W., & Pipp, S. L. (1984). Processes of cognitive development: Optimal level and skill acquisition. In R. J. Sternberg (Ed.), *Mechanisms of Cognitive Development* (pp. 45-80). Prospect Heights, IL: Waveland Press.

Ford, D. H., & Lerner, R. M. (1992). *Developmental systems theory*. Newbury Park, CA: Sage.

Galbicka, G. (1992). The dynamics of behavior. *Journal of the Experimental Analysis of Behavior, 57*, 243-248

Gersten, R. (1991). The eye of the beholder: A response to "Sociomoral Atmosphere... A Study of Teachers' Enacted Interpersonal Understanding". *Early Childhood Research Quarterly*, 6, 529-537.

Gewirtz, J. L. (1991). Social influence on child and parent via stimulation and operant-learning mechanisms. In M. Lewis & S. Feinman (Eds.), *Social influences and socialization in infancy* (pp. 137-163). New York: Plenum Press.

Gewirtz, J. L., & Boyd, E. F. (1977). Does maternal responding imply reduced infant crying?: A critique of the 1972 Bell and Ainsworth report. *Child Development, 48*, 1200-1207.

Gewirtz, J. L., & Pelaez-Nogueras, M. (1990, August). Infant social referencing as an instrumental conditioning process. Paper presented at the annual meeting of the American Psychological Association, Boston, MA.

Gewirtz, J. L., & Pelaez-Nogueras, M. (1991). The attachment metaphor and the conditioning of infant separation protests. In J. L. Gewirtz & W. M. Kurtines (Eds.), *Intersections with attachment* (pp. 123-143). Hillsdale, NJ: Laurence Erlbaum Associates.

Gewirtz, J. L., & Pelaez-Nogueras, M. (1992a). B. F. Skinner's legacy to human infant behavior and development. *American Psychologist, 47*, 1411-1422.

Gewirtz, J. L., & Pelaez-Nogueras, M. (1992b). Social referencing as a learned process. In S. Feinman (Ed.), *Social referencing and the social construction of reality in infancy* (pp. 151-170). New York, NY: Plenum.

Gewirtz, J. L., & Stingle, K. G. (1968). Learning of generalized imitation as the basis for identification. *Psychological Review, 75*, 374-397.

Gibson, J. J. (1979). *The ecological approach to visual perception*. Boston: Houghton-Mifflin.

Gil, D. (1971). Violence against children. *Journal of Marriage and the Family, 33*, 639-648.

Gleick, J. (1987). *Chaos: The making of a new science*. New York: Viking.

Goetz, E. M., & Salmonson, M. M. (1972). The effect of general and descriptive reinforcement on "creativity" in easel painting. In G. B. Semb (Ed.), *Behavior analysis in education, 1972* (pp. 53-61). Lawrence, KS: University of Kansas Support and Development Center for Follow Through.

Goldberg, L. R. (1993). The structure of phenotypic personality traits. *American Psychologist, 48*, 26-34.

Good, T. L., & Brophy, J. E. (1984). *Looking in Classrooms* (Third ed.). New York: Harper & Row.

Good, T. L., & Weinstein, R. S. (1986). Schools make a difference: Evidence, criticisms, and new directions. *American Psychologist, 41*, 1090-1097.

Goodwyn, S. W., Acredolo, L. P., & Novak, G. (1995, March). Accounting for individual differences in maternal interactive reading styles: Mother versus child factors. Presented at the Biennial Convention of the Society for Research in Child Development, Indianapolis, IN.

Gottesman, I. I. (1963). Heritability of personality: A demonstration. *Psychological Monographs, 77.*

Gottfried, A. E., Gottfried, A. W., & Bathurst, K. (1988). Maternal employment, family environment and children's development: Infancy through the school years. In A. E. Gottfried & A. W. Gottfried (Eds.), *Maternal employment and children's development: Longitudinal research* (pp. 11-58). New York: Plenum.

Gottlieb, G. (1991a). Epigenetic systems view of human development. *Developmental Psychology, 27,* 33-34.

Gottlieb, G. (1991b). Experiential canalization of behavioral development: Results. *Developmental Psychology, 27,* 4-13.

Gottlieb, G. (1991c). Experiential Canalization of behavioral development: Theory. *Developmental Psychology, 27,* 4-13.

Gottlieb, G. (1994, May). On the prenatal experiential origin of "innate" behavior in infants. Presented at the 20th international meeting of the Association for Behavior Analysis. Atlanta, GA.

Gottman, J. M., & Parkhurst, J. T. (1980). A developmental theory of friendship and acquaintanceship processes. In A. Collins (Ed.), *Minnesota Symposium on Child Psychology* (Vol. 13). Hillsdale, NJ: Erlbaum.

Grantham-McGregor, S., Powell, C., Walker, S., Chang, S., & Fletcher, P. (1994). The long-term follow-up of severely malnourished children who participated in an intervention program. *Child Development, 65,* 428-439.

Green, L., Fry, A. F., & Myerson, J. (1994). Discounting of delayed rewards: A life-span comparison. *Psychological Science, 5,* 33-36.

Greenberger, E., & Goldberg, W. (1989). Working, parenting, and socialization in children. *Developmental Psychology, 25,* 22-35.

Greenough, W. T. (1991). Experience as a component of normal development: Evolutionary considerations. *Developmental Psychology, 27,* 14-17.

Greenwood, C. R., Delquadri, J., & Hall, R. V. (1984). Opportunity to respond and student academic achievement. In W. L. Heward, T. E. Heron, D. S. Hill, & J. Trapp-Porter (Eds.), *Focus on behavior analysis in education* (pp. 58-88). Columbus, OH: Merrill.

Greenwood, C. R., Delquadri, J. C., Stanley, S. O., Sasso, G., Whorton, D., & Schulte, D. (1981). Allocating opportunity to learn as a basis for academic remediation: A developing model of teaching. *Monograph in Behavior Disorders, Summer,* 22-33.

Greenwood, C. R., Hart, B., Walker, D., & Risley, T. (1994). The opportunity to respond and academic performance revisited: A behavioral theory of developmental retardation and its prevention. In R. Gardner, D.M. Sainato, J.O. Cooper, T.E. Heron, W.L. Heward, J. Eshleman, & T.A. Grossi (Eds.), *Behavior analysis in education: Focus on measurably superior instruction* (pp. 213-223). Pacific Grove, CA: Brooks-Cole.

Greer, R. D. (1992). L'enfant terrible meets the educational crisis. *Journal of Applied Behavior Analysis, 23,* 65-69.

Greer, R. D. (1994). The measure of a teacher. In R. Gardner, D.M. Sainato, J.O. Cooper, T.E. Heron, W.L. Heward, J. Eshleman, & T.A. Grossi (Eds.), *Behavior analysis in education: Focus on measurably superior instruction* (pp. 161-171). Pacific Grove, CA: Brooks-Cole.

Griffiths, P. (1985). The communicative function of children's single-word speech. In M. Bennett (Ed.), *Children's single word speech* (pp. 87-112). New York: Wiley.

Grimwade, J. C., Walker, D. W., Bartlett, M., Gordon, S., & Wood, C. (1971). Human fetal heart rate change and movement in response to sound and vibration. *American Journal of Obstetrics & Gynecology, 109,* 86-90.

Guerin, B. (1990). Gibson, Skinner, and perceptual responses. *Behavior and Philosophy, 18*, 43-54.

Guthrie, R. D. (1976). *Body hot spots: The anatomy of human social organs and behavior*. New York: Van Nostrand Reinhold.

Harlow, H. (1959). Love in infant monkeys. *Scientific American, 202*, 68-74.

Hart, B., & Risley, T. R. (1974). Using preschool materials to modify the language of disadvantaged children. *Journal of Applied Behavior Analysis, 7*, 234-256.

Hart, B., & Risley, T. R. (1975). Incidental teaching of language in the preschool. *Journal of Applied Behavior Analysis, 8*, 411-420.

Hart, B., & Risley, T. R. (1980). *In vivo* language intervention: Unanticipated general effects. *Journal of Applied Behavior Analysis, 13*, 407-432.

Hatano, G. (1991). Commentary. *Early Childhood Research Quarterly, 6*, 519-521.

Hawkins, J. D., & Lishner, D. M. (1987). Schooling and delinquency. In E. H. Johnson (Ed.), *Handbook on crime and delinquency prevention* (pp. 179-221). New York: Greenwood Press.

Hay, D. F., Nash, A., & Pedersen, J. (1983). Interaction between six-month-old peers. *Child Development, 54*, 557-562.

Hayes, S. C. (1986). The case of the silent dog–verbal reports and the analysis of rules: A review of Ericsson and Simon's *Protocol Analysis: Verbal Reports as Data. Journal of the Experimental Analysis of Behavior, 45*, 351-363.

Hayes, S. C. (1987). A contextual approach to therapeutic change. In N. Jacobsen (Ed.), *Psychotherapists in clinical practice: cognitive and behavioral perspectives* (pp. 327-387). New York: Guilford Press.

Hayes, S. C. (1991). A relational control theory of stimulus equivalence. In L. J. Hayes & P. N. Chase (Eds.), *Dialogues on Verbal Behavior* (pp. 19-40). Reno, NV: Context Press.

Hayes, S. C. (1994). Relational frame theory: A functional approach to verbal events. In S. C. Hayes, L. J. Hayes, M. Sato, & O. Koichi (Eds.), *Behavior Analysis of Language and Cognition* (pp. 9-30). Reno, NV: Context Press.

Hayes, S. C., & Hayes, L. J. (1992). Verbal relations and the evolution of behavior analysis. *American Psychologist, 47*, 1383-1395.

Henderson, N. D. (1982). Human behavior genetics. *Annual Review of Psychology, 33*, 403-440.

Hetherington, E. M. (1989). Coping with family transitions: Winners, losers, and survivors. *Child Development, 60*, 1-14.

Hetherington, E. M. (1990). Coping with family transitions: Winners, losers, and survivors. Presidential address at the meeting of the Society for Research in Child Development. In *Annual Progress in child psychiatry and child development* (pp. 221-241). : .

Hetherington, E. M., & Clingempeel, W. G. (1992). *Coping with marital transitions* (Serial No. 227 ed., Vol. 57, nos. 2-3). Chicago, IL: University of Chicago Press.

Hetherington, E. M., Cox, M., & Cox, R. (1982). Effects of divorce on parents and children. In M. Lamb (Ed.), *Nontraditional families* (pp. 233-288). Hillsdale, NJ: Erlbaum.

Hetherington, E. M., Cox, M., & Cox, R. (1985). Long-term effects of divorce and remarriage on the adjustment of children. *Journal of American Academy of Psychiatry, 24*, 518-830.

Hetherington, E. M., Stanley-Hagan, M., & Anderson, E. R. (1989). Marital transitions: A child's perspective. *American Psychologist, 44*, 303-312.

Heward, L. W. (1994). Three "low-tech" strategies for increasing the frequency of active student response during group instruction. In R. Gardner, D. M. Sainato, J. O. Cooper,

T. E. Heron, W. L. Heward, J. Eshleman, & T. M. Grossi (Eds.), *Behavior analysis in education: Focus on measurably superior instruction* (pp. 283-320). Pacific Grove, CA: Brooks-Cole.

Hock, E., & DeMeis, D. K. (1990). Depression in mothers of infants: The role of maternal employment. *Developmental Psychology, 26,* 285-291.

Hoffman, L. W. (1986). Work, family, and the child. In M. S. Pallak & R. O. Perloff (Eds.), *Psychology and work: productivity, change, and employment* (pp. 173-220). Washington, DC: American Psychological Association.

Hoffman, L. W. (1989). Effects of maternal employment in the two-parent family. *American Psychologist, 44,* 283-294.

Holman, J., Goetz, E. M., & Baer, D. M. (1977). The training of creativity as an operant and an examination of its generalization characteristics. In B. C. Etzel, J. M. LeBlanc, & D. M. Baer (Eds.), *New developments in behavioral research theory, methods, and application: In honor of Sidney W. Bijou* (pp. 441-472). Hillsdale, NJ: Erlbaum.

Hopkins, B. L. (1994, October). Behavior analysis and education. Paper presented at the Second International Congress on Behaviorism and the Sciences of Behavior. Palermo, Italy.

Horowitz, F. D. (1989a). Commentary: Process and systems. In *Minnesota Symposium on Developmental Psychology* (pp. 211-218). .

Horowitz, F. D. (1989b). In the interest of the nation: A reflective essay on the state of our knowledge and the challenges before us. *American Psychologist, 44,* 441-445.

Horowitz, F. D. (1992). John B. Watson's legacy: Learning and environment. *Developmental Psychology, 28,* 360-367.

Horowitz, F. D. (Ed.). (1987). *Exploring developmental theories: Toward a structural/behavioral model of development.* Hillsdale, NJ: Erlbaum.

Horton, S. V., & Lovitt, T. C. (1989). Using study guides with three classifications of secondary students. *Journal of Special Education, 22,* 447-462.

Howard, V. F., Williams, B. F., & McLaughlin, T. F. (1994). Children prenatally exposed to alcohol and cocaine: Behavioral solutions. In R. I. I. I. Gardner (Ed.), *Behavior Analysis in Education* (pp. 131-146). Pacific Grove, CA: Brooks Cole.

Hoyert, M. S. (1992). Order and chaos in fixed-interval schedules of reinforcement. *Journal of the Experimental Analysis of Behavior, 57,* 339-363.

Huesman, L. R., Eron, L. D., Lefkowitz, M. M., & Walder, L. O. (1984). Stability of aggression over time and generations. *Developmental Psychology, 20,* 1120-1134.

Huston, A. C. (1983). Sex typing. In E. M. Hetherington (Ed.), *Handbook of child psychology: Socialization, personality, and social development* (Vol. 4). New York: Wiley.

Huston, A. C. (1994). Children in poverty: Designing research to affect policy. *Social Policy Report: Society for Research in Child Development, 8,* 1-12.

Huston, A. C., McLoyd, V. C., & Coll, C. C. (1994). Children and poverty: Issues in contemporary research. *Child Development, 65,* 275-282.

Izard, C., & Malatesta, C. Z. (1987). Perspectives on emotional development I: Differential emotions theory of early emotional development. In J. D. Osofsky (Ed.), *Handbook of Infant Development* (Second ed., pp. 555-578). New York: Wiley.

Jacobson, S. W. (1979). Matching behavior in the young infant. *Child Development, 50,* 425-530.

Johnson, K. R., & Layng, T. V. J. (1994). The Morningside model of generative instruction. In R. Gardner, D. M. Sainato, J. O. Cooper, T. E. Heron, W. L. Heward, J. Eshleman, & T. A. Grossi (Eds.), *Behavior Analysis in Education: Focus on Measurably superior instruction* (pp. 173-197). Belmont, CA: Brooks/Cole.

Jones, M. C. (1924). A laboratory study of fear: the case of Peter. *Pedagogical Seminary, 31*, 308-315.

Kagan, J. (1974). Discrepancy, temperament, and infant distress. In M. Lewis & L. A. Rosenblum (Eds.), *The origins of fear* (pp. 229-248). New York: Wiley.

Kagan, J., Kearsley, R. B., & Zelazo, P. R. (1978). *Infancy: Its place in human development.* Cambridge, MA: Harvard University Press.

Kagel, J. H., Green, L., & Caraco, T. (1986). When foragers discount the future: Constraint or adaptation? *Animal Behaviour, 34*, 271-283.

Kantor, J. R. (1959). *Interbehavioral psychology (Rev. ed.).* Bloomington, Ind.: Principia Press.

Kaye, H., & Levin, G. R. (1963). Two attempts to demonstrate tonal suppression of non-nutritive sucking in neonates. *Perceptual and Motor Skills, 17*, 521-522.

Kazdin, A. E. (1987). Treatment of antisocial behavior in children: Current status and future directions. *Psychological Bulletin, 102*, 187-203.

Kendler, K. S., & Robinette, C. D. (1983). Schizophrenia in the National Academy of Sciences'-National Research Council Twin registry: A 16-year update. *American Journal of Psychiatry, 140*, 1551-1563.

Kimble, G. (Ed.). (1961). *Hilgard and Marquis' conditioning and learning.* New York: Appleton-Century-Crofts.

Klein, S. B. (1987). *Learning: Principles and applications.* New York: McGraw-Hill.

Kolata, G. (1987). Early signs of school age IQ. *Science, 236*, 774-775.

Kolata, G. (1995, March 4). Vitamin can avert birth defect, but message goes unheeded. *New York Times, 144*, 7.

Kroger, R. O., & Wood, L. A. (1993). Reification, "faking," and the Big Five. *American Psychologist, 1993*, 48.

Lack, D., Gibb, J., & Owen, D. F. (1957). Survival in relation to brood-size in tits. *Proceedings of the Zoological Society of London, 128*, 313-326.

Lamb, R. E., & Bornstein, M. H. (1987). *Development in infancy: An introduction (2nd ed.).* New York: Random House.

Layng, T. V. J. (1995, February). Crisis in Education. Remarks made at the Conference of the Northern California Association for Behavior Analysis.

Lazar, I., & Darlington, R. (1982). Lasting effects of early education. *Monographs of the Society for Research in Child Development, 47 (2-3, Serial no. 195).*

Legeland, S. (1993). The case against physicalism in the analysis of behavior. *The Behavior Analyst, 16*, 351-355.

Lempers, J. D., Clark-Lempers, D., & Simons, R. L. (1989). Economic hardship, parenting, and distress in adolescence. *Child Development, 60*, 25-39.

Lerner, R. M. (1991). Changing organism-context relations as the basic process of development: A developmental contextual perspective. *Developmental Psychology, 27*, 27-32.

Levin, G. R. & Kaye, H. (1964). Nonnutritive sucking by human neonates. *Child Development, 35*, 749-758.

LeVine, R. A. (1974). Parental goals: A cross-cultural view. *Teachers College Record, 76*, 226-239.

Lewis, M. (1987). Social development in infancy and early childhood. In J. D. Osofsky (Ed.), *Handbook of infant development (2nd Ed.)* (pp. 419-493). New York: Wiley.

Liebert, R. M., & Wicks-Nelson, R. (1981). *Developmental psychology* (Vol. 3rd Ed.). Englewood-Cliffs,NJ: Prentice-Hall.

Liebman, R., Minuchin, S., & Baker, L. (1974a). An integrated treatment program for anorexia nervosa. *American Journal of Psychiatry, 131*, 432-436.

Liebman, R., Minuchin, S., & Baker, L. (1974b). The use of structural family therapy in the treatment of intractable asthma. *American Journal of Psychiatry, 131*, 535-540.

Lipkens, R., Hayes, S. C., & Hayes, L. J. (1993). Longitudinal study of the development of derived relations in an infant. *Journal of Experimental Child Psychology, 51*, 201-239.

Lipsitt, L. P., & Kaye, H. (1964). Conditioned sucking in the human newborn. *Psychonomic Science, 1*, 29-30.

Lipsitt, L., & Wiener, J. S. (1981). The infancy of human learning processes. In E. S. Gollin (Ed.), *Developmental Plasticity*. New York: Academic Press.

Lore, R. K., & Schultz, L. A. (1993). Control of human aggression: A comparative perspective. *American Psychologist, 48*, 16-25.

Lorenz, K. (1943). Die angegorenen formen moglicher erfahrung. *Zeitschrift fur Tierpsychologie, 5*, 235-409.

Lundin, R. W. (1961). *Personality*. New York: Macmillan.

Lutzker, J. R. (1984). Project 12-Ways: Treating child abuse and neglect from an ecobehavioral perspective. In R. F. Dangel & R. L. Polster (Eds.), *Parent training: Foundations of research and practice* (pp. 260-291). New York: Guilford.

Lutzker, J. R., & Campbell, R. (1994). *Ecobehavioral family interventions in developmental disabilities*. Pacific Grove, CA: Brooks/Cole.

Lutzker, J. R., Campbell, R. V., Newman, M. R., & Harrold, M. (1989). Ecobehavioral interventions for abusive, neglectful, and high risk families. In G. H. S. Singer & L. K. Irvin (Eds.), *Support for caregiving families: Enabling positive adaptation to disability* (pp. pp 313-326). Baltimore: Paul H. Brookes.

Lyberger-Ficek, S., & Sternglanz, S. H. (1975, April). Innate sex differences in neonatal crying: Myth or reality? Paper presented at the meeting of the Society for Research in Child Development, Denver..

MacCorquodale, K. (1969). B. F. Skinner's Verbal Behavior: A retrospective appreciation. *Journal of the Experimental Analysis of Behavior, 12*, 831-841.

MacCorquodale, K. (1970). On Chomsky's review of Skinner's *Verbal Behavior*. *Journal of the Experimental Analysis of Behavior, 13*, 83-99.

Madison, L. S., Madison, J. K., & Adubato, S. A. (1986). Infant behavior and development in relation to fetal movement and habituation. *Child Development, 57*, 1475-1482.

Major, B., Carnevale, P. J., & Deaux, K. (1981). A different perspective on androgyny: Evaluations of masculine and feminine personality characteristics. *Journal of Personality and Social Psychology, 41*.

Marantz, S. A., & Mansfield, A. F. (1977). Maternal employment and the development of sex-role stereotyping in five- to eleven-year-old girls. *Child Development, 48*, 66-673.

Maratos, O. (1973). The origin and development of imitation in the first six months of life.

Margolis, L., & Farran, D. (1981). Unemployment: The health consequences for children. *North Carolina Medical Journal, 42*, 849-850.

Marr, M. J. (1992). Behavior dynamics: One perspective. *Journal of the Experimental Analysis of Behavior, 57*, 249-266.

Massad, C. M. (1981). Sex role identity and adjustment during adolescence. *Child Development, 52*, 1290-1298.

McDonald, M. A., Sigman, M., Espinosa, R. P., & Neumann, C. G. (1994). Impact of a temporary food shortage on children and their mothers. *Child Development, 65*, 404-415.

McGraw, M. (1935). *Growth: A study of Jimmy and Johnny*. New York: Appleton-Century-Crofts.

McLoyd, V. C. (1989). Socialization and development in a changing economy: The effects of paternal job and income loss on children. *American Psychologist, 44*, 293-302.

McNally, S., Eisenberg, N., & Harris, J. D. (1991). Consistency and change in maternal child-rearing practices and values: A longitudinal study. *Child Development, 62,* 190-198.

Mehler, J., & Bever, T. G. (1967). Cognitive capacity of very young children. *Science, 158,* 141-142.

Meltzoff, A. N., & Moore, M. K. (1977). Imitation of facial and manual gestures by human neonates. *Science, 198,* 75-77.

Meltzoff, A. N., & Moore, M. K. (1983). Newborn infants imitate adult facial gestures. *Child Development, 54,* 702-709.

Michael, J. (1993). Establishing operations. *The Behavior Analyst, 16,* 191-206.

Michael, J. L. (1982). Distinguishing between the discriminative and motivational functions of stimuli. *Journal of the Experimental Analysis of Behavior, 37,* 149-155.

Miller, D. B. (1994, May). The development of "instinctive" behavior: Alarm call responsivity of mallard ducklings. Paper presented at the 20th international meeting of the Association for Behavior Analysis. Atlanta, GA.

Miller, D. B., & Hicinbothom, G. (1991). Alarm call responsivity of mallard ducklings: X. ontogenetic adaptation or artifact of arousal? *Bird Behaviour, 9(1-2),* 114-120.

Miller, S. A. (1987). *Developmental research methods.* Englewood Cliffs,NJ: Prentice-Hall.

Minuchin, S., Baker, L., Liebman, R., Milman, L., & Todd, T. C. (1975). A conceptual model of psychosomatic illness in children. *Archives of General Psychiatry, 32,* 1031-1038.

Minuchin, S., Rossman, B. L., & Baker, L. (1978). *Psychosomatic families: Anorexia nervosa in context.* Cambridge, MA: Harvard University Press.

Moerk, E. L. (1986). Environmental factors in early language acquisition. In G. J. Whitehurst (Ed.), *Annals of Child Development* (Vol. 3, pp. 191-235). : JAI Press.

Moerk, E. L. (1989). The LAD was a lady and the tasks were ill-defined. *Developmental Review, 9,* 21-57.

Moerk, E. L. (1990). Three-term contingency patterns in mother-child verbal interactions during first-language acquisition. *Journal of the Experimental Analysis of Behavior, 54,* 293-305.

Morris, E. K. (1993). Mechanism and contextualism in behavior analysis: Just some observations. *The Behavior Analyst, 16,* 255-269.

Moyer, K. E. (1967). Kinds of aggression and their physiological basis. Report No. 67-12. Department of Psychology, Carnegie-Mellon University, Pittsburgh, PA.

Neale, J. M., & Liebert, R. M. (1980). *Science and behavior* (2nd Ed.). Englewood Cliffs, NJ: Prentice-Hall.

Nelson, K. (1973). Structure and strategies for learning to talk. *Monographs of the Society for Research in Child Development, 38.*

Nelson-Wicks, R. & Israel, A. C. (1984) Behavior disorders of childhood. Englewood Cliffs, N. J.: Prentice-Hall.

Neuringer, A. (1994, February). Behavioral variability and behavior analysis. (Presented at the thirteenth annual conference of the Northern California Association for Behavior Analysis, Oakland, CA.

Nevin, J. A. (1992). An integrative model for the study of behavioral momentum. *Journal of the Experimental Analysis of Behavior, 57,* 301-316.

Novak, G. (1987, May). Social cognition: A behavior analysis. Paper presented at the Association for Behavior Analysis, Nashville, TN.

Novak, G. (1992, May). The man behind the mask: J. B. Watson, Little Albert, and Santa Claus. Paper presented at the Association for Behavior Analysis, San Francisco, CA.

Novak, G. (1995, May). Skill learning, dynamical systems, and the development of equivalencing. Paper presented at the 21st Annual Convention of the Association for Behavior Analysis, Washington, D.C.

Novak, G., Staggs, D., & Jones, S. (1993, March). Multilogic Reading with Limited English Proficiency Children. Paper presented at the Biennial Meeting of the Society for Research in Child Development, New Orleans.

Novak. (1993, May). A behavior analysis of multilogic reading. Paper presented at the 19th annual convention of the Association for Behavior Analysis. Chicago, 1993.

Papousek, H., & Papousek, M. (1981). Fruhentwicklund des sozialverhaltens und der komunikation (cited in Papousek & Papousek, 1987). In H. Remschmidt & M. Schmidt (Eds.), *Neuropsychologie des Kindesalters*. Stuttgart: Enke Verlag.

Papousek, H., & Papousek, M. (1987). Intuitive parenting: A dialectic counterpart to the infant's integrative competence. In J. D. Osofsky (Ed.), *Handbook of infant development* (Second ed., pp. 669-720). New York, NY: Wiley.

Parker, S., Greer, S., & Zuckerman, B. (1988). Double jeopardy: The impact of poverty on early child development. *Pediatric Clinics of North America, 35*, 1127-1241.

Patterson, G. R. (1980). Mothers: the unacknowledged victims (Vol. 45(5, Serial No. 186)). : *Monographs of the Society for Research in Child Development.*

Patterson, G. R. (1982). *A social learning approach: Coercive family process* (Vol. 3). Eugene, OR: Castalia.

Patterson, G. R., DeBaryshe, B. D., & Ramsey, E. (1989). A developmental perspective on antisocial behavior. *American Psychologist, 44*, 329-335.

Patterson, G. R., Littman, R. A., & Bricker, W. (1967). Assertive behavior in children: A step toward a theory of aggression. *Monographs of the Society for Research in Child Development, 32.*

Patterson, G. R., Reid, J. B., & Dishion, T. J. (1992). *Antisocial boys*. Eugene, Or: Castalia.

Peckham, G. W., & Peckham, E. G. (1887). Some observations on the mental powers of spiders. *Journal of Morphology, 1*, 383-419.

Pelaez-Nogueras, M., Field, T. M., Hossain, Z., & Pickens, J. (1995). Depressed mothers' touching increases infants' positive affect and attention in still-face interactions. Unpublished manuscript.

Pelaez-Nogueras, M., Field, T., Cigales, M., Gewirtz, J. L., Malphurs, J., Clasky, S., & Sanchez, A. (1993, March). Infant preference for touch stimulation in social interactions. Paper presented at the biennial meeting of the Society for Research in Child Development, New Orleans.

Pelaez-Nogueras, M., Field, T., Cigales, M., Gonzalez, A., & Clasky, S. (1994). Infants of depressed mothers show less "depressed" behavior with their nursery teachers. *Infant Mental Health Journal, 15*, 358-367.

Pelaez-Nogueras, M., Field, T., Gewirtz, J. L., Cigales, M., Gonzalez,, A, Clasky, S., & Sanchez, A. (1995, May). Message-like touching versus poking and tickling in adult-infant face-to-face interactions. Paper presented at the 21st annual convention of the Association for Behavior Analysis, Washington, D.C.

Pennypacker, H. S. (1994). A selectionist view of the future of behavior analysis in education. In R. Gardner, D.M. Sainato, J.O. Cooper, T.E. Heron, W.L. Heward, J. Eshleman, & T.A. Grossi (Eds.), *Behavior analysis in education: Focus on measurably superior instruction* (pp. 11-18). Pacific Grove, CA: Brooks-Cole.

Petersen, G. A., & Sherrod, K. B. (1982). Relationship of maternal language to language development and language delay of children. *American Journal of Mental Deficiency, 86*, 391-398.

Petrovich, S. B. & Gewirtz, J. L. (1991) Imprinting and attachment: Proximate and ultimate considerations. In J. L. Gewirtz & W. M. Kurtines (Eds.) *Intersections with attachment.* Hillsdale, NJ: Erlbaum, 69-93

Phillips, D. A., Voran, M., Kisker, E., Howes, C., & Whitebook, M. (1994). Child care for children in poverty: Opportunity or inequity? *Child Development, 65,* 472-492.

Platt, S. A., & Sanislow, C. A. (1988). Norm-of-reaction: Definition and misinterpretations of animal research. *Journal of Comparative Psychology, 102,* 254-261.

Plomin, R. (1986). *Development, genetics, and psychology.* Hillsdale, NJ: Erlbaum.

Plomin, R. (1988). The nature and nurture of cognitive abilities. In R. J. Sternberg (Ed.), *Advances in the psychology of human intelligence.* (Vol. 4, pp. 1-33). Hillsdale, NJ: Erlbaum.

Plomin, R. (1989). Environment and genes: Determinants of behavior. *American Psychologist, 44,* 105-111.

Plomin, R., & Daniels, D. (1987). Why are children in the same family so different from each other? *Behavioral and Brain Sciences, 10,* 1-16.

Plomin, R., Reiss, D., Hetherinton, E. M., & Howe, G. W. (1994). Nature and nurture: Genetic contributions to measures of the family environment. *Developmental Psychology, 30,* 32-43.

Pollitt, E. (1994). Poverty and child development: Relevance of research in developing countries to the United States. *Child Development, 65,* 283-295.

Poulson, C. L. (1983). Differential reinforcement of other-than-vocalization as a control procedure in the conditioning of infant vocalization rate. *Journal of Experimental Child Psychology, 51,* 267-279.

Poulson, C. L., de Paula Nunes, L. R., & Warren, S. F. (1989). Imitation in Infancy: A Critical Review. In *Advances in child development and behavior* (Vol. 22, pp. 271-298). New York: Academic Press.

Poulson, C. L., Kymissis, E., Reeve, K. F., Andreatos, M., & Richards, L. (1991). Generalized vocal imitation in infants. *Journal of Experimental Child Psychology, 88,* 1-21.

Powers, M. K., Schneck, M., & Teller, D. Y. (1981). Spectral sensitivity of human infants at absolute visual threshold. *Vision Research, 21,* 1005-1016.

Premack, D. (1959). Toward empirical behavior laws: 1. Positive reinforcement. *Psychological Review, 66,* 219-233.

Prosser, C. J., & Hunter, W. S. (1936). The extinction of startle responses and spinal reflexes in the white rat. *American Journal of Physiology, 117,* 609-618.

Rachlin, H. (1976). *Introduction to modern behaviorism* (Second ed.). San Francisco: W. H. Freeman.

Rachlin, H., & Green, L. (1972). Commitment, choice, and self-control. *Journal of the Experimental Analysis of Behavior, 17,* 15-22.

Rachlin, H., Raineri, A., & Cross, D. (1991). Subjective probability and delay. *Journal of the Experimental Analysis of Behavior, 55,* 233-244.

Radke-Yarrow, M., Zahn-Waxler, C., & Chapman, M. (1983). Children's prosocial dispositions and behavior. In P. H. Mussen (Ed.), *Handbook of child psychology* (Fourth ed., Vol. 4: Socialization, personality, and social development). New York: Wiley.

Ramey, C. T., & Watson, J. S. (1972). Nonsocial reinforcement of infants' vocalizations. *Developmental Psychology, 6,* 538.

Ray, W. S. (1932). A preliminary report of a study of prenatal conditioning. *Child Development, 3,* 175-177.

Reese, H. W. (1994). Cognitive and behavioral approaches to problem solving. In S. C. Hayes, L. J. Hayes, M. Sato, & K. Ono (Eds.), *Behavior analysis of language and cognition* (pp. 197-258). Reno, NV: Context Press.

Reich, P. A. (1986). *Language Development.* Englewood Cliffs, NJ: Prentice Hall.

Rheingold, H. L., Gewirtz, J. L., & Ross, H. W. (1959). Social conditioning of vocalizations in the infant. *Journal of Comparative and Physiological Psychology, 52*, 68-73.

Riegler, H. C., & Baer, D. M. (1989). A developmental analysis of rule-following. In H. W. Reese (Ed.), *Advances in child development and behavior* (Vol. 21, pp. 191-219). New York: Academic Press.

Robins, L. N., & Ratcliff, K. S. (1979). Risk factors in the continuation of childhood antisocial behavior into adulthood. *International Journal of Mental Health, 7*, 96-116.

Rogers-Warren, A., & Rogers, S. (1980). Mands for verbalization: Facilitating the display of newly-taught language. *Behavior Modification, 4*, 361-382.

Rondal, J. A. (1979). Mama est au courant: Une etude des connaissances maternelles quant aux aspects formels du language de jeune enfant (Mommy is informed: A study of maternal knowledge about formal aspects of the language of the young child). *Enfance, 2*, 95-105.

Rosales, J., & Baer, D. M. (1994). A behavior-analytic view of development. In E. Ribes & S. W. Bijou (Eds.), *Recent approaches to behavioral development.* Guadalajara, Mexico: Editorial Universidad de Guadalajara.

Ross, A. O. (1976). *Psychological aspects of learning disabilities and reading disorders.* New York: McGraw-Hill.

Ross, A. O. (1980). *Psychological disorders of children: a behavioral approach to theory, research, and therapy* (Second ed.). New York: McGraw-Hill.

Roth, W. E., & Gewirtz, J. L. (1995, May). The role of contingent maternal attention in training jealous initiations in twin infants. Paper presented at the 21st Annual Convention of the Association for Behavior Analysis, Washington, D.C.

Rothbart, M. K., & Maccoby, E. E. (1966). Parents' differential reactions to sons and daughters. *Journal of Personality and Social Psychology, 9*, 353-362.

Rotter, J. (1966). *Psychological Monographs: General and Applied. Generalized expectancies for internal versus external control of reinforcement* (Vol. 80, 1, Whole No. 609).

Rovee-Collier, C. (1987). Learning and memory in infancy. In J.D.Osofsky (Ed.), *Handbook of Infant Development* (2nd ed., pp. 98-148). New York: Wiley.

Rovee-Collier, Griesler, P. C., & Earley, L. A. (1985). Contextual determinants of retrieval in three-month-old infants. *Learning & Motivation, 16*, 139-157.

Rowe, D. C., & Plomin, R. (1981). The importance of nonshared (E1) environmental influences in develop. *Developmental Psychology, 17*, 517-531.

Rubin, J. S., Provenzano, F. J., & Luria, Z. (1974). The eye of the beholder: Parents' views on the sex of newborns. *American Journal of Orthopsychiatry, 5*, 353-363.

Sagan, C. (1980). *Cosmos.* New York: Random House.

Sakabe, N., Arayama, T., & Suzuki, T. (1969). Human fetal evoked response to acoustic stimulation. *Acta Oto-Laryngologica, Supplementum, 252*, 29-36.

Sameroff, A. J., & Chandler, M. J. (1975). Reproductive risk and the continuum of caretaking casualty. In F. D. Horowitz, M. Hetherington, S. Scarr-Salapatek, & G. Siegel (Eds.), *Review of child development research* (Vol. 4). Chicago: University of Chicago Press.

Sampson, R. J., & Laub, J. H. (1994). Urban poverty and the family context of delinquency: A new look at structure and process in a classic study. *Child Development, 65*, 523-540.

Scarr, S., & McCartney, K. (1983). How people make their own environments: A theory of genotype – environment effects. *Child Development, 54*, 424-435.

Scholzman, K. L., & Verba, S. (1978). The new employment: Does it hurt? *Public Policy, 26*, 333-358.

Schantz, C. (1983). Social Cognition. In J. H. Flavell, E. M. Markham (Volume Eds.), & P. H. Mussen (Series Ed..), *Handbook of Child Psychology* (Fourth ed., Vol. IV, pp. 495-555). New York: Wiley.

Schwartz, M. (1984). The role of sound for space and object perception in the congenitally blind infant. In L. P. Lipsitt & C. Rovee-Collier (Eds.), *Advances in infancy research* (Vol. 3, pp. 23-56). Norwood, NJ: Ablex.

Shadel, W. G., & Cervone, D. (1993). The Big Five versus nobody? *American Psychologist, 48*, 1200-1302.

Shaffer, D. B. (1989). *Developmental psychology* (Vol. 2nd Ed.). Monterey: Brooks/Cole.

Sharpless, S. K., & Jasper, H. (1956). Habituation of the arousal reaction. *Brain, 79*, 655-680.

Sheldon, W. H. (1940). *The varieties of human physique*. New York: Harper & Row.

Sheppard, W. C., & Willoughby, R. H. (1975). *Child behavior: Learning and development*. Chicago, IL: Rand McNally].

Sidman, M. (1986). Functional analysis of emergent verbal classes. In T. Thompson & d Zeiler (Eds.), *Analysis and integration of behavioral units* (pp. 231-245). Hillsdale, NJ: Erlbaum.

Sidman, M. (1994). *Equivalence relations and behavior: A research story*. Boston: Authors Cooperative.

Siegler, R. S. (1994). Cognitive variability: A key to understanding cognitive development. *Psychological Science*, 1-5.

Siqueland, E. R. (1964). Operant conditioning of head-turning in four-month-old infants. *Psychonomic Science, 1*, 223-224.

Skinner, B. F. (1938). *The behavior of organisms*. New York: Appleton-Century-Crofts.

Skinner, B. F. (1953). *Science and human behavior*. New York: Macmillan.

Skinner, B. F. (1957). *Verbal Behavior*. New York: Appleton-Century-Crofts.

Skinner, B. F. (1968). *The technology of teaching*. New York: Appleton-Century-Crofts.

Skinner, B. F. (1969). An operant analysis of problem solving. In B. F. Skinner (Ed.), *Contingencies of Reinforcement*. New York: Appleton-Century-Croft.

Skinner, B. F. (1974). *About behaviorism*. New York: Knopf.

Skinner, B. F. (1982). Contrived reinforcement. *The Behavior Analyst, 5*, 3-8.

Skinner, B. F. (1984). The shame of American education. *American Psychologist, 39*, 947-954.

Skinner, B. F. (1989). *Recent issues in the analysis of behavior*. Columbus, OH: Merrill.

Skinner, B. F. (1992). The shame of American education. In R. P. West & L. A. Hemerlynck (Eds.), *Designs for excellence in education: The legacy of B.F. Skinner* (pp. 15-30). Longmont, CO: Sopris West.

Smith, W. I., & Moore, J. W. (1966). *Conditioning and instrumental learning: A program for self-instruction*. New York: McGraw-Hill.

Snow, C. E. (1972). Mothers' speech to children learning language. *Child Development, 43*, 549-565.

Snow, C. E., & Goldfield, B. A. (1983). Turn the page please: situation-specific language acquisition. *Journal of Child Language, 10*, 551-569.

Spelt, D. K. (1948). The conditioning of the human fetus in utero. *Journal of Experimental Psychology, 38*, 338-346.

Spence, J. T. (1982). Comments on Baumrind's "Are androgynous individuals more effective persons and parents?". *Child Development, 53*, 76-80.

Spinetta, J., & Rigler, D. (1972). The child-abusing parent: a psychological review. *Psychological Bulletin, 77*, 296-304.

Sroufe, L. A. (1977). Wariness of strangers and the study of infant development. *Child Development, 48*, 731-746.

Staines, G. L., Pottick, K. J., & Fudge, D. A. (1986). Wive's employment and husbands' attitudes toward work and life. *Journal of Applied Psychology, 71*, 118-128.

Stein, J. (Ed.). (1973). *The Random House dictionary of the English language* (Unabridged ed.). New York: Random House.

Stokes, T. F., Fowler, S. A., & Baer, D. M. (1978). Training preschool children to recruit natural communities of reinforcement. *Journal of Applied Behavior Analysis, 11*, 285-303.

Stone, J. E. (1994). Developmentalism's impediments to school reform: Three recommendations for overcoming them. In R. Gardner, D.M. Sainato, J.O. Cooper, T.E. Heron, W.L. Heward, J. Eshleman, & T.A. Grossi (Eds.), *Behavior analysis in education: Focus on measurably superior instruction* (pp. 57-72). Pacific Grove, CA: Brooks Cole.

Tanner, J. M. (1970). Physical Growth. In P. H. Mussen (Ed.), *Carmichael's manual of child psychology, 3rd. Ed.* (Vol. 1, pp. 77-155). New York: Wiley.

Thelen, E. (1989). Self-organization in developmental processes: Can systems approaches work? In *Minnesota Symposium on Developmental Psychology* (pp. 77-117).

Thelen, E. (1994). Three-month-old infants can learn task-specific patterns of interlimb coordination. *Psychological Science, 5*, 280-285.

Thelen, E., & Ulrich, B. D. (1991). *Hidden Skills* (Serial No. 233 ed., Vol. 36*). Monographs of the Society for Research in Child Development*: University of Chicago Press.

Thelen, E., Kelso, J. A. S., & Fogel, A. (1987). Self-organizing systems and infant motor development. *Developmental Review, 7*, 39-65.

Thomas, A., & Chess, S. (1977). *Temperament and development.* New York, NY: Bruner/ Mazel.

Thomas, A., Chess, S., & Birch, H. G. (1968). *Temperament and behavior disorders in children.* New York, NY: University Press.

Thomas, A., Chess, S., & Birch, H. G. (1982). The reality of difficult temperament. *Merrill-Palmer Quarterly, 28*, 1-20.

Thomas, A., Chess, S., & Korn, S. (1982). The reality of difficult temperament. *Merrill-Palmer Quarterly, 28*, 1-20.

Thomas, A., Chess, S., Birch, H. G., Hertzig, M. E., & Korn, S. (1963). *Behavioral individuality in early childhood.* New York, NY: University Press.

Thomas, R. M. (1985). *Comparing theories of child development* (Second ed.). Belmont, CA: Wadsworth.

Thompson, S. K. C. (1975). Gender labels and early sex role development. *Child Development, 46*, 339-447.

Turkheimer, E., & Gottesman, I. I. (1991). Individual differences and the canalization of human behavior. *Developmental Psychology, 27*, 18-22.

Turkkan, J. S. (1989). Classical conditioning: The new hegemony. *Behavioral and Brain Sciences, 12*, 121-179.

U.S. Bureau of the Census. (1992). *Poverty in the United States, 1991. Current Population Reports (Series P-60, no. 181).* Washington, DC: Government Printing Office.

Underwood, B., & Moore, B. S. (1982). Perspective-taking and altruism. *Psychological Bulletin, 91*, 143-173.

Uzgiris, I. C. (1972). Patterns of cognitive development in infancy. Merril-Palmer Institute Conference on Infant Development, Detroit.

Valdez-Menchaca, M. C., & Whitehurst, G. J. (1992). Accelerating language development through picture book reading: A systematic extension to Mexican Day Care. *Developmental Psychology, 28,* 1106-1114.

Vasta, R. (1982). Physical child abuse: A dual-component analysis. *Developmental Review, 2,* 125-149.

Vaughn, M. E., & Michael, J. L. (1982). Automatic reinforcement: An important but ignored concept. *Behaviorism, 10,* 217-227.

Vorhees, C. V., & Mollnow, E. (1987). Behavioral teratogenesis: Long-term influences on behavior from early exposure to environmental agents. In J. D. Osofsyk (Ed.), Handbook of infant development (second ed., pp. 913-971). New York: Wiley.

Vygotsky, L. S. (1987). *The collected works of L. S. Vygotsky: Vol. 1, Problems of general psychology* (Vol. 1). New York: Plenum.

Waddington, C. H. (1957). *The strategy of the genes.* London: Allen & Unwin.

Walberg, H. J. (1990). Productive teaching and instruction: Assessing the knowledge base. *Phi Delta Kappan,* 470-478.

Walk, R. D., & Gibson, E. J. (1961). A comparative and analytic study of visual depth perception. *Psychological Monographs, 75.*

Watkins, C. L. (1988). Project Follow Through: a story of the identification and neglect of effective instruction. *Youth Policy, 10,* 7-11.

Watson, J. B., & Rayner, R. (1920). Conditioned emotional reactions. *Journal of Experimental Psychology, 3,* 1-14.

Watson, J. S. (1969). Operant conditioning of visual fixations in infants under visual and auditory reinforcement. *Developmental Psychology, 1,* 508-516.

Watson, J. S. (1972). Smiling, cooing, and "the game". *Merrill-Palmer Quarterly, 18,* 323-339.

Watson, J. S., & Ramey, C. T. (1972). Reactions to response-contingent stimulation in early infancy. *Merrill-Palmer Quarterly, 18,* 219-227.

Weinraub, M., Clemens, L. P., Sockloff, A., Ethridge, T., Gracely, E., & Myers, B. (1984). The development of sex-role stereotypes in the third year: Relationships to gender labeling, gender identity, sex-typed toy preferences, and family characteristics. *Child Development, 55,* 1493-1503.

Weisberg, P. (1963). Social and nonsocial conditioning of infant vocalizations. *Child Development, 34,* 377-388.

Weisberg, P. (1988). Direct instruction in the preschool. *Education and Treatment of Children, 11,* 349-364.

Weisberg, P. (1994). Helping preschoolers from low -income backgrounds make substantial progress in reading through direct instruction. In R. Gardner, D.M. Sainato, J.O. Cooper, T.E. Heron, W.L. Heward, J. Eshleman, & T.A. Grossi (Eds.), *Behavior analysis in education: Focus on measurably superior instruction* (p. 115=129). Pacific Grove, CA: Brooks Cole.

Wellman, H. M., & Lempers, J. D. (1977). The naturalistic communicative abilities of two-year-olds. *Child Development, 48,* 1052-1057.

Werner, E., & Smith, R. (1982). *Vulnerable but invincible: A study of resilient children.* New York: McGraw-Hill.

Whitehurst, G. J., & Novak, G. (1973). Modeling, imitation training, and the acquisition of sentence phrases. *Journal of Experimental Child Psychology, 16,* 332-345.

Whitehurst, G. J., & Valdez-Menchaca, M. (1988). What is the role of reinforcement in language acquisition? *Child Development, 59,* 430-440.

Whitehurst, G. J., Falco, F., Lonigan, C., Fischel, J., DeBaryshe, B., Valdez-Menchaca, M., & Caufield, M. (1988). Accelerating language development through picture book reading. *Developmental Psychology, 24*, 4.

Wicks-Nelson, R., & Israel, A. C. (1984a). *Behavior disorders of childhood* (First ed.). Englewood Cliffs, NJ: Prentice-Hall.

Wildavsky, B. (1995). Cal State Students Lag in Basic Skills: Angry debate over remedial classes. *San Francisco Chronicle, January 2*, 1,11.

Willett, W. C. (1992). Folic acid and neural tube defect: Can't we come to closure? *American Journal of Public Health, 82*, 666-669.

Williams, R. D. (1994). FDA proposes folic acid fortification. *FDA Consumer, 28*, 11-114.

Wilson, D. S., & Sober, E. (1994). Reintroducing group selection to the human behavioral sciences. *Behavioral and Brain Sciences, 17*, 585-654.

Wilson, E. O. (1985). *Sociobiology: The new synthesis.* Cambridge, MA: Harvard University Press.

Wilson, J. G. (1973). *Environment and birth defects.* New York: Academic.

Wilson, J. Q., & Herrnstein, R. J. (1985). *Crime and human nature.* New York: Simon & Shuster.

Wilson, M. N. (1989). Child development in the context of the black extended family. *American Psychologist, 44*, 380-385.

Winokur, S. (1976). *A primer of verbal behavior: An operant view.* Englewood Cliffs,NJ: Prentice-Hall.

Wolff, P. H. (1966). The causes, controls, and organizations of behavior in the newborn. *Psychological Issues, 5*, 1-105.

Wolff, P. H. (1969). The natural history of crying and other vocalizations in early infancy. In B. M. Foss (Ed.), *Determinants of infant behavior* (Vol. 4). London: Methuen.

Wynne-Edwards, V. C. (1962). *Animal dispersion in relation to social behavior.* Edinburgh: Oliver & Boyd.

Zebrowitz, L. A., & Montepare, J. M. (1992). Impressions of babyfaced individuals across the life span. *Developmental Psychology, 28*, 1143-1152.

Zentall, T. R., & Urcuioli, P. J. (1993). Emergent relations in the formation of stimulus classes by pigeons. *Psychological Record, 43*, 795-810.

Zentall, T., Edwards, C. A., & Hogan, D. E. (1983). Pigeon's use of identity. In M. L. Commons, R. J. Herrnstein, & A. R. Wagner (Eds.), *Quantitative analyses of behavior* (Vol. 4, Discrimination processes, pp. 273-294). Cambridge, MA: Ballinger.

Zettle, R. D., & Hayes, S. C. (1982). Rule-governed behavior: A potential framework for cognitive-behavioral therapy. In P. C. Kendall (Ed.), *Advances in cognitive-behavioral research and therapy* (Vol. 1, pp. 73-119). New York: Academic Press.

Zigler, E., & Seitz, V. (1982). Social policy and intelligence. In R. J. Sternberg (Ed.), *Handbook of human intelligence* (pp. 568-641). Cambridge, England: Cambridge University Press.

Zigler, E., & Styfco, S. J. (Eds.). (1993). *Head Start and beyond: A national plan for extended childhood intervention.* New Haven: Yale University Press.

Zimmerman, B. J., & Whitehurst, G. J. (1979). Structure and function: A comparison of two views of the development of language and cognition. In G. J. Whitehurst & B. J. Zimmerman (Eds.), *The functions of language and cognition* (pp. 1-22). New York: Academic Press.

Glossary

Compiled by - Emily Branscum and L. Gena Martella

Contributions by - Mike Higuera and Margaret Walker

Ability: Knowing how to do things. An operant sequence in a certain order, or an operant with a characteristic response topography cued by certain classes of discriminative stimuli.

Accommodation: The modification of existing mental structures in accordance with newly assimilated information. One of Piaget's mental adaptation processes.

Acquired Reinforcers: Stimuli that acquire the ability to reinforce behavior through being paired with primary reinforcers and other acquired reinforcers. Cf. SECONDARY REINFORCERS, CONDITIONED REINFORCERS.

Activity Reinforcers: A behavior class of common acquired reinforcers which encompasses physical and mental stimuli.

Adaptation: In Piaget's theory, changes in mental structures occurring through the processes of assimilation and accommodation. Assimilation + accommodation = adaptation.

Adenine: One of four chemical bases which make up D.N.A. Along with Cytosine, Guanine, and Thymine, the are basis of genetic code.

Age of Viability: Occurs around the 26th week of prenatal development when the baby's structure has sufficiently developed to sustain life outside the womb.

Aggression: Intentional injurious behavior towards other organism(s). Consequences of aggression may become reinforcing to the aggressor.

Allantois: A structure that becomes the umbilical cord (the conduit for substances between child & placenta).

Allele: Any sequences of bases determining the form of the gene at a given site on a chromosome.

Altruism: The principle or practice of unselfish concern for or devotion to the welfare others.

Amnion: An inner membrane surrounding the embryo and containing amniotic fluid.

Animism: Giving human characteristics to inanimate objects.

Antecedent: A stimulus that precedes some contingency; usually, a discriminative stimulus in a four-term contingency.

Anti-social children: Cf. CHILD ANTI-SOCIAL TRAIT.

Assimilation: The modification of incoming information so that it will fit existing mental structures. Another component in Piaget's theory.

Attachment: Organized social bonding pattern that develops between infant and primary caregiver(s).

Attractor (dynamic attractor or attractor state): Molar regularities of behavior patterns that are the cumulative and emergent products of moment-to-moment relations among events defined over brief periods of time.

Autoclitic: A unit of verbal behavior based upon or dependent upon other verbal behavior by modifying the effects of that other verbal behavior on the listener.

Automatic Reinforcement: a reinforcer related to a response in such a way that it is produce automatically by that response. For example, when sounds made by parents in their native language are presented with other reinforcers, resulting in the sounds acquiring the ability to reinforce behavior which produces them. Thus, infant motor behavior that produces these sounds is automatically reinforced by the ability to hear the sounds. Cf. INTRINSIC or PRIMARY REINFORCEMENT.

Autonomic Arousal: Physiological responses that may act as reinforcing stimuli. Such responses could include; increase heart rate and breathing.

Autosome: Chromosome that is identical in length and carries the same gene location. (22 pairs) Any chromosome other than a sex chromosome.

Backward Chaining: Chaining procedure which begins with teaching the last behavior in a behavioral chain, and continues to teach each behavior in the reverse order that it occurs within the chain.

Backward Conditioning: Type of conditioning that occurs when the unconditioned stimulus precedes the neutral stimulus.(Respondent)

Behavioral Analysis: A field of psychology that is concerned with the environmental influences that change behavior. The breaking down of complex behavior into its functional parts.

Behavioral Contrast: A change in a behavior pattern which is the result of a change in a second behavior pattern. This change can be seen as a setting event – the fourth term.

Behavioral Gerontology: Field of study concerned with continuing developmental issues involving the aging process and the elderly.

Behavioral Pediatrics: The application of psychological research findings to prevent and deal with developmental problems in medical settings.

Behavioral Scheme: Child first mental representation of stimulus-response reflexive reaction (Piaget).

Behavior Chain: A set of discrete behaviors sequenced in a particular order.

Behaviors: The actions or changes of an organism.

Biparental Reproduction: Assures variability by having the organism receive half its genetic make-up from its father and the other half from its mother.

Blastocyst: Inner mass of cells within the blastula from which the child originates.

Blastula: Hollow sphere of cells formed during the germinal period of prenatal development.

Canalized (Phenotype): A deeply entrenched path of development from which it is difficult to deviate. The more highly canalized the phenotype, the more genetics has limited the environment's influence on the development of a given trait or environment.

Cephalo-Caudal Law of Development: Principle of developmental direction stating that development occurs from head to tail (toe).

Chaining: Process that involves the reinforcement of a set of discriminated operants sequenced in a particular order.

Chaos: A branch of science dealing with nonlinear systems. Behavior can be consider a nonlinear system. Such systems is sensitive to initial conditions, which means even small changes may have drastic effects. ie. Butterfly effect.

Child-Antisocial Trait: An organized pattern of responding seen in aggressive children. This pattern is a result of active and evocative person–> environment interactions.

Child Development: The study of the psychological, physiological, and social development of humans between conception and adulthood.

Chorion: The protective membrane that surrounds the embryo/fetus and amnion.

Chromosome: Strands of DNA. 23 pairs of threadlike bodies within the cell nucleus that carry the genes in a linear order.

Circular Explanation: Occurs when a description merely labels the behavior but offers no cause and effect relationship clarification. (e.g., The child cannot read because he has dyslexia. We know the child has dyslexia because he cannot read.).

Circular Reactions: In Piaget's view, the process of reflexes turning into other stimulus-response (operant) relationships.

Clinical Method: An approach to the study of psychology that is concern with or based on actual observation and treatment of patients rather than artificial experimentation or theory.

Coalescent Organization: The dynamical process by which factors bring together coherent patterns of behavior. These factors include; genetics, physical structure, previous experiences and the task at hand.

Co-dominance: Occurs when two alleles are of equal strength. Characteristics of both alleles are expressed in the phenotype.

Coercive Family Process: Breakdown of the parental effectiveness in disciplinary conflict which allows the development of aggressive behavior patterns which include lying, whining, and threatening.

Cognition: The process of thinking. Cognitive processes can only be measure indirectly.

Cognitive Development: Progressive changes in one's knowledge and thinking processes over the lifespan.

Communication: Function of language. To communicate means to change via verbal behavior (spoken, written, or gestured) the relationship between a person's behavior and some part of the environment.

Comparative Psychology: The study of the evolution of behavior across species.

Concordance Rate: Commonly used measure of heritability. The concordance rate is the degree to which one individual's measure on a given test (e.g., IQ or personality test) correlates with another individual's measure on the same test. The more similar, the higher the concordance rate.

Concrete Operations Stage (7-11 years)**:** In Piaget's model, the stage of cognitive development characterized by the ability to engage in inductive reasoning, conservation, and seriation.

Conditioned Reinforcers: Stimuli that becomes reinforcing due to the pairing with primary or secondary reinforcers. Cf. SECONDARY OR ACQUIRED REINFORCERS.

Cones: Receptor cells in the retina responsible for color vision.

Confluence of Research Methodologies: Approach to the study of development which involves, 1) naturalistic observation to identify the existence of the problem and potential causal variables in the real world, 2) bringing the phenomena under control in the laboratory environment to identify the processes involved, 3) returning to the real world to verify that the processes found in the laboratory function in the outside world.

Consequence: An event produced by some other event. The effect of consequences will be to strengthen or weaken behavior. It is the second term in the four-term contingency.

Conservation: This is a characteristic of Piaget's concrete operations stage of cognitive development. Specifically, this is the ability to recognize that the quantity or volume of an object does not change when the form of the object has been altered.

Contingency: An if-then relationship which involves a response and a consequence. (if response A occurs, then consequence A will happen). The effect of the response, the consequence, the discriminative stimulus and the setting event produces the contingency.

Contingency Shaped Behavior: Patterns of behavior that has been learned through the consequences resulting from that behavior, in opposition to rule-governed behavior.

Continuous Reinforcement (CRF): A schedule of reinforcement in which every response within the operant class is reinforced. This leads to most rapid acquisition of a response.

Control Parameters: A property of dynamical systems in which organismic and environmental variables determine changes in behavior. Small changes in control parameters may produce phase shifts. (e.g. bone length, muscle strength, time of day)

Continuum of Caretaking Casualty: The influence of the environmental dimensions mediated by the care taker. This theoretical perspective suggests that interactions of environmental (caretaking), genetic, and historical bases are crucial on developmental outcome.

Cooing: The production of vowel like sounds usually occurring under pleasant setting events, most often seen in infants around the second month of life.

Correlation: The degree of relationship between two or more variables.

Counterimitation: OCRs when an observer does not follow a modeled behavior. In fact, the opposite behavior of the modeled may be seen. The modeled behavior serves as a discriminative stimulus that signals a matching behavior could have unwanted consequences.

Creative behavior: In dynamical systems, creative behavior emerges in an attractor state. This attractor state is a result of knowledge and ability and a history of being reinforced for unique combinations of responding.

Critical Mass: A property of dynamical systems, important to phase shifts. Specifically, it is the accumulation of a significant number of functionally equivalent components that leads to an attainment of a critical mass which is necessary for a shift to a new state.

Crossing Over: Occurs during meiosis. It involves the actual exchange of parts of genetic material, as segments of one chromosome in a pair changes place with segments of its compliment. Crossing over ensures genetic variability.

Cytosine: Cf. ADENINE

Deep Structure: According to Chomsky, this is the underlying meaning of an utterance.

Delayed Conditioning: The most effective type of conditioning. Respondent conditioning in which the CS is presented for some fixed, extended time period before the US is presented.

Developmental Momentum: The principle of dynamical systems that states behavior moving in a particular direction at a particular rate will continue on its trajectory unless their is some disturbance. (ie. Newton's Law of Motion.)

Developmental Ontogenesis: The study of the development or life history of an individual organism.

Developmental Phylogenesis: The study of the development or evolutionary history of a species.

Developmental Psychology: The study of the progressive changes in the relationships between an organism and its environment over its lifespan.

Differentiation: In reproduction, differentiation occurs when the cells of a zygote begin to divided into cells for specific functions.

Differential Reinforcement of Other Behavior (DRO): A reinforcer that is delivered after a set time with no responding. DRO's are often used to reduce undesirable attention seeking behavior with reinforcement of another incompatible (desirable) behavior.

Difficult Child: Characteristic behaviors such as negative mood and short attention span, which produces nonadaptability reactions. These reactions evoke environments (setting events) that are nonfacilitative.

Discrimination: Differences in responding to different stimuli as the result of the contingency histories. Discrimination is a learning process in which an individual is said to discriminate among relevant stimuli.

Discriminative Stimulus: An antecedent stimulus which cues or signals a response. The third term of the four-term contingency.

Disequilibrium: A principle of Piaget's cognitive development theory. This occurs when functional knowledge is lacking for the current environment. In dynamical systems, the imbalance between functional knowledge and environment sets the stage for a phase shift.

Disphoria: A negative mood state.

Dizygotic Twins: Developed from two fertilized ova (fraternal twins).

Dominant: Term used to describe alleles that are stronger than other alleles and more likely to express themselves in the phenotype.

Dual Component Model of Child Abuse: Model offering an explanation of child abuse by identifying the transactions among the genetic, historical, and environmental factors of both the parents and the child. This model places emphasis on the significance of respondent and operant behaviors.

Dynamical Systems Approach: The analysis of development into bi-directional, inseparable, and interlocking systems. It emphasizes a nonlinear model of change in which initial interactions have been reorganized so that their effects on other components of the system is ever-changing.

Dyslexia: An impairment of the ability to read.

Easy Child: Child whose characteristics, such as moderate activity level, rhythmicity in biological functions, positive mood and others, make it easy to care for him/her.

Echoic: Formal verbal class in which the response matches the form of its verbal controlling stimulus.

Echolalic Babbling: Babbling with the intonation of adult language. Occurring near the end of the baby's babbling period.

Ecological Stimulus: Environmental objects, social stimuli, or biological stimuli that are the property of intrinsic reinforcers. Ecological stimuli are discussed through the natural reinforcers occuring in exploratory behavior.

Ectoderm: Outer layer of the embryo from which develops the hair, nails and the central nervous system.

Ectomorph: One of Sheldon's three body types. These individuals are thin, frail, and intellectual.

Edible Reinforcers: A class of common acquired reinforcers.

Egocentrism: Thinking or acting with one's self as the major concern or point of view.

Elicitation: The reliable production of a response by a stimulus in unconditioned or conditioned reflexes.

Emergent Properties: Higher organized behavior that develops from less complex behaviors. Emergent properties are qualitatively different from the previous behaviors and occur as the early behaviors become less adaptive to the current environment.

Emitted: The occurrence of operant behavior. A response that occurs without an eliciting stimulus.

Empiricism: The view that experience, especially of the senses, is the only source of knowledge.

Enactive Representation: Bruner's term for the mental representation of the world by physical activity. A behavioral schemata.

Endoderm: Innermost layer of the embryo from which the inner organs develop (e.g., digestive tract, respiratory system, pancreas, and liver).

Endomorph: One of Sheldon's body types. These individuals are round, plump, and seek pleasurable activity.

Equifinality: Characteristic of development in which common milestones are reached for most individuals even though the environmental interactions of the individuals differs.

Equilibrium: Jean Piaget's term for a temporary mental state occurring when there is a match between what the child knows and what he/she needs to know.

Establishing Operation (EO)**:** Any operation or situation which influences the status of a stimulus as a reinforcer or punisher. For example, the temperature of the room is an establishing operation for the consequence of a window being opened.

Experimental Method: The manipulation of a variable, while controlling extraneous variables, and the measuring of changes in another variable in order to detect a cause-and-effect relationship between the variables.

Exploratory Behavior: A sequence of operant interactions that is strengthened and maintained by contingent ecological stimuli under specifiable setting factors.

External Locus of Control: Attributing the cause of one's behavior to someone or something that is external to the individual.

Extinction: Cf. OPERANT EXTINCTION, RESPONDENT EXTINCTION.

Extinction Burst: An initial, temporary increase in responding, resulting from the withholding of reinforcement.

Extroversion: The psychological state of a person who is interested more in what happens outside him than in his own emotions.

Extrinsic Reinforcers: Responses delivered from the environment (not from intrinsic sources) that strengthen a behavior.

Facilitative/Non-facilitative Continuum: Continuum pertaining to the degree to which the environment is conducive to optimal development. At the facilitative extreme, the environment is conducive to an optimal developmental outcome. At the nonfacilitative extreme, the environment is conducive to a less functional developmental outcome.

Fixed Action Patterns: Elaborate patterns of unlearned behavior elicited by particular environmental stimuli.

Fixed Interval Schedule: A schedule of intermittent reinforcement where a reinforcer follows the first response after a specific time interval (e.g., 30 minutes, 24 hours) has elapsed. FI schedule produces a scalloping response pattern.

Fixed Ratio Schedule: A schedule of intermittent reinforcement where a reinforcer follows a specific number of responses (e.g., every fourth response is reinforced).

Formal Operations Stage (12 years and up)**:** Piaget's last stage of cognitive development characterized by the ability to engage in abstract reasoning.

Forward Chaining: Chaining procedure which begins with teaching the first behavior in the chain, and continues teaching each behavior in the order that it occurs within the behavioral chain.

Four Term Contingency: Contingent relationship involving four terms: 1) a response, 2) a consequence (reinforcement or punishment), 3) a discriminative stimulus, and 4) a setting event. The discriminative stimulus limits the response, which in turn is reinforced or punished by its consequence. The setting event is the context in which the contingency occurs.

Functional Environmental Surround: The portion of the environment that affects the individual's behavior.

Functional Knowledge: The ability to combine pieces of information to produce a desired outcome. Even when information regarding the specifics of the singular pieces is not known.

Functional Response Classes: The grouping of responses based on their consequences. (Operant)

Functional Stimulus Classes: The grouping of stimuli according to their effects on behavior. A set of stimuli that emit common behaviors. (Operant)

Gametes: The sex cells involved in biparental reproduction (the female's ovum and male's sperm).

Gender Consistency: When sex roles are identified across settings.

Gender Identity: Knowledge of one's sex. The ability to identify with one's own sex.

Gender Stability: Knowledge that one's sex is not going to change.

Generalization: The occurance of similar responding to stimuli that differ along one or more dimensions from the originally trained conditioned stimuli.

Generalized Imitation: Occurs when the child's imitation of certain behaviors is reinforced and the child's imitation of other behaviors that were not reinforced for imitating increases as well.

Generalized Reinforcers: Acquired reinforcers which have been associated with many other secondary and primary reinforcers, so that they are generally reinforcing.

Generative Nature of Language: Language is not merely imitative or rote, but characterized by an infinite number of grammatical utterances.

Genes: Locations along a chromosome that determine physical or behavioral characteristics.

Genetic-Constitutional make-up: That which is inherited at conception, including gross physiological characteristics such as: gender, physique, and race.

Genotype: The code of an individuals DNA.

Genotype / Environment Interactions: Two factors responsible for individual differences in development. There are three types: passive, evocative, and ductive.

Gross-Fine Law of Development: Principle of developmental direction stating that general, unrefined characteristics develop into specific, refined characteristics.

Guanine: One of four amino acids that are the chemical bases of a DNA molecule.

Habituation: A reduction in responding to a particular stimulus as a result of repeated exposure to that stimulus.

Heritability: Statistical concept pertaining to the amount of the individual variability, of specific characteristics, that can be attributed to genes.

Heterozygous: Two alleles from the same pair of chromosomes that are of different values (one is dominant and the other recessive).

Hierarchical: A type of organization in which earlier behaviors must develop into organized patterns before more complex behaviors can develop.

History of Interactions: All past interactions one has had with his/her environment.

Holophrastic Stage: Stage of language development during which children use single words to stand for entire concepts.

Homozygous: Two alleles from the same pair of chromosomes that are of the same value (both are dominant or both are recessive).

Iconic Representation: Bruner's term for the mental representation of the world in the form of an image.

Identical Twins: Twins possessing the same genetic make-up because they originated from the same zygote. Identical twins are called "monozygotic" or "paternal" twins.

Impaired-Unimpaired Continuum: Continuum pertaining to the physiological integrity of the individual. At the impaired extreme of the continuum, the individual has severe physiological defects. At the unimpaired extreme, the individual has no physiological defects.

Implantation: The embedding of the blastula into the uterus.

Incompatible Behavior: A behavior that can not occur during the presence of a different behavior.

Incompatible Response Technique: Employing a reinforcement schedule to a behavior in order to extinguish an incompatible negative behavior. Also called differential reinforcement of other behavior (DRO).

Incomplete Dominance: Some of the characteristics of an allele showing incomplete dominance are expressed in the phenotype. A phenotype characteristic that does not follow the recessive/dominant rule of traits.

Individual Differences: Theories which assume that personality is part of the biological nature of the individual.

Inductive Reasoning: Reasoning going from the specific to the general.

Innate Releasing Mechanisms: Stimuli that elicit Fixed Action Patterns.

Instrumental Aggression: Operant aggressive behavior that is controlled by its consequences.

Interactional model: Model of development which views development as the product of reciprocal interactions, involving mutual actions.

Intermittent Reinforcement(Partial Reinforcement)**:** Schedules in which reinforcement does not follow every response. This schedule produces high frequent response patterns.

Internal Locus of Control: Attributing the cause of one's behavior to a relatively stable characteristic one possesses.

Interval Schedules: Intermittent reinforcement schedules (Fixed or Variable) in which the first response following the lapse of a time interval is reinforced.

Intraverbal: A verbal behavior whose controlling stimulus is the speaker's prior verbal behavior.

Intrinsic Reinforcers: Strengthening stimuli that are naturally related to the consequences they produce (sniffing a flower produces a smell).

Introversion: An Eysenck personality trait which includes non-engaging behaviors as strong influences in interaction patterns.

Intuitive Period (4-7 years)**:** The second half of the preoperational stage of cognitive development. The intuitive period is characterized by egocentrism, simple reasoning, and an inability to perform tasks involving conservation or class inclusion.

Invariant: Resistant to change.

Irritable Aggression: Respondent aggressive behavior, usually displayed during intense autonomic arousal, that is elicited by noxious child behaviors.

Karyotyping: Genetic analysis technique which measures the degree to which genetic make-up contributes to the development of a given characteristic.

Knowledge: Having the ability to recognize information that has been previously trained.

Language: System of symbols forming the structure of verbal behavior.

Language Acquisition Device (LAD): Hypothetical mental construct believed by psycholinguists to be responsible for the child's acquisition of language. Term coined by Norm Chomsky.

Law of Least Effort: Principle stating that one engages in the least effortful or difficult behavior that is reinforced.

Leading Parts: Elements of a system, such as a mother in a nuclear family, which have the power to disproportionately affect the system.
Learning: A relatively permanent change in behavior in relation to the environment that is due to experience.
Learning History: Past interactions with the environment that influence current behavior.
Life-Span Developmental Psychology: The study of the psychological development of humans from birth to death.
Linear Model: Theoretical model which assumes that development is an additive process.
Linguistic Competence: Structural approach to language development that focuses on a child's capability rather than on observable behavior.
Linguistic Universals: Aspects of language shared by all members of the human species due to the structure of human thought.
Literality: Belief that concurrently occurring thoughts, behaviors, and physiological conditions are one in the same.
Locus of Control: Personality trait regarding a person's tendency to avoid or engage in behaviors.
Mand: Operant behavior under the control of a setting event such as deprivation or aversive stimulation and reinforced by the stimulus that reduces this deprivation or aversive situation.
Matching Law: States that people will closely match their behavior to the value of the consequences of each behavior.
Maturation: Physical and behavioral changes due to biological growth.
Meiosis: Cell divisions that take place in reproductive organs and bring about the reduction of the number of chromosomes for the formation of gametes.
Mesoderm: Middle layer of the embryo from which the muscles, bones, and circulatory system develop.
Mesomorph: Body type of individuals who are muscular, strong, athletic, and energetic.
Mitosis: Process involving the division of a cell into two new cells. Chromosomes are duplicated, during this process, so that each new cell has exactly the same genetic code as the original cell.
Molar Levels: Level of analysis that encompasses large portions of behavior.
Molecular Levels: Levels of analysis that focus on the specific individual units of behavior (e.g., S-R analysis).
Monozygotic Twins: Identical twins which develop from same ovum and sperm.
Multifactorial Gene Influence: Type of genetic influence on behavior involving many genes, each of which has a small effect by itself. Also called polygenic inheritance patterns.
Multiple Determination: The influence of many factors on the development of behavior. There are 3 categories of multiple determinants: organism conditions, environmental conditions, and control parameters.
Mutation: The product of a proofreading error that resulted in the wrong sequence of DNA bases being formed during mitosis or meiosis.
Nativism: Proposes that perception is present at birth.
Natter: Universal term for nagging, whining or other aversive behavior.
Naturalistic Approach: Approach to the study of development focusing on the observation and description of development in its natural surroundings.

Natural Selection: Process-based theory of overproduction, genetic variability, and survival of the best adapted organisms in a particular environment. This process shows effect through the maintenance or alteration of gene pools.

Negative Punishment (Punishment by Loss)**:** A response is weakened due to the removal of a stimulus following the response.

Negative Reinforcement: Occurs when a response removes, terminates, or avoids a stimulus event; and the response increases in strength. Negative reinforcement is NOT punishment.

Negative Reinforcer: A stimulus that strengthens a response by the removal, avoidance, or termination of an aversive stimulus.

Neonatal Imitation: A newborns ability to appreciate equivalencies between what they do, and what they see.

Neonate: Newborn to about two weeks of age.

Neuroticism: Having to do with functional nervous disorders that have no apparent physical origins.

Nonlinear Model: A model of development which emphasizes bi-directional (reciprocal) interactions which result in a continuous reorganization of the system.

Nonshared Environmental Effects: The unique effects the environment has on the individual.

Non-Universal Behaviors: Behaviors that are the result of learning opportunities determined by cultural values and variations in functional environments.

Observational Learning: Learning based on observing the responding at another individual and/or its consequences.

One Trial Conditioning: Responding to a neutral stimulus which became conditioned from a single pairing of an unconditioned stimulus of high magnitude or frequency.

Ontogenic Contingencies: Environmental influences including genetic factors, which shape the behavioral development of individuals over their lifespans.

Operant: Behavior that operates on the environment and thereby effects and is effected by it.

Operant Extinction: The weakening of behavior through the withholding of its reinforcement.

Operational Schemata: Logical rules used to perform problem solving tasks (Piaget).

Optimal Discrepancy: Process that produce the changes in schemata, which causes cognitive development to occur when there is a difference between what the child knows and what the child needs to know.

Organismic Characteristics: The result of the organism's genetic make-up and repertoire of behavior.

Osmosis: The flowing of substances from a location of high concentration to one where concentration is low.

Paternal Twins: See Identical Twins.

Partial Reinforcement: Reinforcing only some of the desired responses. Results in high response rates (See Intermittent Reinforcement).

Perception: An integrated response to a sensation that results in a functional response.

Period of the Embryo: The second of three prenatal periods, beginning with implantation and ending when all of the basic bodily organs have developed.

Period of the Fetus: The third of three prenatal periods, beginning when all the bodily organs have developed and ending with birth. This period is characterized by growth and refinement of the fetus.

Period of the Ovum (Germinal Period): The first of three prenatal periods, beginning with the establishment of the fertilized ovum (zygote) and ending with implantation of the blastula.

Person/Environment Interactions: Transactions that produce developmental outcomes.

Personality: The organization of unique behavioral patterns or systems an individual has acquired under the special conditions of his development.

Phagocytosis: Process used by blastula to absorb nutrients through the cell membrane.

Phase Shifts: A factor in dynamical systems approach. These shifts are sudden changes in behavior that occur as a result of the organizing of behaviors into an emergent behavior that is topographically unrelated to the previous behaviors.

Phenotype: The physical characteristic that is produced from a genetic trait.

Phoneme: A basic unit of sound.

Phylogenic Contingencies: Environmental influences, including genetic factors, which shape the development of a species over evolutionary time.

Placental Barrier: A semi-permeable membrane which serves as an interface between the blood supply of the mother and that of the fetus. It is the point of contact for the passage of nutrients into the fetus and the outflow of waste products from the fetus.

Positive Punishment (Punishment by Hurt): The process of a response being weakened due to the addition of an aversive stimulus following the response (operant principle).

Positive Reinforcement: The process of a response being strengthened due to the addition of a stimulus following the response (operant principle).

Positive Reinforcer: The actual stimulus that is delivered when the desired response occurs. It's production strengthens the response.

Pragmatics: The functional study of language. Analysis of different language styles through the consequences of it's exchange.

Preconceptual Period (ages 2-4 years): First part of the preoperational stage of cognitive development. The preconceptual stage is characterized by transductive reasoning, animism, egocentrism, and a poor understanding of cause-and-effect relationships.

Prelinguistic Sounds: Sounds produced by infants prior to their production of words (e.g., crying, cooing, and babbling).

Premack Principle: Operant principle stating that any high frequency behavior can be used to reinforce any low frequency behavior.

Preoperational Stage of Development (ages 2-7 years): The second stage of Piaget's cognitive development theory. The preoperational stage consists of two substages: 1) the preconceptual period, and 2) the intuitive period.

Primary Circular Reactions: Behaviors centered on pleasant sensations to the child's own body that occur first by chance but become repetitive due to their intrinsic reinforcing qualities.

Primary Reinforcers: Universal reinforcers that are functioning at birth and are not contingent upon a relation to another reinforcer.

Principles of Developmental Direction: Generalizations that state the order in which characteristics develop. Contains 3 specific developmental laws: 1) cephalo-caudal; 2) proximo-distal; and 3) gross-fine.

Private Events: Behaviors that are observable only to the individual emitting the behaviors (e.g., thinking).

Pro-social Development: The development of the individual's behavior in social transactions.

Proximo-Distal Law of Development: Principle of developmental direction stating that things nearer to the center of the body (e.g., heart) develop before things that are more extreme (e.g., fingers).

Psycholinguists: Nativists who invoke biology as the primary mechanism for language acquisition. These theorists believe that a type of language acquisition device in the child's head is responsible for language development.

Psychological Androgyny: Sex role flexibility characterized by an individual's ability to identify with both masculine and feminine traits.

Psychological Development: Progressive changes in the interactions between the behaviors of a person and the events in his/her environment.

Psychology: The science of mind and behavior.

Psychoticism: The state of being psychotic.

Public/Private Events: Behaviors occuring both inside and outside the skin.

Punishment: An operant principle in which a response is weakened by its consequence.

Random Assortment: The chance sorting of chromosomes into 23 pairs, during meiosis. Random assortment ensures genetic variability.

Range of Reaction: Range set by one's genotype within which a particular characteristic can develop. The level of development obtained within the range of reaction is determined by environmental influences.

Reactional Biography: One's entire history of interactions that influence moment-to-moment behavior.

Recessive: Term used to describe an allele that is masked by a dominant allele. Recessive traits are expressed in the phenotype only when both alleles in a pair carry a homogenous recessive code.

Reductionism: The reducing of a phenomenon to a lower level of analysis. Attempts to explain behavior in terms of physiological mechanisms, rather than through person/ environment interactions.

Reflexes: Relationship involving the eliciting of an unconditioned response by an unconditioned stimulus.

Reinforced Behavior: Behavior that has an increased probability of occuring because of the consequence that behavior produces.

Reinforcement: Any operation which strengthens behavior.

Reinforcement Trap (involving negative reinforcement)**:** Type of transaction whereby the mother's termination of behaviors that are aversive to the child is negatively reinforced by the child's cessation of behaviors that are aversive to the mother. (There are also positive reinforcement traps.)

Reinforcer: A stimulus which strengthens the behavior that it immediately follows.

Relativistic View of Science: View that one's conclusions, and even basic observations, are colored by his/her own world view.

Repertoire of Behaviors (Behavioral Repertory)**:** The sum total of response classes a person has emitted in the past.

Reproductive Risks: Exposure to teratogens, or other nonfacilitative conditions, which are harmful to ontogenic and phylogenic development.

Resistance to Extinction: The ability for a behavior to continue once a consequence no longer occurs. (operant principle).

Resistance to Temptation: The ability to abstain from a behavior which results in a small, immediate consequence in order to obtain a larger, delayed consequence.

Respondent Conditioning: The pairing of an initially neutral stimulus with an unconditioned stimulus which results in the neutral stimulus becoming a conditioned stimulus. Through learning trials, conditioned stimulus comes to elicit the same response as the unconditioned stimulus in the absence of the unconditioned stimulus.

Respondent Extinction: Occurs when the repeated presentation of the conditioned stimulus, in the absence of the unconditioned stimulus, results in the conditioned stimulus becoming a neutral stimulus which no longer elicits the conditioned response.

Response: Any action or change that an individual produces. The behavior of interest when analyzing a four term contingency.

Rods: Visual receptors which respond to small changes in light.

Rubber Band Hypothesis: Metaphor pertaining to the role of the environment with various genotypes. The rubber band represents different genotypes, varying according to their flexibility (range of reaction). The stretching of the rubber band is done by the environment. The more a characteristic can be influenced by the environment the more stretchable the rubber band.

Rule-Governed Behavior: Behavior that is under the influence of verbal instruction.

Schedules of Reinforcement (Reinforcement Schedules): The pattern of response that occurs as a result of the timing of reinforcer. The basic schedules are Fixed Ratio, Fixed Interval, Variable Ratio, and Variable Interval.

Schemata: Term coined by Piaget as mental representations of the world.

Secondary Circular Reactions: Functional repetitive behaviors that produce consequences from the external environment.

Secondary Reinforcers: Stimuli that acquire the ability to reinforce behavior by being paired with primary or other secondary reinforcers.

Selective Imitation: Behavior that matches some dimension of the model's utterance but is novel on another dimension.

Selectivism: An adaptation process where new forms of behavior emerge and are selected by natural environmental contingencies. This process influences both phylogenic and ontogenic adaptations.

Self-As-Knower: The you that you know.

Self-As-Known: Your personality as you think others see you.

Self-Concept: The sum of all the self-statements an individual makes.

Self-Control: The ability to alter a behavior due to the anticipated consequences.

Self-Efficacy Beliefs: Self-statements about the ability to succeed in accomplishing specific behaviors.

Self-Esteem: Evaluative statements about what we can do and how we appear to others.

Semantics: Study of how meaning is effected by the situation or context in which it occurs.

Sensation: The stimulation of sensory receptors and their connections to neurons traveling to the sensory center in the central nervous system.

Sensorimotor Stage: (birth to 2 years) First stage of Piaget's theory of cognitive development. Learning occurs through reflexive behavior.

Setting Event: Context in which the four term contingency occurs. It influences an interactional sequence by altering the strength and characteristic of the particular stimulus response function involved in an interaction.

Sex Chromosomes: Chromosomes that determine the sex of the individual (XX for females and XY for males).

Sex-Linked Characteristics: Characteristics that occur more frequently in males than females. The Y chromosome of the male lacks sites for dominant genes that would mask the expression of recessive genes on the X chromosome.
Shaping: An operant procedure in which successive approximations of a terminal behavior are reinforced.
Shared Environmental Effects: Facets of the environment that affect all persons within that environment equally.
Single Gene Inheritance: Occurs when a characteristic is the result of the presence of one gene, rather than many genes.
Slow-to-Warm Child: Child whose withdrawal, and unpredictability in moods and biological patterns evokes less detrimental reactions from the environment than the difficult child.
Social Behaviors: The responses of an individual which are strengthened or weakened by the reciprocal actions of other individuals or group.
Social Cognition: The development of reasoning and social knowledge.
Social Referencing: Viewing a model's bodily expressions as a discriminative stimulus for one's own behavior.
Social Reflex: Reflexes with the function of evoking parental caretaking.
Social Reinforcers: Acquired reinforcers which develop because they are associated with many primary reinforcers or previously established secondary reinforcers (e.g., physical contact, proximity, and verbal statements).
Somatotypes: The ectomorph, mesomorph, and endomorph body types which were named after the embryological layer from which they are presumed to have originated.
Species-Typical Environment: Environment that is normal for a given species.
Stable/Unstable Traits: A learned attribute that views the source of control as being either internal or external.
Stimulus: Any environmental change or event that has a functional relationship to a particular behavior.
Structural Equation Models: Models which show the degree of relationship between variables and their direction of influence over time .
Structural Knowledge: Knowledge about what aspects of development there are and how they relate to each other even if the outcome of the knowledge is not present.
Supernormal Stimulus: Increases intensity of at least one dimension of a stimulus.
Surface Structure: The actual ordering of words as spoken.
Symbolic Representation: Mental representation of the world in the form of symbols or language.
Symbolic Schemata: Representations of the things they stand for, not the things themselves.
Syntax: The order of words in a sentence or phrase
Systematic Desensitization: Common treatment used for phobias which involves the exposure to feared stimuli starting with the least feared and gradually progressing to the most feared. With each exposure, extinction of the fear elicited by the stimuli occurs.
System Level I: First level at which development can be analyzed. Development is analyzed into basic processes and components (e.g., studying genetics or learning processes).
System Level II: At this level of analysis new units emerge from System Level I processes. A combination of basic units analyzed at Level I are organized and reorganized (e.g., stages of development and personality characteristics).
System Level III: Nonlinear reciprocal interactions between the individual and his/her environment are the focus of analyses conducted at this system level.

System Level IV: Analyses conducted at this level examine the influence of society and culture on development.

Tact: A class of verbal operants in which a response of a given form is evoked by a particular object or event or property of an event.

Tangible Reinforcers: Objects which derive their reinforcing effects because they can be touched, viewed, smelled, or manipulated in a variety of ways.

Task Analysis: Procedure used to teach a behavioral chain. The discrete behaviors comprising the chain and the sequence in which these behaviors occur are identified by the task analysis.

Telegraphic Stage: Stage of language development following the Holophrastic stage. This stag is characterized by the use of as few words as possible to convey a message.

Temperament: Style of behaving present at birth. Such characteristics become strengthened and organized into what we call personality.

Teratogens: Substances present during the prenatal period such as disease or drugs that cause physical or psychological abnormalities.

Teratology: The study of birth defects.

Tertiary Circular Reactions: Piaget's third type of circular reactions marked as the beginning of curiosity. The child accidentally produces a consequence and then varies the response to determine what behaviors produce the same consequence.

Textual: A verbal response to a written or printed discriminative stimulus.

Thymine: One of four amino acids that are the chemical bases of a DNA molecule.

Time-Out: Type of punishment by loss where an undesired behavior is immediately consequated by removing the child from reinforcement.

Topography as A Response Class: The grouping of responses based on their common form.

Trace Conditioning: Occurs when the neutral stimulus is presented and terminated prior to the onset of the unconditioned stimulus (respondent principle).

Trajectory: System of behaviors that organize into one of three patterns: remaining stable, continuing to develop on the same linear or curvilinear path, or shifting suddenly (phase shifting).

Transaction: Process involving reciprocal interactions in which the result of previous interactions influence current interactions.

Transductive Reasoning: Thinking from specific to specific, unable to make generalizations due to the lack inductive or deductive abilities.

Transformational Rules: Simple rules for changing a sentence into another form (e.g., statement to question).

Trophoblast: Outer protective layer of the blastula which develops into the membranes surrounding the child (e.g, the amnion, chorion, placenta, umbilical cord, and allantois).

Umbilical Cord: The conduit for substances between the child and placenta.

Unconditioned Response: A response that is elicited and not the result of learning (i.e., reflexes). A respondent learning principle.

Unconditioned Stimulus: Stimulus which elicits an unlearned (reflexive) response. A respondent learning principle.

Universal I Behaviors: Hard-wired behaviors present at birth, requiring only a species typical environment for their development (e.g., reflexive and perceptual responses).

Universal II Behaviors: Inherited behavioral capabilities (e.g., walking and talking). UII behaviors differ from UI behaviors in that UII behaviors: are more variable in form and quality, are less hard -wired, have a more variable level of development that can be obtained, take longer to develop, and are influenced to a greater extent by learning.

Variability: A characteristic of the action of objects.

Variable Interval Schedule: A schedule of intermittent reinforcement in which the first behavior occuring after a variable amount of time has elapsed is reinforced.

Variable Ratio Schedule: An intermittent reinforcement schedule in which the number of responses before reinforcement varies around an average. This schedule results in high constant rate of responding.

Verbal Behavior: Behavior involving words that are reinforced through the mediation of other persons. Verbal behavior is not just spoken words. Skinner developed six verbal categories.

Vicarious Consequences (vicarious reinforcement /punishment): Principle of observational learning where behavior changes without direct consequation of responses.

Visual Cliff: A large glass covered table with a shallow and deep end used to study the infants' development of depth perception and fear.

Vocables: Unique sounds of an infant which function as words.

Vulnerable-Invulnerable Continuum: Continuum pertaining to the degree of resiliency of an individual to an aversive environment. At the vulnerable extreme, a harmful environment will have the most detrimental effect on development. At the invulnerable extreme, the same harmful environment will have a much less damaging effect on development.

Yolk Sac: The initial source of embryo blood cells.

Zygote: Single-cell fertilized ovum.

Author Index

D

E

F

S

T

U

V

W

Z

Subject Index

G

H

I

R

S

Other Books from Context Press

Scientific Standards of Psychological Practice: Issues and Recommendations
Steven C. Hayes, Victoria M. Follette, Robyn M. Dawes, & Kathleen E. Grady (288 pp.; 1995)

Changing Cultural Practices: A Contextualist Framework for Intervention Research
Anthony Biglan (464 pp.; 1995)

Acceptance and Change: Content and Context in Psychotherapy
Steven C. Hayes, Neil S. Jacobson, Victoria M. Follette, and Michael J. Dougher (272 pp.; 1994)

Analyzing Social Behavior: Behavior Analysis and the Social Sciences
Bernard Guerin (400 pp.; 1994)

Behavior Analysis of Language and Cognition
Steven C. Hayes, Linda J. Hayes, Masaya Sato, and Koichi Ono (Eds.) (320 pp.; 1994)

Ethical Issues in Developmental Disabilities
Linda J. Hayes, Gregory J. Hayes, Stephen L. Moore, and Patrick M. Ghezzi (Eds.) (208 pp.; 1994)

Outline of J. R. Kantor's Psychological Linguistics
Sidney W. Bijou and Patrick M. Ghezzi (79 pp.; 1993)

Varieties of Scientific Contextualism
Steven C. Hayes, Linda J. Hayes, Hayne W. Reese, Theodore R. Sarbin (Eds.) (320 pp.; 1993)

Radical Behaviorism: Willard Day on Psychology and Philosophy
Sam Leigland (Ed.) (208 pp.; 1992)

Understanding Verbal Relations
Steven C. Hayes and Linda J. Hayes (Eds.) (224 pp.; 1992)

Dialogues on Verbal Behavior
Linda J. Hayes and Philip N. Chase (Eds.) (349 pp.; 1991)

To order write to: Context Press
933 Gear St., Reno, NV 89503-2729
or call (702) 746-2013